Idiotypy in Biology and Medicine

Idiotypy in Biology and Medicine

Edited by

Heinz Köhler
Department of Molecular Immunology
Roswell Park Memorial Institute
Buffalo, New York

Jacques Urbain
Département de Biologie Moléculaire
Laboratoire de Physiologie Animale
Université Libre de Bruxelles
Bruxelles, Belgium

Pierre-André Cazenave
Département d'Immunologie
Institut Pasteur
Paris, France

1984

ACADEMIC PRESS, INC.
(Harcourt Brace Jovanovich, Publishers)
Orlando   San Diego   San Francisco   New York   London
Toronto   Montreal   Sydney   Tokyo   São Paulo

ACADEMIC PRESS, INC.
Orlando, Florida 32887

United Kingdom Edition published by
ACADEMIC PRESS, INC. (LONDON) LTD.
24/28 Oval Road, London NW1 7DX

Library of Congress Cataloging in Publication Data

Main entry under title:

Idiotypy in biology and medicine.

Includes index.
1. Immunoglobulin idiotypes. I. Köhler, Heinz,
Date   . II. Urbain, Jacques. III. Cazenave, Pierre-
André. [DNLM: 1. Antigenic determinants. 2. Antibody
specificity. QW 573 I19]
QR186.7.I34 1984   599'.029   83-19702
ISBN 0-12-417780-8

PRINTED IN THE UNITED STATES OF AMERICA

84 85 86 87   9 8 7 6 5 4 3 2 1

Contents

4. The Uniqueness and Boundaries of the Idiotypic Self
Nelson M. Vaz, Carlos Martinez-A., and António Coutinho

Section II: Idiotypes in the Immune System

5. Structural Properties and Genetic Control of an Idiotype Associated with Antibodies to the p-Azophenylarsonate Hapten
Michael F. Gurish and Alfred Nisonoff

6. Idiotype-Specific T Helper Cells

M. McNamara and H. Köhler

7. Manipulating an Idiotypic System with Asymmetric Circuitry: Antiidiotypic Antibodies versus Idiotype-Recognizing T Cells

Eli E. Sercarz and Christopher D. Benjamin

8. Biochemical, Functional, and Genetic Aspects of T-Cell Idiotypes

Bent Rubin

9. Ontogeny of the HA-Responsive B-Cell Repertoire:
Interaction of Heritable and Inducible Mechanisms
in the Establishment of Phenotype

*Michael P. Cancro, Mary Ann Thompson, Syamal Raychaudhuri,
and David Hilbert*

10. Ontogeny of Antilevan and Inulin Antibody Responses

Constantin A. Bona and Carol Victor

14. Idiotypes of Anti-MHC Monoclonal Antibodies

Jeffrey A. Bluestone, Hugh Auchincloss, Jr., Suzanne L. Epstein, and David H. Sachs

Section III: Idiotypes in Other Biological Systems

15. Production of Monoclonal Antibodies to Integral Membrane Transport and Receptor Proteins and Their Use in Structural Elucidation

J. Craig Venter, Barbara Eddy, Ursina Schmidt, and Claire M. Fraser

16. Studies on Idiotypes Shared by Neuronal and Lymphoid Cells
John H. Noseworthy and Mark I. Greene

17. Idiotypy in Autoimmune Central Nervous System Demyelinating Disease: Experimental Allergic Encephalomyelitis and Multiple Sclerosis
Robert B. Fritz

18. Idiotypes in Myasthenia Gravis
Donard S. Dwyer, Ronald J. Bradley, Shin J. Oh, and John F. Kearney

19. Antiidiotypic Antibodies as Immunological Internal Images of Hormones

A. D. Strosberg

20. Immunization to Insulin Generates Antiidiotypes That Behave as Antibodies to the Insulin Hormone Receptor and Cause Diabetes Mellitus

Irun R. Cohen, Dana Elias, Ruth Maron, and Yoram Shechter

21. Induction of Protective Immunity Using Antiidiotypic Antibodies: Immunization against Experimental African Trypanosomiasis

David L. Sacks

22. The Idiotype Network: Theoretical and Practical Implications for Autoimmune Disease

Michael Fischbach and Norman Talal

23. Human Antiidiotypic Antibodies

H. G. Kunkel

Contributors

Numbers in parentheses indicate the pages on which the authors' contributions begin.

Hugh Auchincloss, Jr.[1] (243), Transplantation Biology Section, Immunology Branch, National Cancer Institute, National Institutes of Health, Bethesda, Maryland 20205

Christopher D. Benjamin[2] (101), Department of Microbiology, University of California, Los Angeles, Los Angeles, California 90024

Jeffrey A. Bluestone (243), Transplantation Biology Section, Immunology Branch, National Cancer Institute, National Institutes of Health, Bethesda, Maryland 20205

Constantin A. Bona (29, 173), Mount Sinai School of Medicine, One Gustave L. Levy Place, New York, New York 10029

Ronald J. Bradley (347), Department of Psychiatry, The University of Alabama in Birmingham, Birmingham, Alabama 35294

Michael P. Cancro (144), Department of Pathology and Laboratory Medicine, University of Pennsylvania Medical School, Philadelphia, Pennsylvania 19104

Irun R. Cohen (385), Department of Cell Biology, The Weizmann Institute of Science, Rehovoth 76100, Israel

António Coutinho[3] (43), Laboratory of Immunobiology, Pasteur Institute, Paris, France

Donard S. Dwyer (347), Max Planck Gesellschaft, Klinische Forschungsgruppe für Multiple Sklerose, D-8700 Würzburg, Federal Republic of Germany

[1]Present address: Massachusetts General Hospital, Boston, Massachusetts 02114.

[2]Present address: Department of Microbiology, Naval Medical Research Institute, National Naval Medical Center, Bethesda, Maryland 20814

[3]Present address: Unité d'Immunobiologie, Institut Pasteur, 75724 Paris, Cedex 15, France, and Avd. för Immunologi, Universitet, S-901 85 Umeå, Sweden.

Barbara Eddy (274), Department of Molecular Immunology, Roswell Park Memorial Institute, New York Department of Health, Buffalo, New York 14263

Dana Elias (385), Department of Hormone Research, The Weizmann Institute of Science, Rehovoth 76100, Israel

Suzanne L. Epstein (243), Transplantation Biology Section, Immunology Branch, National Cancer Institute, National Institutes of Health, Bethesda, Maryland 20205

Michael Fischbach (417), University of Texas Health Science Center, and Audie L. Murphy Veterans' Administration Hospital, San Antonio, Texas 78284

Claire M. Fraser (274), Department of Molecular Immunology, Roswell Park Memorial Institute, New York State Department of Health, Buffalo, New York 14263

Robert B. Fritz (329), Department of Microbiology/Immunology, Emory University School of Medicine, Atlanta, Georgia 30322

Mark I. Greene (303), Department of Pathology, Harvard Medical School, Boston, Massachusetts 02254

Michael F. Gurish (64), Rosenstiel Research Center, Department of Biology, Brandeis University, Waltham, Massachusetts 02254

David Hilbert (144), Department of Pathology and Laboratory Medicine, University of Pennsylvania Medical School, Philadelphia, Pennsylvania 19104

John F. Kearney (187, 347), Cellular Immunobiology Unit of the Tumor Institute, The Comprehensive Cancer Center, and Department of Microbiology, University of Alabama in Birmingham, Birmingham, Alabama 35294

Heinz Köhler (3, 89), Department of Molecular Immunology, Roswell Park Memorial Institute, New York Department of Health, Buffalo, New York 14263

H. G. Kunkel[4] (429), The Rockefeller University, 1230 York Avenue, New York, New York 10021

Georg Lehle (203), Faculty of Biology, University of Konstanz, D-7750 Konstanz, Federal Republic of Germany

O. Leo (15), Department of Molecular Biology, Laboratory of Animal Physiology, University of Brussels, B1640 Rhode-St-Genese, Belgium

B. Mariamé (15), Department of Molecular Biology, Laboratory of Animal Physiology, University of Brussels, B1640 Rhode-St-Genese, Belgium

[4]Deceased.

Ruth Maron (385), Department of Hormone Research, The Weizmann Institute of Science, Rehovoth 76100, Israel

Carlos Martinez-A.[5] (43), Laboratory of Immunobiology, Pasteur Institute, Paris, France

M. McNamara (89), Department of Molecular Immunology, Roswell Park Memorial Institute, New York Department of Health, Buffalo, New York 14263

Alfred Nisonoff (64), Rosenstiel Research Center, Department of Biology, Brandeis University, Waltham, Massachusetts 02254

John H. Noseworthy (303), Department of Pathology, Harvard Medical School, Boston, Massachusetts 02254

Shin J. Oh (347), Department of Neurology, University of Alabama in Birmingham, Birmingham, Alabama 35294

Brian A. Pollok[6] (187), Cellular Immunobiology Unit of the Tumor Institute, The Comprehensive Cancer Center, and Department of Microbiology, University of Alabama in Birmingham, Birmingham, Alabama 35294

Syamal Raychaudhuri (144), Department of Pathology and Laboratory Medicine, University of Pennsylvania Medical School, Philadelphia, Pennsylvania 19104

Bent Rubin (113), Centre d'Immunologie INSERM-CNRS, de Marseille-Luminy, 13288 Marseille, Cedex 9, France

David H. Sachs (243), Transplantation Biology Section, Immunology Branch, National Cancer Institute, National Institutes of Health, Bethesda, Maryland 20205

David L. Sacks (401), Immunology and Cell Biology Section, Laboratory of Parasitic Diseases, National Institute of Allergy and Infectious Diseases, National Institutes of Health, Bethesda, Maryland 20205

M. Slaoui (15), Department of Molecular Biology, Laboratory of Animal Physiology, University of Brussels, B1640 Rhode-St-Genese, Belgium

Ursina Schmidt (274), Department of Molecular Immunology, Roswell Park Memorial Institute, New York State Department of Health, Buffalo, New York 14263

Eli E. Sercarz (101), Department of Microbiology, University of California, Los Angeles, Los Angeles, California 90024

Yoram Shechter (385), Department of Hormone Research, The Weizmann Institute of Science, Rehovoth 76100, Israel

---

[5]Present address: Clinica Puerta de Hierro, Departamento de Immunologia, San Martin de Porres 4, Madrid 35, Spain.

[6]Present address: Institute for Cancer Research, Fox Chase Cancer Center, Philadelphia, Pennsylvania 19111.

Robert Stohrer (187), Cellular Immunobiology Unit of the Tumor Institute, The Comprehensive Cancer Center, and Department of Microbiology, University of Alabama in Birmingham, Birmingham, Alabama 35294

A. D. Strosberg (366), Laboratory of Molecular Immunology, Institut Jacques Monod Institut de Recherche en Biologie Moléculaire, Centre National de la Recherche Scientifique and University Paris VII, Cedex 05, 75251 Paris, France

Norman Talal (417), The University of Texas Health Science Center at San Antonio, and Audie L. Murphy Memorial Veterans' Administration Hospital, San Antonio, Texas 78284

Mary Ann Thompson[7] (144), Department of Pathology and Laboratory Medicine, University of Pennsylvania Medical School, Philadelphia, Pennsylvania 19104

Jacques Urbain (15, 219), Départment de Biologie Moléculaire, Laboratory of Animal Physiology, Université Libre de Bruxelles, B1640 Rhode-St-Genèse, Belgique

Nelson M. Vaz[8] (43), Laboratory of Immunobiology, Biomedical Institute, UFF, Niteroi, Brazil

J. Craig Venter (274), Department of Molecular Immunology, Roswell Park Memorial Institute, New York State Department of Health, Buffalo, New York 14263

Carol Victor (173), Department of Microbiology, Mount Sinai School of Medicine, New York, New York 10029

Eberhardt Weiler[9] (203), Faculty of Biology, University of Konstanz, D-7750 Konstanz, Federal Republic of Germany

Ivan Jeanne Weiler (203), Faculty of Biology, University of Konstanz, D-7750 Konstanz, Federal Republic of Germany

Maurice Wikler (219), Département de Biologie Moléculaire, Laboratory of Animal Physiology, Université Libre de Bruxelles, B1640 Rhode-St-Genèse, Belgique

Joachim Wilke (203), Faculty of Biology, University of Konstanz, D-7750 Konstanz, Federal Republic of Germany

[7]Present address: Institute for Cancer Research, Philadelphia, Pennsylvania.

[8]Present address: Laboratorio de Immunologia, Instituto Biomédico, UFF, Rua Hernani Mello 101, 24.210 Niteroi, RJ, Brasil.

[9]Present address: Institute for Cancer Research, Fox Chase Cancer Center, Philadelphia, Pennsylvania 19111.

Preface

In 1963 Jacques Oudin and Henry Kunkel described for the first time idiotypic specificities on rabbit and human antibodies, but for many years their finding remained largely a curiosity. When in the early 1970s the antibody structure and the genetics of immunoglobulins had become better understood, idiotypes turned out to be useful as genetic markers for antibodies. In 1972 the first idiotype suppression experiments were reported demonstrating that antiidiotypic antibodies might be extremely specific and powerful reagents to modulate or control immune responses. A few years later the first reports on auto-antiidiotypic responses and on the idiotypes on T cells appeared. These findings completed the scenario of an immune system consisting of a network of interacting complementary idiotypes as proposed by Niels Jerne.

Today a new dimension in idiotypy is developing, which has the potential of broad applications in biology medicine. Idiotypic reagents are used in standard immunological procedures, and the immune network is unfolding through intensive and numerous studies. New findings, predicted from Jerne's network, that antibodies (idiotypes) can be used as vaccines or that antibodies (idiotypes) can mimic biologically active molecules like hormones are already confirmed.

The purpose of this book is to serve the increasing interest and involvement in the practical aspects of idiotypy in biological systems. In the first section, the original concepts of idiotypic manipulations are discussed. Köhler reviews old and recent data important for the concept of an idiotype network and reports on attempts to deal with the T-cell receptor paradox. Urbain and colleagues explain the immune system in terms of a circular idiotype network that can be demonstrated by sequential immunization. Bona emphasizes the need for restrictions in network interactions. His "regulatory idiotypes" are specialized idiotypes that are involved in the control of the immune system.

In the second section, the role and activity of idiotypic and antiidiotypic antibodies in the regulation of the immune system are addressed. Nisonoff and colleagues summarize the ARS system, one of the classical immune responses in which idiotype regulation was demonstrated. Köhler and colleagues present new data on the role of T helper cells in the PC system and present evidence that T cells recognize B-cell idiotypes otherwise than B cells recognize idiotypes. This idiotype recognition difference is further discussed by Sercarz and Benjamin, who present data on the network response to lysozyme. A summarizing overview on the serology and structure of alloreactive T cells and their idiotypic receptors by Rubin follows. A model is proposed in which the T-cell receptor has a structural analogy to Ig.

In the next four chapters the effects of idiotype, antiidiotype, and antigen on the maturation of the B-cell repertoire are discussed. Cancro and colleagues show how neonatal exposure to the antigen modulates the expression of the inherited B-cell repertoire against influenza hemagglutin. Bona and Victor present results that show that neonatal exposure to idiotype induces the expression of a normally silent antibody idiotype for bacterial levan or inulin antigens. Kearney and his group report on the profound alterations of the idiotype repertoire for PC and dextran, which can be induced by administration of monoclonal antiidiotypic antibodies. Weiler and colleagues, also working on the idiotypically restricted antidextran response, emphasize the need of using isogeneic antiidiotypic antibodies in attempts to understand the physiological role of idiotype network interactions.

The last two contributions in this section deal with attempts to manipulate the adult idiotype expression. Sachs and colleagues show that xenogenic antiidiotype can effectively act across species to induce alloantibody-associated idiotypes. Wikler and Urbain present their elegant experiments on sequential immunizations in rabbits and demonstrate that outbred rabbits share a universal idiotype repertoire.

In the last section, the issue of idiotype-antiidiotype is taken out of the realm of the immune system and discussed as a new principle to analyze and manipulate biological systems in general.

Venter and colleagues discuss their work on monoclonal antireceptor antibodies for neurotransmitter receptors. This work demonstrates clearly that antibodies (idiotypes) can be made and used to characterize and isolate cellular receptors that exist in minute quantities.

Greene and Noseworthy discuss some provocative findings on idiotypic cross-reactions between reovirus receptors, specific T-cell receptors, and neuronal cell receptors. These data demonstrate the general sharing of receptor structures among different biological systems.

The role of antiidiotypic reactions in experimental allergic encephalomyelitis is discussed in the contribution by Fritz. In this animal model, general procedures are developed that may be adapted for therapy of human neurological autoimmune diseases such as multiple sclerosis.

The problem of human autoimmune diseases and possible manipulation via idiotypy is directly addressed in the contribution by Kearney and colleagues. They describe a naturally occurring antiidiotypic antibody in myasthenia gravis and suggest that the antiidiotypic antibodies are somehow involved in the regulation of this disease.

The next three chapters give convincing evidence for the general usefulness of the idiotype approach to immunotherapy. Strosberg discusses antiidiotypic antibodies as internal images of hormones. Cohen and colleagues describe experiments on antiidiotypic antibodies against antiinsulin. Sacks reports on successful attempts to immunize mice against trypanosomiasis using antiidiotypic antibodies.

The last two chapters review the present knowledge on auto-antiidiotypic immunity in humans. Fischback and Talal summarize critically the evidence of auto-antiidiotypic immunity in autoimmune disease. Finally, Kunkel, one of the discoverers of idiotypy, summarizes the evidence for human antiidiotypic antibodies. The finding of auto-antiidiotypic antibodies in the maternal–fetal situation indicates a possible significant physiological role in the survival of the fetal transplant.

The editors would like to express their appreciation to the authors for their exciting and stimulating contributions, which contain many original data and ideas. The concept of idiotypy has received wide recognition and interest far beyond the area of immunology. Experiments and interpretation of findings, reported here, clearly support the general nature of the idiotype concept in manipulating biological systems to correct pathological conditions or to improve the immune adaptation to environmental factors.

Idiotype Concepts

Chapter 1

The Immune Network Revisited

Heinz Köhler

Department of Molecular Immunology
Roswell Park Memorial Institute
(A unit of the New York State Department of Health)
Buffalo, New York

I. Introduction

The network hypothesis of immune regulation approaches its tenth anniversary (1, 2). Numerous findings on the response and regulation of the immune system have been interpreted with the network theory, and many experiments have been specially designed to test this hypothesis. Among the early key supportive data are idiotype suppression (3, 4), neonatally induced idiotype suppression (5), the finding of auto-antiidiotypic responses (6), and the induction of mirror imaging antibodies (7–9).

II. The B-Cell Idiotype Network

For the B-cell portion of the immune network, specific tools are available; these include monoclonal antiidiotypic reagents, synthetic idiotypic peptides, idiotypes of myelomas and hybridomas that are expressed dominantly, and the genes coding for heavy and light chains of idiotypes. Far less is known about T-cell idiotypes; this limits the analysis of T-cell-mediated interactions and has often led to controversial data.

3

The sequence of interaction steps in an experimentally induced idiotype network chain can now be described with some precision mainly because of the work in the laboratories of Cazenave and Urbain (8, 9). Starting with an antibody, Ab1, induced by immunization or produced by a myeloma or hybridoma cell line, an antiidiotypic antibody, Ab2, is induced. This Ab2 can have very different specificities for Ab1, that is, it can recognize different idiotopes on Ab1. If an idiotope distant from the antigen-binding site of Ab1 is recognized by one type of Ab2, then antigen binding does not interfere with the Ab1-Ab2 interaction. This antiidiotypic antibody is thus not site related or hapten inhibitable. Jerne had termed this part of the network the specific antiidiotype set, or recently, the α-type antiidiotype (10).

If, on the other hand, the antiidiotype Ab2 recognizes a determinant near the antigen-binding site of Ab1, hapten or hapten-conjugates can interfere with the Ab1-Ab2 binding. This Ab2 antiidiotype is, therefore, site related or hapten inhibitable. Important biological consequences for such site-related Ab2s have been implied. It is important to view this type of Ab1-Ab2 binding in three-dimensional space. There it becomes evident that two cavities of two antibodies, Ab1 and Ab2, cannot form complementary structures with their binding sites. Thus, the site-related Ab2 must simply recognize an idiotope on the rim or periphery of the binding site of Ab1. By this definition, this Ab2 is a special antiidiotype set that defines the antigen specificity of Ab1. We shall term this set the γ type.

The third type of Ab2, called by Jerne the β type, is of considerable theoretical and practical interest. The binding site of Ab1 not only binds antigen but can also recognize determinants on other antibodies that mimic the structure of antigen. Thus, the antigen-binding site of Ab1 can bind to the internal image of antigen present on a totally unrelated antibody. Ab2, which carries the internal image of antigen, can be stimulated by Ab1. Also, Ab2 can be used for immunizing another animal, and because it carries the antigen image, it can induce a very special Ab3 type which can bind the original antigen. However, although Ab3 is similar to Ab1 in its antigen-binding capacity, it may have different idiotopes which make it distinct from Ab1. Thus, this Ab3 has been called Ab1' (8, 9). The similarity of Ab1 and Ab1' and that of Ab2 and the next step in the idiotype cascade, Ab4, has led to the concept of a circular network (8, 9, 11).

Immunization with antigen thus induces a cascade of idiotope expression. The crossroad is at the Ab2 step (Fig. 1). Ab1 carries idiotopes that can stimulate different Ab2 types. The α type is an antiidiotypic antibody in the original sense of Oudin (12). The γ type

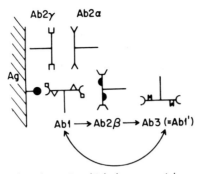

Fig. 1. A minimal network is shown in which the sequential appearance of three complementary antibodies is described. Ab1 is induced by antigen. Ab1 carries at least two different idiotypes; one is remote from the binding site and can induce an antiidiotope, Ab2, which is of the α type. If antiidiotype Ab2 is directed against an idiotope near the binding site of Ab1, then its binding to Ab1 can be inhibited by Ag; this Ab2 is the γ-type Ab2. Ag is minced by an idiotope (internal image of antigen), and thus Ab1 will bind to that idiotope on a given antibody. This antibody now becomes a part of the minimal network and is designated Ab2β. Ab2β can induce Ab3, which is directed against the internal image idiotope of Ab2β. Therefore, this Ab3 will also bind antigen and is called Ab1'. However, Ab1' is different from Ab1 because it has a different set of idiotopes. Ab2α, anti-id antibody; Ab2β, carrying internal image antibody; Ab2γ, antisite anti-id antibody.

is essentially a special case of the α type. The unique feature of Ab2γ is that it binds to an idiotope close to the antigen-binding site of Ab1, thus interfering with the antigen-binding function of Ab1. Both types, α and γ, are part of the immune network which cannot be easily traced experimentally much farther beyond Ab2. Ab2β is different because it mimics the antigen determinant. Therefore, Ab3 raised against Ab2β can bind antigen and acts like Ab1. The likeness and identical antigen specificity of Ab1 and Ab1' (which is a subset of Ab3) produce a circular, closed functional network created by the interactions of complementary binding site structures. The principal element of this Ab1-Ab2-Ab3 (Ab1') network was formulated by us earlier (13, 14) using the concept of a reciprocal complementary network. More importantly for the following discussion on the T-cell receptor repertoire, it defines Ab2β as the internal image of antigen.

III. T-Cell Idiotypes

There is agreement that T cells are specific for antigen, which indicates T cells have receptors for antigen. However, there is great uncertainty regarding the chemical nature of T-cell receptors and the genes coding for the receptor structures. The consistent failure to detect rearranged Ig V_H genes in T-cell clones argues against the hypothesis that T-cell receptors are immunoglobulin like. On the other hand, genes coding for B- and T-cell idiotypes have been mapped to the same *Igh-V* locus (15), and idiotypic cross-reactions between T and B cells have been observed in several systems (15–17).

Assuming that T-cell receptors and factors are not encoded by immunoglobulin genes or gene segments does not invalidate data showing that T cells can recognize B-cell idiotypes or that T cells can be generated which have antigen specificities similar to those of antibodies. This T-cell property has been most clearly demonstrated in studies where T helper cells interact with an idiotype to which a hapten has been coupled. The hapten-idiotype is used as hapten-carrier antigen for a B-cell antihapten response (18). The specificity of this idiotype recognizing T helper is, however, distinctly different from that of antiidiotypic antibodies. If antigen priming is used to induce this helper cell, it recognizes an idiotope that is on the binding site of the idiotype. The T-cell specificity differs from the conventional antiidiotype specificity by a different kind of idiotype recognition. T helper cells do not distinguish between idiotype-positive and idiotype-negative antibody carrier; they recognize the majority of PC binding myelomas and hybridomas (19).

Two important differences between the B-cell and T-cell recognition repertoires appear. First, the antigen and idiotope specificity of T cells is different, and at least in certain cases, less specific. For example, T cells recognize complex determinants created by a combination of a hapten coupled to a particular carrier molecule (19–21). In one case (22), it was clearly shown that T cells recognized determinants contributed by both the hapten and the carrier, i.e., T cells showed conjugate specificity. In other experiments (23, 24), T cells and antibodies were shown to be directed against different epitopes on multideterminant antigens. Second, effective T-cell function occurs only if self-recognition of MHC determinants is included (25, 26). These differences lead to the hypothesis that the T-cell repertoire is secondarily developed and selected; the effective T-cell repertoire is generated not by selection through antigen but by idiotypes mimicking antigens.

Thus, the internal idiotope images shape a second repertoire of complementary T-cell receptor structures that resembles a complementary internal image of B-cell idiotopes (Fig. 2). This hypothesis deals with several findings otherwise difficult to reconcile; T-cell receptors do not have to be immunoglobulins or be encoded by the

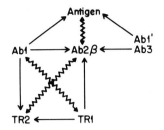

Fig. 2. Relation of B-cell idiotypes to T-cell receptors. The minimal B-cell idiotype network, as shown in Fig. 1, provides the internal image of Ag for T-cell selection. T cells are selected in the thymus by Ab2β, which carries the internal image of Ag. The receptor of this T cell has the complementary TR1 receptor. TR1 is also the internal image of Ab1, whereas TR2 shares the internal image of Ag with AB2β. The important feature of this model is that T cells are selected or educated by idiotope representing the internal images of Ag and not directly by antigen. B-cell idiotypes, internal Ag images; T-cell receptors, complementary internal idiotype images; binding direction, → [—◁ ●⊣]; image sharing, ⤳ [⊢●≅◁].

same genes that code for Ig because their specificity for antigens rests on mimicry of idiotopes. This explains the idiotypic cross-reaction between B- and T-cell idiotypes. The specificity of T-cell receptors (TR) is different from and "looser" than that of antibodies. Because, according to this hypothesis, the T-cell repertoire is selected and expanded by idiotopes and their internal images of antigen, the selected T-cell repertoire appears in genetic linkage with immunoglobulin genes. Thus, the finding of T-cell responses and specificities linked to the Igh locus can be explained by the priming and selection of T-cell function by B-cell idiotype internal images, which occurs in the thymus early in ontogeny. And finally, because the selecting idiotopes present as surface Ig on B cells are associated with self-MHC(Ia determinants), the recognition of self-Ia becomes part of the T-cell antigen specificity.

The distinction made between B- and T-cell receptors, whereby T-cell receptors are internal images of B-cell idiotypes, is essential for our hypothesis (Fig. 2). The important consequence of the internal image character of T-cell receptors is their different specificity. Because images are not perfect copies but more or less blurred pictures, the specificity will be lower and may include parts of the background in the picture. Idiotypes exist in solution and as cell-bound receptors on B cells, and therefore are associated with self-Ia. These cell surface expressed idiotypes appear in ontogeny before circulating idiotypes and thus are the first molds used by T cells to generate or select internal images. Therefore, it is not unexpected that antigen images produced by B-cell idiotypes include portions of the MHC and that T-

cell receptors require for recognition the presence of self-MHC determinants. Thus, T cells are more efficient and more specific, if they are
operating under MHC restriction.

IV. The Immune Network as an Evolutionary Factor

As outlined above, the existence of mirror images of external antigens in the B-cell and T-cell repertoires is an essential feature of the
network. If T-cell receptors are indeed not Ig related, then the interaction of B and T cells is entirely based on the mimicry of B-cell idiotypes by T-cell receptors and T-cell factors. The interaction of the immune system using the B- and T-cell arms with the external antigen
universe is, of course, a decisive factor in survival, and any genetic
deficiency in this system would impair the existence of the species.
This postulates that the internal antigen image must be fairly complete and accurate. Failure of a given antigen to be represented in the
internal image catalog could exert a negative selective pressure by
prohibiting the interaction of B and T cells in a particular response.
Some time ago (27), we postulated that the clonal diversity of
germline genes has evolved by evolution and that this basic diversity
is maintained in the absence of external antigenic stimulation. Thus,
the immune system appears to be preadapted to antigenic exposure.
The idiotype network therefore becomes a necessity for evolution (28)
because encounters with external antigen are too infrequent to be a
sufficiently strong selective force (26). Although the repertoires of B
and T cells are degenerate and are in themselves "complete," difficul-
ties in communication between them can be expected because the B-
cell repertoire is constantly changing through the development of
new variants. Furthermore, the regulation of B- and T-cell function
appears to be accomplished by a restricted number of recurrent
idiotopes that had been called regulatory idiotypes (29, 30).

To avoid network "holes" in the internal image repertoire, selective
pressure is exerted on the B- and T-cell genes to maintain a complete
repertoire. However, by the same reasoning, selective pressure could
be working on the external antigen universe to eliminate a given
antigenic structure for which a response gap or a B-T interaction problem has developed. This is certainly a nonconventional way of looking
at the evolutionary relationship between the immune system and its
targets, the external antigens. There is some indirect support for the
selective influence of the immune system on antigenic structures in
the auto-response of rabbits against different amino acid sequence

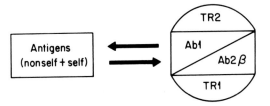

Fig. 3. A model for the evolution and interactions of antigenic structures and the immune system. The immune system consists of antibodies, produced by B cells, and specific T-cell receptors (TR) and factors. The structures of antigens are copied by the immune system as internal images. In this model, a mutual evolutionary surveillance of changes in the antigen repertoire and the antigen-recognizing immune system is proposed. Changes in one system must be met by adaptive changes in the other system, and vice versa.

positions in cytochrome C (31). A relationship between the evolutionary appearance of given amino acid substitutions and the potential to recognize such substitutions in an auto-response has been described. It will be necessary to search for other examples in the phylogenetic tree for a relationship of immune responsiveness and evolutionary age of the given antigenic determinants. Virus-encoded antigens would be a good choice for establishing such relationships because of the high evolutionary instability of these antigens. If this concept of an evolutionary surveillance (Fig. 3) by the immune system is valid, this would be a substantive addition to Darwin's theory subsequent to its formulation.

V. Idiotopes on Non-Ig Molecules

Idiotopes on T-cell receptors that are not necessarily chemically or genetically related to immunoglobulins are only one example of the general phenomenon of idiotope mimicry. Cross-reaction of anti-idiotypic antibody with non-Ig molecules has already been described in several instances. This cross-reaction evidently provides a direct link between the immune system and other biological systems. This link is probably of great biological significance. Idiotope mimicry has practical consequences in experimental biology and has already been used to characterize and isolate nonimmunological receptors (32, 33; also see Chapters 15, 16, 19 and 20). We can expect this approach to develop into a new hybrid of research between immunology and receptor biology.

Idiotypic cross-reaction with non-Ig idiotopes has been observed in the immune system. The cross-reactive nature of the immune system is detected classically with antigens but is also manifested with anti-idiotypic antibodies. In particular, idiotypic cross-reactivity can be clearly demonstrated if monoclonal hybridoma antiidiotypic antibodies are used where the signal-to-noise ratio is very high. Antiidiotypic antibodies may react with their primary targets, idiotypic determinants (idiotopes). Antiidiotypic antibodies also react with nonimmunoglobulin structures that mimic the shape of idiotopes. Examples of this idiotopic cross-reaction are (a) the T15 idiotype on the T15 myeloma, which is also detected on the Thy1 antigen (33), and (b) the finding that antibodies specific for the idiotype of anti-insulin receptor antibodies mimic hormone receptors (7, 32, 34). Thus, immunoglobulin idiotopes and nonimmunoglobulin idiotopes are both targets for recognition by the immune system.

The biological significance of idiotypic determinants detected on nonimmunoglobulin molecules is obscure. These "unconventional" idiotypes are polyclonally distributed because they are not present on immunoglobulins that are allelicly excluded. If these non-Ig idiotypes are found on lymphocytes, they may represent receptors for mitogens, as proposed by Coutinho et al. (35).

Several years ago, Coutinho and co-workers detected cells in fetal and neonatal mouse livers and spleens that reacted with both monoclonal and polyclonal heterologous antiidiotypic antibodies (anti-Id). Furthermore, these anti-Id antibodies were able to induce polyclonal differentiation of murine liver and spleen lymphoid cells (36). It was therefore proposed that receptor molecules involved in the differentiation of antibody-secreting cells possess structural determinants similar to those of common idiotopes. This concept, however, creates constraints that could significantly alter the network theory. In this situation, antiidiotypic antibodies would possess many properties of hormones, reacting with a potentially heterogeneous group of receptor molecules on different lymphocytes. Each receptor would bear a similar epitope. These interactions would allow the same antibody to modify the functional potential of a large number of cells committed to producing different immunoglobulin idiotypes but possessing determinants on their surface that react with idiotypic or antiidiotypic antibodies. Further specificity might also be obtained by reactivity of groups of antiidiotypic antibodies with various receptors or fragments of receptor molecules on cells (37). In these situations, antiidiotypic antibodies would react specifically with the complementary epitope on an Ig molecule, as well as non-Ig molecules on lymphocyte surfaces.

In cases in which it has been investigated, immunization with molecules bearing multiple epitopes can induce both specific antibody formation and nonspecific (polyclonal) antibody production (38–40). Because polyclonal antibody synthesis after immunization is rarely evaluated and usually not deemed significant, its etiology and function in immune regulation have been poorly investigated. Certainly, various microorganisms contain substances that induce polyclonal antibody production after infection (41–43). The role of these polyclonal antibodies in protection against infection is unclear; however, the occurrence of polyclonal antibody production *in vivo* is unquestioned.

A role for the polyclonal nonspecific antibodies produced by mitogenic stimulation can be envisioned within the concept of idiotype networks. Polyclonal stimulation could simply raise the level of network interactive activities and lower the threshold of activation for specific responses. Regardless of the positive effects of nonspecific stimulation, excess polyclonal antibodies may account for the abnormal amounts of immunoglobulins in the serum of some humans and mice with autoimmune disorders (44, 45).

Because Coutinho and Moller (46) have postulated that the mitogen receptor accepts the essential trigger signal from antigenic mitogenic properties, the question arises whether the mitogenic signal can be delivered by antiidiotypic interaction with non-Ig receptors. We have discussed this idea in a previous article (47). It seems, therefore, that the classical concept of complementary idiotype interactions based on Ig expression needs to be expanded to include response interactions with non-Ig cell-bound receptors.

With the increasing availability of monoclonal antiidiotopic reagents produced by cell fusion, the resolution in the analysis of idiotypic interactions is improving rapidly. Monoclonal antiidiotopic antibodies define single, individual epitopes. By this analysis, each classical idiotype may be further characterized by multiple determinants (idiotopes). The expression of these determinants on antibody molecules is being explored (48, 49).

VI. The Need for a Network

Generally, the existence of the complex immune network is explained by the need for an effective fine-tuning control of immune responses. However, it seems that for control purposes a simplified network would be more effective and certainly more "economical." Networks of high connectivities tend to become unstable (50) if disturbed by even specifie and restricted stimulation. Thus, there is probably another biological reason for developing and maintaining a complex immune network. The need for complexity stems from the way the immune system achieves target specificity. Because the antigen binding sites of B-cell receptors and antibodies and possibly those of T-cell receptors are restricted in terms of the size of target determinant, the probability exists that a given target determinant is present on two totally unrelated antigens. This means that if the immune system produced only one antibody (a monoclonal response), this antibody would not be very antigen specific, although it would be very determinant specific. The immune system reduces the effective determinant cross-reactivity with different antigens by evoking a heterogeneous antibody response. A mixture of different antibodies reacts with different determinants on the same antigen. This recognition pattern of determinants by a heterogeneous antibody response increases the overall specificity of the immune response because the probability that a similar or identical determinant pattern might be present on other antigens is very low.

The same need for a heterogeneous external antigen-specific response exists also for the internal antigens, that is, the idiotypes. It follows that the need for a heterogeneous antigen response creates a complex network of idiotopes which is regulated by balanced network interactions. Balance and stability are achieved by establishing a hierarchy of idiotope interactions whereby so-called regulatory idiotopes (29, 30) provide the framework for regulation. Private or rare idiotopes function mainly as internal images for antigen. The role of internal images in evolution is to create and maintain the size of the network repertoire. The large size is necessary to produce functioning network circuits and to maintain the immune system preadapted for external antigen encounters.

References

1. Lindenmann, J. (1973). *Ann. Immunol.* (*Paris*) **124C**, 171.
2. Jerne, N. K. (1974). *Ann. Immunol.* (*Paris*) **125C**, 373.
3. Cosenza, H., and Kohler, H. (1972). *Proc. Natl. Acad. Sci. U.S.A.* **69**, 2701.
4. Hart, D. A., Wang, A.-L., Pawlak, L. L., and Nisonoff, A. (1972). *J. Exp. Med.* **135**, 1293.
5. Strayer, D. S., Lee, W., Rowley, D. A., and Kohler, H. (1975). *J. Immunol.* **114**, 728.

6. Kluskens, L., and Kohler, H. (1974). *Proc. Natl. Acad. Sci. U.S.A.* **71**. 1508.
7. Sege, K., and Peterson, P. A. (1978). *Proc. Acad. Natl. Sci. U.S.A.* **75**, 2443.
8. Cazenave, P.-A. (1977). *Proc. Natl. Acad. Sci. U.S.A.* **74**, 5122.
9. Urbain, J., Wikler, M., Fransson, J. P., and Collingnon, T. (1977). *Proc. Natl. Acad. Sci. U.S.A.* **74**, 5126.
10. Jerne, N. K., Roland, J., and Cazenave, P.-A. (1982). *EMBO J.* **1**, 243.
11. Wikler, M., Franssen, J. D., Collignon, C., Leo, O., Marriame, P., Van de Walle, D., Degroote, D., and Urbain, J. (1979). *J. Exp. Med.* **150**, 182.
12. Oudin, J., and Michel, M. (1963). *C.R. Hebd. Seances Acad. Sci.* **257**, 805.
13. Kohler, H. (1975). *Transplant Rev.* **27**, 26.
14. Kohler, H., Rowley, D. A., DuClos, T., and Richardson, B. (1972). *Fed. Proc., Fed. Am. Soc. Exp. Biol.* **36**, 221.
15. Eichmann, K. (1970). *Adv. Immunol.* **26**, 195.
16. Binz, H., and Wigzell, H. (1975). *J. Exp. Med.* **142**, 197.
17. Cosenza, H., Julius, M., and Augustin, A. (1977). *Immunol. Rev.* **34**, 3.
18. Gleason, K., Pierce, S. K., and Kohler, H. (1981). *J. Exp. Med.* **153**, 926.
19. Pierce, S. K., Speck, N. A., Gleason, K., Gearhart, P., and Kohler, H. (1981). *J. Exp. Med.* **154**, 1178.
20. Paul, W. F. (1970). *Transplant. Rev.* **5**, 130.
21. Janeway, C. A., Jr. (1976). *Transplant. Rev.* **29**, 164.
22. Bikoff, E. (1982). *Proc. Natl. Acad. Sci. U.S.A.* **79**, 4156.
23. Maizels, R. M., Clarke, J. A., Harvey, M. A., Miller, A., and Sercarz, E. E. (1980). *Eur. J. Immunol.* **10**, 509.
24. Infante, A., Atassi, M. Z., and Forthman, C. G. (1981). *J. Exp. Med.* **154**, 1342.
25. Zinkernagel, R. M., and Doherty, P. C. (1975). *J. Exp. Med.* **141**, 1427.
26. Shearer, G. M., Rehn, T. G., and Carbarino, C. A. (1975). *J. Exp. Med.* **141**, 1348.
27. Kohler, H., and Rowley, D. A. (1977). *In* "Autoimmunity" (N. Talal, ed.), p. 267. Academic Press, New York.
28. Urbain, J., and Winlmart, C. (1982). *Immunol. Today* **3**, 88.
29. Bona, C. A., Heber-Katz, E., and Paul, W. (1981). *J. Exp. Med.* **153**, 951.
30. Gleason, K., and Kohler, H. (1982). *J. Exp. Med.* **156**, 539.
31. Jemmerson, R., and Margoliash, E. (1979). *Nature (London)* **282**, 468.
32. Wassermann, N. H., Penn, A. S., Freimuth, P. I., Treptow, N., Wentzel, S., Cleveland, W. L., and Erlanger, B. F. (1982). *Proc. Natl. Acad. Sci. U.S.A.* **79**, 4810.
33. Pillemer, E., and Weissman, I. L. (1981). *J. Exp. Med.* **153**, 1068.
34. McLachlan, S. M., Rees-Smith, B., Petersen, Y. B., Davies, T. F., and Hall, R. (1977). *Nature (London)* **270**, 447.
35. Coutinho, A., Forni, L., and Blomberg, B. (1978). *J. Exp. Med.* **148**, 862.
36. Coutinho, A., Forni, L., Martinez, A. C., Bernabe, R. R., Larsson, E. L., Reth, M., Augustin, A. A., and Cazenave, P. A. (1980). *Prog. Clin. Biol. Res.* **42**, 279.
37. Hood, L., Huang, H. V., and Dreyer, W. J. (1977). *J. Supramol. Struct.* **7**, 531.
38. Rosenberg, Y. J., and Chiller, J. M. (1979). *J. Exp. Med.* **150**, 517.
39. Moticka, E. J. (1974). *Immunology* **27**, 401.
40. Antoine, J. C., and Avrameas, S. (1976). *Immunology* **30**, 573.
41. Rosen, A., Grengely, P., Jandel, M., Klein, G., and Brittan, S. (1977). *Nature (London)* **267**, 52.
42. Biberfeld, G., and Gronowicz, E. (1976). *Nature (London)* **261**, 238.
43. Pryjma, J., Munoz, J., Galbraith, R. M., Fudenberg, H. H., and Virella, G. M. (1980). *J. Immunol.* **124**, 656.

44. Fauci, A. J. (1980). *J. Allergy Clin. Immunol.* **66**, 5.
45. Theofilopoulos, A. N., and Dixon, F. J. (1981). *Immunol. Rev.* **55**, 179.
46. Coutinho, A., and Moller, G. (1975). *Adv. Immunol.* **21**, 113.
47. Kohler, H., Levitt, D., and Bach, M. (1981). *Immunol. Today* **2**, 58.
48. Geha, R. S. (1980). *Clin. Res.* **128**, 471.
49. Wittner, M. K., Bach, M. A., and Kohler, H. (1982). *J. Immunol.* **128**, 595.
50. McMurtie, R. E. (1975). *J. Theor. Biol.* **50**, 1.

Chapter 2

Idiotypy and Internal Images

J. Urbain, M. Slaoui, B. Mariamé, and O. Leo

Department of Molecular Biology
Laboratory of Animal Physiology
University of Brussels
Rhode-St-Genèse, Belgium

I. Introduction

As stated by Niels Jerne in his introduction to the Basel workshop on idiotypes (17), the research on idiotypes is entering a state of crisis, a state of crisis being proof of the importance of and the interest in the subject. On the other hand, a crisis leads to confusion, paradoxes, and misunderstandings. The idiotype crisis is explained by several reasons, among them the flood of papers on the subject. This information overflow is difficult to grasp by "bystander" immunologists, those not specialized in this field. And although it may seem ironic that we want to add one more work on idiotypes, it actually is not. More seriously, different phenomena are designated by the same words. The real missing link—at the bottom of the idiotype crisis—is our poor understanding of the chemical basis of idiotopes. The major problem involves the genetic conclusions that can be drawn from serological data. This problem is the subject of this chapter. We intend to discuss idiotypes "à la Oudin," recurrent idiotypes, and internal images.

Before dealing with the problem itself, we would like to look at the history of immunological ideas. Immunology was once primarily a part of microbiology, devoted to the establishment of bacterial serotypes and vaccination. It was gradually realized that the immune repertoire is infinite and complete. The immune system is able to respond to an enormous array of unforeseen antigenic stimuli (newly synthesized haptens, "exotic" antigens such as crocodilian albumin, spinach carboxylase, etc.). Therefore, as has happened so many times in science, instructive theories were put forward. Immunologists were flirting with Larmackian concepts. Then came Niels Jerne, with his foreshadowing of the clonal selection theory (15). The distinction between instructive and selective theories is approximately the same as the distinction, in philosophy, between essentialism and existentialism. By an elegant extension of Darwinism to the cellular level, Burnet postulated the theory that is still the basis of much immunological thinking, the clonal selection theory (8). After this era of elegant simplicity (a kind of "lost paradise" for some immunologists), immunology dropped into darkness. The discovery of thymus–bone marrow cooperation (11), the so-called hapten-carrier phenomenon (22), forced the conclusion that regulation of the immune response relied on interlymphocytic communications.

Antigens displaying distinct epitopes can link lymphocytes of different specificities (associative recognition). Is this really the basis of immune regulation, as proposed by Bretscher and Cohn (7), or is it merely the visible tip of the iceberg? After all, the immune system cannot know which epitope is linked to another epitope. Perhaps some more basic and subtle principle underlies immune regulation. The discovery of idiotypy by J. Oudin, H. Kunkel, and A. Kelus (20, 21, 23) paved the way for the idiotype network hypothesis (16). One immunoglobulin molecule is not just an antibody to an epitope, but is also an antigen able to elicit specific antiantibodies or antiidiotypic antibodies. The immune system is not only able to cover the external antigenic universe but is also recognizing itself. Therefore, if we suppose that idiotypes and antiidiotypes coexist in the repertoire of one individual (and this has been proven), a new form of interlymphocytic communication can be imagined.

The antigen is not just selecting and amplifying preexisting clones but is also disturbing some kind of equilibrium between different clones displaying complementary receptors (recognizing each other). Taking into account the H-2 restriction phenomenon (35) and the fact that idiotypes are involved in clonal interactions (32), we arrive at a strange and fascinating picture of lymphocyte interactions. The most extreme forms of polymorphism known are idiotypy and histocompatibility, and the molecules mainly involved in and responsible for lymphocyte interactions are precisely those exhibiting these polymorphisms. This is perhaps not so surprising if we consider that the immune system is able to evolve in anticipation of future needs. Immunoglobulin and histocompatibility antigens seem to derive from common ancestor genes; therefore, it is quite possible that a still more basic and subtle phenomenon is underlying lymphocyte interactions. Self-recognition is the secrete of a system whose purpose is to recognize non-self.

It is common to oppose antigenic and idiotypic regulation. We believe that there is no contradiction or paradox. Antigen can bridge sets of lymphocytes that are able to interact by virtue of their idiotypic specificities. We shall refer to these sets as idiotypic communities. In the absence of antigen, these communities ignore each other. Antigens associate some of these communities, and this is important because activated lymphocytes can release "nonspecific" factors physiologically active in their vicinity.

Let us consider idiotypes à la Oudin. A series of rabbits is injected with the same antigen [*Salmonella*, tobacco mosaic virus (TMV), etc.]. All rabbits make specific antibodies, but if one antibody prepared from one rabbit is injected into another rabbit (allotype matched with the first), the second rabbit will make antibodies (antibody 2, or Ab2) specific for antibodies from the first rabbit. Antibody 2 is usually called an antiidiotypic antibody, or antibody of the second generation. Generally, antibody 2 recognizes antibody 1 but does not recognize the antibodies from other rabbits immunized with the same antigen at all. Antibody 2 is therefore able to discriminate between many antibodies, despite the fact that all these antibodies were raised against the same antigen. These antiidiotypic antibodies therefore recognize epitopes associated with hypervariable regions (these epitopes are called *idiotopes*). By virtue of their high discriminatory power, antiidiotypic antibodies can probably be used as "genetic probes," although idiotopes are complex three-dimensional epitopes of variable regions. The frequency of recurrency of these idiotypes is in the range of 2–5% (measured by immunodiffusion with (PEG) and radioimmunoassay).

A simple yet important question which has not yet been addressed is, How many idiotypes exist in one species and for one antigen? From the frequency of idiotypic cross-reactions, a reasonable guess would be 20–50.

In several systems (that have been thoroughly investigated for obvious reasons), a different picture is emerging. Antibody 1 (Ab1) is taken from one mouse. Antibody 2 (Ab2) is raised against Ab1; this Ab2, contrary to the previous explanation, now recognizes all Ab1 made against the same antigen by all individuals from the same strain. These idiotypes have been called public, major, or cross-reactive. We have proposed the term recurrent. From this recurrency, it would be tempting to draw the conclusion that all the mice from one strain use the same germline gene when immunized with the same antigen. Idiotypes à la Oudin would appear as the amplification of different somatic variants which have arisen in different individuals from a few germline genes. However, the recurrency of a given idiotype is *not* a sufficient observation from which to draw direct genetic conclusions. This is because, in the set of possible Ab2 against an Ab1, there is a subset of Ab2 that behaves as an "internal image" of one epitope of the antigen (16). In other words, these Ab2 display an idiotope, which mimics structurally one antigenic determinant. These Ab2 (Jerne called them Ab2β) that behave like antigen do not discriminate between different Ab1. Just as the fact that antigen elicits specific antibodies in different individuals does not allow us to draw conclusions at the genetic level, no genetic conclusions can be drawn if Ab2β antibodies are present in one serum.

To clarify further the notion of an internal image, we shall use an example furnished by the superb and elegant work of Atassi (1). Atassi located and defined precisely several epitopes from myoglobin, lysozyme, etc. He then produced a synthetic peptide containing the contact amino acid residues of the antigenic determinants, respecting the distance measured between the different contact amino acid residues by the use of appropriate spacers. The synthetic peptide obtained, when attached to carrier and injected into animals, elicits the synthesis of antibodies that recognize the native antigen. Atassi then synthesized "a synthetic active site" by making a complementary peptide to the antigenic site peptide (see the example). The synthetic active site is able to bind to lysozyme. Furthermore, the injection of the artificial antibody binding site promotes the appearance of antibodies that recognize specifically antilysozyme antibodies from goats immunized with lysozyme. These "anti-binding site" antibodies thus behave as antiidiotypic antibodies of the β type, as internal images of the antigenic determinant.

Example (from Atassi, 1980)

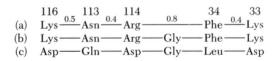

(a) Amino acid residues from the third antigenic site of lysozyme. The distance between amino acids is in nanometers.
(b) Synthetic antigenic site.
(c) Simulated complementary site.

Therefore, we come to the provisional conclusion that Ab2 à la Oudin, by their high power of discrimination, can be used as genetic probes, whereas the apparent recurrency of some idiotopes could be caused either by the use of the same germline gene or by the presence of Ab2β antibodies in the idiotypic serum. However, it should be strongly emphasized that, on the basis of amino acid sequence data and nucleotide sequences, many recurrent idiotopes correspond to the fact that the same set of germline genes is exploited during immunization with the same antigen in different individuals. This is obvious from amino acid sequence data, from nucleotide sequences, and from studies showing linkage of idiotype expression with the Ig C_H locus (32).

Before considering data concerning idiotypes à la Oudin, recurrent idiotypes, and internal images, we shall discuss briefly another potential source of ambiguity in idiotype research. This ambiguity could become a source of information for future work in immunology.

We are now all acquainted with the clonal selection theory. The immune system is viewed as a library of unipotential precommitted lymphocytes waiting for antigen. The repertoire size is commonly estimated to be of the order of 10^7–10^8 clones. Let us consider the frequency of B lymphocytes able to respond to a given antigen. Using the splenic focus assay, Klinman and his collaborators have found that the frequency of antigen-reactive B cells was about 1 in 10^5 (30).

However, if the same frequencies are measured under conditions of polyclonal activation, which bypasses normal regulatory mechanisms (that push one-third of the B lymphocytes toward terminal differentiation), quite different numbers are found. For SRBC, the frequency of B cells is 1 in 10^3 (12). We might say that SRBC is an antigen displaying a large array of epitopes. But similar experiments reveal that the frequency remains the same for the A5A idiotype and the MOPC 460 idiotope (assayed by monoclonal antiidiotypic antibodies). If we want to adhere to the clonal selection theory (one cell–one antibody), multipotentiality must be introduced at the level of the immunoglobulin molecule itself. One immunoglobulin must be able to bind to many different antigens. The end of Fab should be a "sticky" end (Hoffman), with several idiotopes behaving as multiple potential binding sites. This was proposed by Jerne at the Basel meeting (17, 18), by Gershon (13), and earlier by Richards (27). If this is true, intriguing questions arise regarding the mechanism of natural tolerance, "connectance" in idiotypic networks, interactions between T and B lymphocytes, etc.

These frequencies also indicate that the repertoire available for antigen is usually ~1% of the potential repertoire. To summarize before illustrating these ideas, any so-called antiidiotypic serum Ab2 can contain true antiidiotypic antibodies (called Ab2α by Jerne), which recognize idiotopes of antibody 1, and antiidiotypic antibodies displaying idiotopes mimicking one epitope. Jerne called the latter Ab2β. We shall denote these Ab2 internal images as Ab2ε (for epitope related).

II. A Recurrent Idiotype (6, 26)

One of the nicest examples of a recurrent idiotype is the Np system, which was discovered by Olli Mäkelä and T. Imanishi-Kari. The Rajewsky group has done a beautiful characterization of this idiotype. After immunization with the 4-hydroxy-3-nitrophenylacetyl hapten (Np) coupled to a carrier, mice belonging to the IgH b haplotype produced a recurrent idiotype that is made up of a family of closely related but nonidentical anti-Np antibodies. This idiotype is usually present in the early immune response, is associated with λ_1 light chains, and disappears in the sera of hyperimmune mice. The heavy chain genes that are responsible for this family have been characterized. They form a cluster of seven genes, two of which seem to be nonfunctional pseudogenes. The seven genes are highly homologous (they differ by 15 nucleotides at most). Of the seven genes, only one (perhaps two) is responsible for the recurrent idiotype. The large family of Ig molecules with anti-Np specificity seems to be generated by somatic mutations. The Np system is therefore a recurrent idiotype in the genetic sense (6).

Interestingly, one of the seven genes (102) seems to encode an immunoglobulin which shares idiotopes with the recurrent idiotype but which does not bind antigen (this gene therefore seems to be a good candidate for what we call an Ab3; see below). Different strains of mice were injected with monoclonal Ab2 coupled to hemocyanin. Injection of Ab2 can, in principle, induce true anti-antiidiotypic antibodies which recognize idiotopes on Ab2 but also B cells bearing idiotopes recognized by Ab2. (The situation is actually more complex because of the existence of silent clones inhibited by suppressive mechanisms; see the discussion of the immunization cascade). In the Np system, idiotypic molecules will probably be associated with the λ chain, whereas anti-antiidiotypic immunoglobulins should be associated with the κ light chain (which is the predominant form of light chain in mice).

In brief, injection of Ab2 coupled to KLH into strains that do not normally express the recurrent idiotype after antigen alone promotes the expression of immunoglobulins bearing idiotopes shared with the recurrent idiotype. Depending on the Ab2, some are Np-binding and some are non-Np-binding. These results are in good agreement with our results in rabbits. The repertoire available to one antigen is smaller than the potential repertoire of one individual (see following section).

III. Classical Idiotypes

Let us consider the *Micrococcus luteus* antigenic system in the rabbit. This system elicits strong immune responses of restricted heterogeneity and is made up of at least two distinct antigenic specificities, the carbohydrate moiety (CHO) and the peptidoglycan specificity (Pg). Antiidiotypic antibodies can easily be raised in allotype-matched rabbits. These antiidiotypic antibodies are strictly specific for the antigen (one Ab2 made against an anti-CHO Ab1 does not react with the anti-Pg Ab1 made in the same rabbit) and specific for one or a few individuals (the frequency of idiotypic cross-reactions is 2%).

The first question that comes to mind is, What is the basis of this phenomenon? Do different rabbits express different idiotypes because they possess different repertoires (e.g., different somatic mutations could occur in different individuals, leading to different repertoires), or do all rabbits possess the same idiotypic potential repertoire, from which different expressed repertoires are selected? Let us consider two rabbits, X and Y. When injected with *Micrococcus*, different idiotypes IdX and IdY are expressed. Is it possible to orient the repertoire toward a predetermined goal in order to guide the immune response of rabbit Y to the synthesis of idiotype X?

If we suppose that IdX is not produced in rabbit Y, because the clones precommitted to the synthesis of IdX are kept silent by suppressive mechanisms, it must be assumed that the suppressor has the capacity to discriminate between IdX and IdY. This suppressor therefore cannot be antigen-like or an Ab2ε (internal image). It resembles a classical Ab2. If we suppress the suppressors (by inducing an immune response against Ab2, or an Ab3 response), we would expect to free the silent IdX from suppression in rabbit Y. This was the basis of our immunization cascade: making sequential sets of antiidiotypic anti-

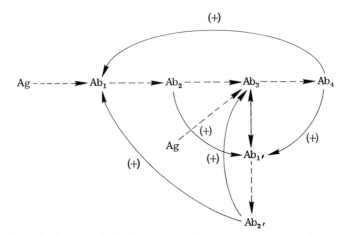

Fig. 1. Immunization cascade. Broken arrows indicate immunizations. Full arrows labeled (+) indicate specific recognition. Note that Ab3 and Ab1' antibodies are synthesized in the same rabbit. Ab1, idiotype; Ab2, antiidiotype; Ab3, anti-antiidiotype; Ab4, anti-anti-anti-idiotype; Ab2', antibodies are antiidiotypic to Ab1' antibodies.

bodies (5, 9, 10, 31–33). The results are summarized in Fig. 1. The main conclusions drawn are the following:

1. The potential repertoire of one individual is much greater than the repertoire expressed after antigen injection alone.

2. The immune response of one animal does not rely only on antigenic selection but also depends on the previous idiotypic history of the animal.

3. There is no need to consider idiotypic networks *ad infinitum*. Diversity does not increase along the immunization chain because a large part of Ab3 shares idiotopes with Ab1 and Ab4 behaves like Ab2. A large part of Ab3 are not anti-antiidiotypic antibodies *sensu stricto* but are idiotypic immunoglobulins. Ab4 resembles classical Ab2 and are totally different from Ab2ε or Ab2β. Although induced by Ab3, they recognize Ab1 and Ab1' antibodies; they do not recognize other Ab1 induced by the same antigen in other individuals.

4. The potential idiotypic repertoire of all rabbits is more or less the same. This does not necessarily imply that different rabbits have the same V genes. In the absence of sequence data, it is difficult to draw definite conclusions. However, in view of the discriminatory power of classical Ab2, it is difficult to escape the conclusion that Ab1 and Ab1' antibodies are probably strongly similar in sequences.

5. A part of Ab3 (50–70%) shares idiotypic specificities with Ab1

but does not bind antigen. This suggests strongly the existence of idiotypic families made up of immunoglobulins sharing some idiotopes, but not all. Although they share some idiotopes, these immunoglobulins can bind to different antigens. The genes 186.1 and 102 of the Np cluster are probably examples of this phenomenon (26).

6. The immunization cascade can be replaced by maternal Ab3 immunoglobulins (34).

7. Because only a few percent, at most, of Ab3 bind antigen, it seems that antiidiotypic antibodies of the ε type play no role in this immunization cascade when the antigen is TMV, *Micrococcus,* nuclease, ribonuclease, β-galactosidase, etc. Different results are obtained when the antigen is an alloantigen such as H-2 (2) or a rabbit allotype such as (28).

8. Induction of silent idiotypes can also be performed with polyclonal B-cell activators (25) and by injection of antiidiotypic antibodies into neonates (14).

9. The studies of Bona and Paul (3, 4) have shown that the expression of idiotype MOPC 460 is hampered by "naturally occurring" suppressors displaying receptors of antiidiotypic specificity. These suppressor T cells seem to recognize idiotopes in association with "allotypic markers." Furthermore, these suppressors are undetectable in Ab3 mice and can be blocked by Ab3 passively injected into normal mice. These results fit well with our initial hypothesis (31–33).

10. So far, the immunization cascade has led to the synthesis of the expected idiotype in all cases using polyclonal antiidiotypic antibodies. The procedure is expected to work with some monoclonal antiidiotypic antibodies, but not all. Some idiotopes may be absent from the germline repertoire (genetic polymorphism). Some idiotopes could be the result of somatic mutations. Others could be unconnected in the functional idiotypic network.

11. We have induced Ab1′ antibodies which are idiotypically very similar but derive from distinct germline genes. For example, it is possible to manipulate BALB/c mice so that they can later express the cross-reactive antiarsonate idiotype of A/J mice (despite the fact that the corresponding germline gene seems to be absent from the BALB/c genome) (22a).

IV. Internal Images

We shall end by considering some cases of recurrency from which probably no genetic conclusions can be drawn. Antibodies against

TMV in rabbits behave like antibodies against *Salmonella, Micrococcus,* etc. The frequency of idiotypic cross-reactions is on the order of 2–3%. Nonetheless, in some rabbits producing Ab2 antibodies, some bleedings contain antiidiotypic antibodies with strange properties.

1. These antibodies react with the antigen (Ab1) as expected, but also react with all anti-TMV antibodies from all rabbits (whatever the allotypic formula: a1, a2, a3, etc.).
2. These peculiar antibodies also react with anti-TMV antibodies from mice, goats, horses, and chickens.
3. However, they do not recognize antibodies raised against other antigens (DNP, *Micrococcus,* bungarotoxin, hemocyanin, etc.). They are therefore exquisitely specific for anti-TMV antibodies.
4. These special Ab2 from rabbits, when injected into mice, elicit the synthesis of anti-TMV antibodies in the absence of antigen. Therefore, in this case, Ab3 does recognize antigen.

The most obvious explanation is that some antiidiotypic antibodies display some idiotopes that mimic conformationally one epitope of TMV. They behave as the internal images of TMV or, more precisely, TMV behaves as the external image of some idiotopes. These data are illustrated in Figs. 2 and 3. The occurrence of these special AB2 in the TMV system is sporadic and rare. This is also true of antiidiotypic antibodies in the insulin and alprenolol systems.

An interesting example comes from the study of b6 antigen by J. Roland and P. A. Cazenave. When antiidiotypic antibodies are raised against antiallotypic antibodies (anti-b6), an apparent recurrency is found. One Ab2 recognizes all anti-b6. Furthermore, Ab3 antibodies regularly react with immunoglobulins bearing b6 allotopes. In this case, the phenomenon is not at all sporadic. The authors have proposed that some antiidiotypic antibodies behave as the internal image of b6 antigen. The appearance of internal images is more frequent in alloantigenic systems (28).

A final and important question concerning internal images is, Do they have a special meaning in functional idiotypic networks, or do they simply show that the immune system is able to respond to unforeseen antigenic stimuli because it already contains the imprevisible in the form of imperfect internal images? A clue to the answer can perhaps be furnished by experiments measuring the frequency of Ab2ε (Ab2β) in the set of possible Ab2 and by identifying the parameters promoting the appearance of classical Ab2 or the so-called internal images.

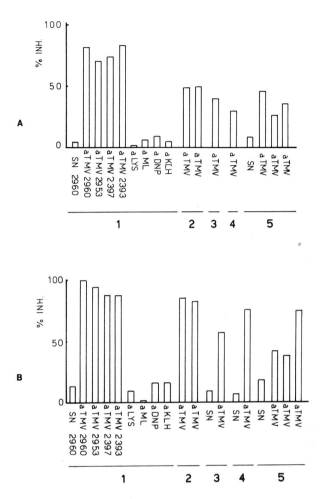

Fig. 2. (A) A rabbit antiidiotypic antiserum (2880) was raised, in the usual way, against the anti-TMV antibodies from rabbit 2960. This rabbit Ab2 serum, as explained in the text, has an unusual behavior. The figure shows the inhibition of the heterologous binding of this special Ab2 to radiolabeled anti-TMV antibodies from rabbit 2393 by 5 μl of putative inhibitory sera from (1) rabbit, (2) goats, (3) horses, (4) chickens, and (5) mice. SN, normal serum: a TMV, anti-TMV antibodies; aKLH, antihemocyanin antibodies; aDNP, anti-DNP antibodies; aML, anti-*Micrococcus luteus* antibodies; aLys, antilysozyme antibodies. (B) Inhibition of the heterologous binding between radiolabeled purified goat anti-TMV antibodies to the "special" antiidiotypic serum. As in (A), the lines below the bars indicate the species origin of tested sera: (1) rabbit, (2) goat, (3) horses, (4) chicken, and (5) mice.

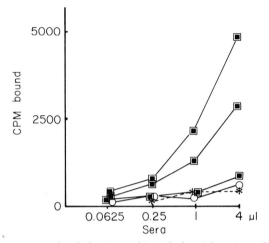

Fig. 3. Mice were injected with the "special" purified antiidiotypic antibodies from rabbit 2880 (■), with other conventional antiidiotypic antibodies raised against the rabbit anti-TMV idiotype 2953 (○), or with normal rabbit immunoglobulins (∗). Sera from injected mice were incubated with 96 wells of trays previously coated with TMV. Bound antibodies are revealed with iodinated protein A from *Staphylococcus aureus*. Results are given for individual mice in immunization with the internal image. For the other immunizations, the numbers given represent the mean of three mice. It should be noted that these mice have never been injected with TMV. The magnitude of the response is comparable to that of a primary response to TMV.

Finally, it is our hope that this chapter will not add more confusion to the growing field of idiotypic studies but will be of some help in clarification and interpretation.

References

1. Atassi, Z. (1980). Precise determination of protein antigenic structures has unravelled the molecular immune recognition of proteins and provided a prototype for synthetic mimicking of other protein binding sites. *Mol. Cell. Biochem.* **32,** 21–43.
2. Bluestone, J. A., Epstein, S. L., Ozato, K., Sharrow, S. D., and Sachs, D. (1981). Antiidiotypes to monoclonal anti-H2 antibodies. *J. Exp. Med.* **159,** 1305–1318.
3. Bona, C., and Paul, W. E. (1979). Cellular basis of expression of idiotypes. *J. Exp. Med.* **149,** 532–539.
4. Bona, C., Hooghe, R., Cazenave, P.-A., Le Guern, C., and Paul, W. E. (1979). Cellular basis of regulation of expression of idiotype II. Immunity to anti-MOPC 460 idiotypic antibodies increases the level of anti-trinitrophenyl antibodies bearing 460 idiotypes. *J. Exp. Med.* **149,** 815–823.
5. Bona, C., Heber-Katz, H., and Paul, W. E. (1981). Idiotype-antiidiotype regulation.

I. Immunization with a levan-binding myeloma protein leads to the appearance of autoanti-(anti-Id) antibodies and to activation of silent clones. *J. Exp. Med.* **153**, 951–967.

6. Bothwell, A., Paskind, M., Reth, M., Imanishi, T., Rajewsky, K., and Baltimore, D. (1981). Heavy chain variable region contribution to the NP^b family of antibodies somatic mutation evident in a γ2 a variable region. *Cell* **24**, 625–637.

7. Bretscher, P., and Cohn, M. (1970). A theory of self-nonself discrimination. *Science* **169**, 1042–1049.

8. Burnet, M. F. (1959). "The Clonal Selection Theory of Acquired Immunity." Cambridge Univ. Press, London and New York.

9. Cazenave, P.-A. (1977). Idiotypic-antiidiotypic regulation of antibody synthesis in rabbits. *Proc. Natl. Acad. Sci. U.S.A.* **74**, 5122–5125.

10. Cazenave, P.-A., and Le Guern, C. (1979). Regulation of the immune system by idiotype-anti-idiotype interaction in the rabbit and the mouse. *In* "Cells of Immunoglobulin Synthesis" (B. Pernis and H. J. Vogel, eds.), pp. 343–355. Academic Press, New York.

11. Claman, H. N., Chaperon, E. A., and Triplett, R. F. (1966). Thymus-marrow cell combinations. Synergism in antibody production. *Proc. Soc. Exp. Biol. Med.* **122**, 1167–1171.

12. Eichmann, K., Coutinho, A., and Melchers, F. (1977). Absolute frequencies of lipopolysaccharide reactive B cells producing A5A idiotype in unprimed, anti-A5A sensitized and anti-A5A idiotype suppressed A/J mice. *J. Exp. Med.* **146**, 1436–1449.

13. Gershon, R. K. (1981). On the primacy of antigen as a perturbent and mediator of immunological homeostasis. *UCLA Symp. Mol. Cell. Biol.* **20**, 581–594.

14. Hiernaux, J., Bona, C., and Baker, P. J. (1981). Neonatal treatment with low doses of anti-idiotypic antibodies leads to the expression of a silent clone. *J. Exp. Med.* **153**, 1004–1008.

15. Jerne, N. K. (1955). The natural selection theory of antibody formation. *Proc. Natl. Acad. Sci. U.S.A.* **41**, 849–856.

16. Jerne, N. K. (1974). Towards a network theory of the immune system. *Ann. Immunol. (Paris)* **125C**, 373–389.

17. Jerne, N. K. (1982). *In* "Idiotypes-Antigens on the Inside" (E. Westen-Schnurr, ed.), pp. 12–15. Editions Roche, Basel, Switzerland.

18. Jerne, N. K., Roland, J., and Cazenave, P.-A. (1982). Recurrent idiotopes and internal images. *EMBO J.* **1**, 243–247.

19. Juy, D., Primi, D., and Cazenave, P.-A. (1982). Idiotype regulation: Evidence for the involvement of Igh-C-restricted T cells in the M460 idiotype suppressive pathway. *Eur. J. Immunol.* **12**, 24–30.

20. Kelus, A. S., and Cell, P. G. H. (1968). Immunological analysis of rabbit anti-antibody system. *J. Exp. Med.* **127**, 215–234.

21. Kunkel, H. G., Mannick, M., and William, R. C. (1963). Individual antigenic specificities of isolated antibodies. *Science* **140**, 1218–1219.

22. Mitchison, N. A. (1971). The carrier effect in the secondary response to hapten-protein conjugates. *Eur. J. Immunol.* **1**, 10–17.

22a. Moser, M., Leo, O., Hiernaux, J., and Urbain, J. (1983). *Proc. Natl. Acad. Sci. U.S.A.* **80**, 4474–4478.

23. Oudin, J., and Michel, M. (1963). Une nouvelle forme d'allotypie des immunoglobulines du sérum de lapin. *C.R. Hebd. Seances Acad. Sci.* **257**, 805–808.

24. Oudin, J., and Cazenave, P.-A. (1971). Similar idiotypic specificities in immunoglobulin fractions with different antibody functions or even without detectable antibody function. *Proc. Natl. Acad. Sci. U.S.A.* **68**, 2616–2620.
25. Primi, D., Juy, D., and Cazenave, P.-A. (1981). Induction and regulation of silent idiotype clones. *Eur. J. Immunol.* **11**, 393–398.
26. Rajewsky, K., and Takemori, T. (1983). Genetics, expression and function of idiotypes. *Annu. Rev. Immunol.* **7**, 569–607.
27. Richards, F. F., and Konigsberg, W.H. (1973). Speculations. How specific are antibodies? *Immunochemistry* **10**, 545–553.
28. Roland, J., and Cazenave, P.-A. (1981). Rabbits immunized against b6 allotype express similar anti-b6 idiotopes. *Eur. J. Immunol.* **11**, 469–474.
29. Schreiber, A. B., Couraud, P. O., André, C., Vray, B., and Strossberg, A. D. (1980). Anti-alprenolol anti-idiotype antibodies bind to beta adrenergic receptors and modulate catecholamine-sensitive adenylate cyclase. *Proc. Natl. Acad. Sci. U.S.A.* **77**, 7385–7389.
30. Sigal, N. H., and Klinman, N. R. (1978). The B cell clonotype repertoire. *Adv. Immunol.* **4**, 255–337.
31. Urbain, J., Wikler, M., Franssen, J.-D., and Collignon, C. (1977). Idiotypic regulation of the immune system by the induction of antibodies against anti-idiotypic antibodies. *Proc. Natl. Acad. Sci. U.S.A.* **74**, 5126–5130.
32. Urbain, J., Wuilmart, C., and Cazenave, P.-A. (1981). Idiotypic networks in immune regulation. *Contemp. Top. Mol. Immunol.* **8**, 113–148.
33. Wikler, M., Franssen, J.-D., Collignon, C., Leo, O., Mariamé, B., Van de Walle, P., De Groote, D., and Urbain, J. (1981). Idiotypic regulation of the immune system. *J. Exp. Med.* **150**, 184–195.
34. Wikler, M., Demeur, C., Dewasme, G., and Urbain, J. (1980). Immunoregulatory role of maternal idiotypes. *J. Exp. Med.* **152**, 1024–1035.
35. Zinkernagel, R. M., and Doherty, P. (1977). *Contemp. Top. Immunobiol.* **7**, 179–214.

Chapter 3

Regulatory Idiotopes[1]

Constantin A. Bona
Department of Microbiology
Mount Sinai School of Medicine
New York, New York

I. Introduction

Soon after the discovery of idiotypy by Kunkel *et al.* (20) and Oudin and Michel (27), idiotypic determinants were located on Fv fragments of immunoglobulin (Ig) molecules (13) and were therefore considered to be phenotypic markers of the V region gene (21). An immunoglobulin molecule bears several idiotopes, i.e., idiotopes associated with the combining site (paratope) or framework segments of the V region, cross-reactive idiotypes (IdX) shared by various Ig molecules, and individual idiotypes (IdI) characteristic of a monoclonal protein. Antibodies specific for these antigenic determinants can be obtained by xeno- or alloimmunization. By contrast, syngeneic and auto-anti-Id antibodies are restricted to a few idiotopes, suggesting that not all antigenic determinants of the V region are immunogenic in an autologous system.

We have previously proposed that only a few idiotopes play a role in idiotype-regulated immune responses, and we have called these regulatory idiotopes (7). Therefore, regulatory idiotopes represent a cate-

[1] This work was supported by U.S. Public Health Research grants AG/A10271601 Ai and Grant PCM81105788 from the National Science Foundation.

gory of antigenic determinants of Ig molecules that can be defined by several criteria as follows: (a) regulatory idiotopes function as autoimmunogens and are able to induce the synthesis of auto-anti-Id antibodies; (b) they are shared by several members of an idiotype network pathway and could be shared by antibodies with different antigenic specificities (i.e., parallel sets); and (c) they possess the potential of becoming dominant idiotypes, because these determinants are capable of eliciting idiotype-specific T-cell regulation during the course of an immune response.

The concept of regulatory idiotopes emerged from a study of the antigen binding properties of various members of an idiotype network pathway. A series of anti-Id antibodies, mimicking a cascade of the Id-anti-Id chain comprising Ab2 (i.e., anti-Id antibodies), Ab3 (i.e., anti-anti-ID antibodies), and Ab4 (i.e., anti[anti(anti-Id)] antibodies), were induced by the immunization of syngeneic mice with the β2-6 fructosan binding A48 monoclonal protein (7), as well as by immunization of allotype-matched rabbits with polyclonal anti-*Micrococcus lyso-deikticus* polysaccharide antibodies (35).

II. Immunochemical Properties of Syngeneic Ab1, Ab2, Ab3, and Ab4 Antibodies

The immunochemical properties of various anti-Id antibodies of the A48 idiotype pathway were studied using hemagglutination assays (HA) and radioimmunoassays (RIA).

ABPC48 is a β2-6 fructosan binding IgA$_k$ myeloma protein of BALB/c origin. This protein bears several idiotopes, some of them shared with UPC-10, another IgG$_2$a β2-6 fructosan binding myeloma protein. Neither protein expresses the IdXs, i.e., IdX-G, -A, and -B of β2-1 fructosan binding myeloma proteins. Syngeneic anti-A48Id antibodies (Ab2) produced in response to immunization with an A48-KLH conjugate agglutinated both Ab1-SRBC and Ab3-SRBC. The Ab1-SRBC agglutinating activity of Ab2 antibodies was completely removed by prior absorption with A48-Sepharose beads and largely, although not completely, with Ab3-Sepharose beads. Ab3 antiserum, as expected, agglutinated Ab2-SRBC. The syngeneic Ab4 antiserum agglutinated Ab3-SRBC, but interestingly it also agglutinated Ab1-SRBC. The ability of Ab4 antiserum to agglutinate Ab1-SRBC was completely removed by absorption with Ab3-Sepharose beads and only partially with Ab1-Sepharose beads (Table I).

TABLE I

HA Titers of Ab2, Ab3, and Ab4 Antisera[a]

	HA titers[b] on SRBC coated with						
	Ab1			Ab2		Ab3	
	Unadsorbed	Ab1[c]	Ab3	Unadsorbed	Ab2	Unadsorbed	Ab3
Nonimmune	0	ND[d]	ND	0	ND	0	ND
Anti-A48-KLH (Ab2)	10	0	2	0	0	9	2
Anti-(anti-A48)-KLH (Ab3)	0	0	ND	10	0	0	0
Anti-[anti-(anti-A48)-KLH] (Ab4)	3	2	0	0	0	4	0
Rabbit antimouse κ	>12	ND	ND	>12	ND	>12	ND

[a] From Bona et al. (7).

[b] HA titers in $\log_2$ units.

[c] Sera adsorbed with Sepharose 4B conjugated with Ab1, purified Ab2, or purified Ab3.

[d] Not done.

These results suggested that Ab4 resembles Ab2 because both bind to Ab1, although the binding affinity of Ab4 for Ab1 was lower than that of Ab4 for Ab3. In order to investigate the affinity of Ab4 for Ab1, we studied the binding of labeled Ab1 and Ab3 to Ab2- or Ab4-coated microplates, and estimated the concentration of Ab1 required to inhibit the binding of labeled Ab1 and Ab3 to Ab4 microplates.

We observed that labeled Ab1 and Ab3 bound to both Ab2 and Ab4 plates. Controls using BALB/c Ig and Ab3 plates attested to the specificity of this binding. The ratio of the concentration of labeled Ab1 bound by Ab2 and Ab4 plates and the ratio of labeled Ab3 bound by these plates were similar (Table II).

Because all Ab1 and Ab3 molecules should be specific for Ab2, the similarity of this ratio suggests that the fraction of the Ab4 molecules specific for Ab1 is similar to the fraction of the Ab3 molecules specific for Ab4. The relative affinity of Ab4 for Ab1 was estimated from the concentration of Ab1 required to inhibit the binding of labeled Ab1 and Ab3 to Ab4-coated plates. We found that 2.2 μg/ml of Ab1 was needed to inhibit 50% of the binding of labeled Ab3 to Ab4 plates, whereas only 0.006 μg/ml of Ab3 was needed for comparable inhibition (Table III). This result suggested that Ab4 binds to Ab3 with substantially greater affinity than it binds to Ab1.

The study of the β2-6 fructosan binding ability of various members

TABLE II

Binding of Radioactive Ab1 and Ab3 to Plates Coated with Ab2 and Ab4[a]

	Bound ligand	
Microplates coated with	^{3}H-Labeled Ab1 (cpm)	^{125}I-Labeled Ab3 (cpm)
BALB/c Ig (10 μg/ml)	105	1130 ± 111
Ab3 (10 μg/ml)	110 ± 8	ND[b]
Ab2 (10 μg/ml)	1386 ± 142	22,944 ± 1374
Ab4 (150 μg/ml Ig)	524 ± 19	8173 ± 271
Specific binding to Ab4/specific to Ab2[c]	0.33	0.32

[a] From Bona et al., (7).

[b] Not done.

[c] Binding to Ab4 plate; binding to control plates/binding to Ab2 plate; binding to control plates.

of the A48Id network pathway has shown that Ab1 agglutinated BL-SRBC, whereas Ab3 did not. Thus, our results, as well as those reported by Winkler *et al.* (35), indicate an apparent asymmetry of the network because Ab2 and Ab4 bind to Ab1, whereas Ab3 does not bind to BL. The analysis of the binding activity of monoclonal antibodies secreted by hybrid cells obtained by the fusion of SP2/0 cells with spleen cells obtained from BALB/c immunized with Ab2-KLH and then with BL indicated that some of these Ab3 antibodies exhibited β2-6 fructosan binding activity. Interestingly, we have found that

TABLE III

Inhibition of Binding of Radioactive Ab1 and Ab3 to Plates Coated with Ab2 and Ab4[a]

Microplate coated with	Ligand	[Inhibitor] for 50% inhibition (μg/ml)		
		Ab1	Ab3	MOPC-384
Ab2 (10 μg/ml)	^{3}H-labeled Ab1	0.003	ND[b]	>100
Ab2	^{125}I-labeled Ab3	0.007	ND	>100
Ab4 (150 μg/ml Ig)	^{3}H-labeled Ab1	0.03	ND	>100
Ab4	^{125}I-labeled Ab3	2.2	0.006	>100

[a] From Bona et al. (7).

[b] Not done.

TABLE IV

Antigenic Binding Properties of Monoclonal Antibodies
Obtained from BALB/c Mice Producing Ab3 and
Immunized with Bacterial Levan

| Monoclonal antibody | Antigen binding specificity | | | |
| | Bacterial levan | | Inulin | |
	HA[a]	RIA[b]	HA	RIA
ABPC48	11	4829 ± 694	0	171 ± 296
W3082	9	2529 ± 102	23	7016 ± 806
MOPC-21	0	0	0	0
76-Ab3-1	2	ND[c]	1	ND
76-Ab3-12	1	2516 ± 181	0	0
76-Ab3-29	0	3914 ± 94	1	1839 ± 156
76-Ab3-38	6	7502 ± 406	2	5608 ± 137
76-Ab3-42	0	1537 ± 256	1	444 ± 171

[a] HA titer $\log^2$ units.
[b] RIA-cpm. Microtiter plates coated with bacterial levan on inulin BSA were incubated with monoclonal antibodies and then with ^{125}I-labeled goat antimouse Ig.
[c] Not done.

some Ab3 monoclonal antibodies bound to β2-1 fructosan, whereas the A48 monoclonal protein itself lacks β2-1 fructosan binding activity (Table IV). These results demonstrate that injection of Ab2 antibodies profoundly alters the expression of clones because they can activate three different types of clones: (a) clones specific for idiotypes of Ab2 antibodies representing true Ab3; (b) clones that express A48 idiotopes and bind only β2-6 fructosan, representing a true Ab1; and (c) clones that express A48 idiotopes and bind both β2-6 and β2-1 fructosan, similar to Inulin binding myeloma proteins. These clones represent a parallel set that we did not encounter in the conventional antibody response induced subsequent to immunization of normal BALB/c mice with BL.

III. Functional Properties of Syngeneic Ab1, Ab2, Ab3, and Ab4 Antibodies

The concept of a regulatory idiotype predicts not only an immuno-chemical similarity between even and odd members of a given idiotypic pathway but also a functional resemblance between various members. Functional similarities between various members of the A48 idiotype network pathway were studied by investigating the effect of Ab1, Ab2, Ab3, and Ab4 on the anti-β2-6 fructosan response, as well as on the growth of ABPC48 myeloma cells.

A. EFFECT ON THE ANTIBACTERIAL LEVAN RESPONSE

Immunization with BL, which is a β2-6 polyfructosan with β2-1 branch points, leads to the development of a significant titer of anti-BL antibodies and anti-BL plaque-forming cell response (PFC). As we have previously shown, A48Id$^+$ anti-BL antibodies are not detected in this response (6), indicating that A48Id$^+$ clones represent a minor or silent clone of the anti-BL repertoire in IghC^a mice. However, we succeeded in activating A48Id$^+$ clones in IdX-suppressed nude BALB/c mice. Therefore, the effects of Ab2, Ab3, and Ab4 antibodies on both the anti-BL response and the expression of A48Id clones were studied.

Immunization of mice with Ab1 or Ab3-KLH conjugates led to the production of Ab2 and Ab4 antibodies. The study of the kinetics of production of anti-BL antibodies in mice producing Ab2 and Ab4 showed that the titer of anti-BL antibodies in Ab2-producing mice did not approach normal levels until 20 days after immunization with BL. Ab4-producing mice showed a degree of suppression of their total anti-BL response that was at least as pronounced as that of Ab2-producing mice.

BALB/c mice that had been immunized with Ab2-KLH developed a vigorous response upon immunization with BL, and a substantial fraction of these antibodies expressed the A48Id. Therefore, immunity to Ab1, Ab2, or Ab3 in mice has a significant effect on the amount and nature of the antibody response to BL, the antigen that is the putative initiator of the Id-anti-Id chain. In mice producing Ab3, either because of immunization with Ab2-KLH or after immunization with Ab1, a major fraction of their anti-BL antibodies expressed A48Id.

It is interesting to consider why immunity to Ab2 leads to the expression of A48Id. Three hypotheses can be entertained.

1. One obvious possibility is that Ab3, which is an anti(anti-A48Id)-specific antibody, could eliminate suppressor T cells which share the idiotype of Ab2. We have shown in the MOPC-460 trinitrophenyl (TNP) system that mice immunized with Ab2 lack 460Id-

TABLE V

Persistence of A48Id Clones Subsequent to Pretreatment at Birth of BALB/c Mice with 10 ng Anti-A48Id Antibodies

Age of mice (in weeks) when immunized with 20 μg BL	Normal mice		Mice treated at birth	
	BL-Specific PFC[a]	A48Id + PFC (%)	BL-Specific PFC	A48Id + PFC (%)
4	3,290 ± 0.111	6 ± 3	3431 ± 0.081	52 ± 7
5	3,600 ± 0.125	6 ± 3	3518 ± 0.123	46 ± 14
6	3,114 ± 0.02	14 ± 2	2669 ± 0.137	79 ± 10
7	3,704 ± 0.192	6 ± 2	4025 ± 0.121	47 ± 9
12	10,486 ± 0.144	11 ± 3	3510 ± 0.238	47 ± 12

[a] Mean ± SEM for $\log_2$ PFC/spleen detected for five mice 5 days after immunization.

specific suppressor T cells, which occur naturally in normal BALB/c mice (2). We have no evidence, however, that anti-A48Id antibodies share idiotopes with putative A48Id-specific T cells. Moreover, if elimination of suppressor T cells is the only mechanism by which immunity to Ab2 leads to expression of A48Id clones, one might anticipate that nude mice immunized with BL should express A48Id. We have already reported that this is not the case (22).

2. A second possibility is that Ab3 represents a set of antibodies that belong to the Ab1 family and bind to Ab2 via their A48-like idiotopes as well as β2-6 fructosan epitopes. Whether these antibodies are encoded by germline genes or represent somatic variants remains to be established.

3. The third possibility is that Ab2 antibodies express β2-6 fructosan-like determinants because their idiotopes represent the internal image of the antigen. If idiotopes of Ab2 represent the internal image of β2-6 fructosan epitopes, then they can expand β2-6 fructosan-specific clones because they can function as BL. Having previously observed that the production of large amounts of Ab2 inhibited the production of anti-BL antibodies, we studied the effects of administration at birth of small amounts of Ab2. Surprisingly, the injection of 10 ng of Ab2 at birth led to a long-lasting activation of A48Id silent clones, which can be turned on to produce anti-BL antibodies subsequent to immunization with BL 4–12 weeks after birth (14) (Table V). This response can be transferred into lethally irradiated BALB/c mice by the infusion of B cells originating from BALB/c mice pretreated at birth with minute amounts of anti-A48Id antibodies.

B. ANTITUMOR PROPERTIES OF Ab2, Ab3, AND Ab4

Because A48 monoclonal protein is secreted by ABPC48 myeloma cells, we have studied the growth of tumor cells in Ab2-, Ab3-, and Ab4-producing mice subsequent to immunization with Ab1-, Ab2-, and Ab3-KLH conjugates, respectively. The growth of the tumor was monitored by measuring [3H]thymidine incorporation of spleen cells originating from animals injected with 10^3 myeloma cells (previously adapted to growth in spleen), as well as determining, by RIA, the serum BL titer and IgA level. The rationale of this study is based on the observation of Lynch *et al.* (24), who showed that anti-Id immunity can prevent the growth of myeloma cells carrying the corresponding idiotype. We observed a substantial delay in the growth of ABPC48 myeloma cells in BALB/c mice producing Ab2 and Ab4 antibodies subsequent to immunization with A48 or Ab3-KLH conjugates, whereas mice immunized with BL or Ab2-KLH conjugate died 12–15 days after the injection of 10^3 ABPC48 myeloma cells.

These results suggest that Ab2 and Ab4 display a functional similarity, and reinforce serological evidence indicating that Ab4 resembles Ab2 in that it too binds to Ab1.

IV. Regulatory Idiotype Network

Niels Jerne, in his network theory of the immune system (17), viewed the immune system as a collection of clones, each capable of recognizing antigens through their paratopes (i.e., combining sites) and each capable of being recognized by the other clones because they express idiotopes on their antigen binding receptors. A key factor in this concept is the potential importance of receptor-specific regulation of the immune system in contrast to antigen-specific regulation, as postulated by clonal theory. Network theory predicts a vectorial character in these paratope–idiotype interactions. Indeed, it was predicted that Ab1 bearing a paratope (designated p1) and an idiotope (termed i1) can elicit the production of Ab2 which expresses p2 (specific for i1) and an idiotope (i2). This, in turn, can elicit the synthesis of Ab3 (p3i3), which when used as an immunogen can induce the production of Ab4 (p4i4), etc. This linear pathway is the one to be anticipated on the basis of Jerne's postulate that the interaction of an idiotope (i_n) and its complementary paratope (pn + 1) stimulates production of pn + 1-bearing molecules, which in turn suppresses the production of these i_n-bearing molecules. However, recent data have shown that immunization with Ab2 can also exert the opposite effect. We have shown that immunization with syngeneic anti-460Id and anti-A48Id led to a dramatic increase of the 460Id component of anti-TNP antibody (3) or to the activation of A48Id anti-BL silent clones (14), respectively. In mice, it was shown that injection of heterologous (pig) anti-Id against antinuclease or anti-H-2 antibodies elicited the production of antinuclease or anti-H-2 antibodies (1, 26). In the rabbit, it was also shown that the injection of antiidiotypic antibodies against anti-polysaccharide (33), antibovine RNase (8), and anti-allotype (16) elicited the production of so-called Ab1, i.e., antipolysaccharide, anti-RNase, or antiallotype antibodies. Furthermore, immunization of mice or allotype-matched rabbits with syngeneic or allogeneic Ab3 elicited the production of Ab2 antibodies displaying serologic and functional properties of a true Ab2 antibody. To explain these results, we postulated that Ab1 molecules express a particular set of idiotopes—regulatory idiotopes (ri)—as well as other conventional idiotopes. Regulatory idiotopes function as immunogens in an autologous system, and they elicit synthesis of Ab2 which are anti-ri antibodies. Ab2 lack regulatory idiotopes, and immunization with Ab2 leads to the production of a very limited number of true Ab3 antibodies (p3i3), probably specific for the IdI of Ab2; thus, they will activate mainly the production of cells bearing ri. Therefore, the population of Ab3 will be composed primarily of cells bearing ri molecules which belong to the Ab1 family, with only a limited number of cells bearing i3 molecules. Therefore, Ab4 produced in response to immunization with Ab3 is principally made up of anti-ri molecules rather than anti-i3 antibodies (Fig. 1).

A prediction based on the regulatory idiotopes concept is that they can be present at high levels in the sera of animals that have not been intentionally immunized with antigens and can emerge as dominant idiotopes subsequent to immunization. Their expression can be favored by genetically or environmentally determined selection. Examples of these idiotopes include the idiotypic determinants of the T15Id normally expressed on antiphosphocholine antibodies, J558IdX on anti-α-1-3 dextran antibodies, W3129 on anti-α1-3 dextran antibodies, X24 on antigalactan antibodies, E109 found on the majority of anti-β2-1 fructosan antibodies, and IdX Z, W of anti-LPS (lipopolysaccharide) antibodies.

Regulatory idiotopes, in addition to being present at higher concen-

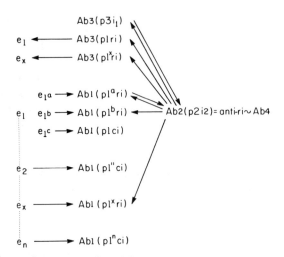

Fig. 1. Regulatory idiotype network model: e, epitype e_{1a}, e_{1b}, e_{1c} epitopes; p, paratope; i = idiotope; ri, regulatory idiotopes; ci, conventional idiotopes; Ab1, antibody; Ab2, anti-Id antibody; Ab3, anti(anti-id)antibody; Ab4, anti[anti(anti-id)]antibody.

trations than conventional idiotopes, should also be found on antibodies displaying many distinct paratopes (i.e., antigenic specificities). This postulate is supported by the following findings:

1. Shared idiotypes were observed among the antibodies specific for distinct antigenic determinants borne by the same antigen (Table VI).

2. Shared idiotopes were identified on monoclonal antibodies specific for galactose and glucose immunodominant sugars of *Escherichia coli* 113 LPS, as well as on MOPC384 and MOPC870 monoclonal proteins specific for α-methyl-β-galactoside, the immunodominant sugar of *Salmonella tranaroa* LPS (15).

3. We have investigated the ability of 198 murine myeloma proteins to inhibit the binding of labeled A48 protein to anti-A48Id antibody-coated plates. We have found that MOPC167, which is a phosphocholine (PC) binding myeloma protein, inhibited 50% of this binding (Table VII). This result is based on a small sample of murine myeloma proteins and suggests a frequency of 0.5% of shared idiotypes. Interestingly, this frequency is comparable to the percentage (0.5–1.0%) of B cells from normal mice stained with various syngeneic and homologous anti-Id antibodies (34). Obviously, the high percentage of cells in which the staining of anti-Id antibodies was associated with the concomitant staining of monoclonal anti-μ or anti-δ antibod-

TABLE VI

Shared Idiotypes among Antibodies Specific for Different Epitopes Borne by the Same Antigen or Antigen-Related Molecules

Antigen specificity	Species of immunized animal	Idiotype	Antigen specificity of antibodies sharing idiotypes	References
Hen ovalbumin	Rabbit	Id of antiova	Duck and turkey ova	28
Sickle cell hemoglobin	Goat	Val Id	Adult hemoglobin	19
IgG_{2a}^b allotype	Mouse	IdX of anti-b allotype	CH_2 and CH_3 domains of IgG_{2a}^b	5
Egg white lysozyme	Mouse	HEL-IdX	L II and N-C fragments of HEL	25
GTGL	Mouse	GTGL-Id	GT and GL	18
PR8 hemagglutinin	Mouse	IdX of anti-PR8	Different domains of PR8 HA	23

ies probably can be explained more by the sharing of idiotypes by the Ig receptor of B clones specific for various antigens. Because an ri is expected to be found on the Ig receptor of many different specificities, the activation of regulatory T cells can lead to the expression of B-cell clones sharing ri and therefore to the occurrence of parallel sets of antibodies. The appearance of so-called nonspecific immunoglobulins during bacterial, viral, and parasitic infections is well known. Molecules bearing E109 IdX A and B devoid of anti-β2-1 fructosan activity

TABLE VII

Ability of MOPC-167 to Inhibit the Binding of A48 Monoclonal Protein to Anti-A48Id Antibodies

Monoclonal protein	Binding activity	HI	RIA	ELISA
ABPC48	β2-6 fructosan	8[a]	5[b]	96[c]
W3082	β2-6 and β2-1 fructosans	0	>5000	0
MOPC-167	Phosphocholine	0	500	52
Other 198 monoclonal proteins	Various and unknown	ND[d]	>5000	0

[a] HI titer $\log_2$ units.
[b] Nanograms required for 50% inhibition.
[c] Percentage of inhibition obtained with 5 μg monoclonal protein.
[d] Not done.

(4), and molecules bearing 460Id which lack TNP binding specificity (11) in unintentionally immunized mice, are clear examples of parallel sets.

Finally, we postulated that B- and T-cell clones bearing such regulatory idiotopes may be especially selected to participate in immune responses to various foreign epitopes, because the preexisting idiotype-specific regulatory T cells might favor their expansion.

There are several reported results that can be interpreted as regulatory idiotopes.

1. Rubinstein *et al.* (30) have shown that administration at birth of A48Id-bearing monoclonal antibodies led to the dominance in A48Id of an anti-BL response. The increased A48Id response was related to the expansion of A48Id-specific helper T cells.

2. In the T15-Id system using the frequency analysis method, the existence of precursors of T15-Id-specific T cells was shown (29). These precursors can be expanded by stimulation with T15 or PC-conjugates subsequent to parenteral administration (10, 32) or during a conventional immune response induced by phosphocholine (9). These Id-specific T cells probably are needed for clonal dominance and are involved in the cyclical appearance of T15-Id during the PC immune response in mice. Gleason and Kohler (12) have shown that the frequency of helper cells that recognize T15 and M167 used as carriers for an anti-TNP B-cell response is similar despite the fact that M167-Id is not detected among anti-PC antibodies. This suggested that T15-Id-specific T cell also recognizes a similar structure on M167. Indeed, MOPC167 inhibited T-cell recognition of TNP-T15, and PC did block the help for T15-TNP and M167-TNP. These results suggested that Id-specific helper cells recognize a shared determinant associated with the PC binding site of T15 and M167 monoclonal proteins. This determinant exhibited by T15 and M167 may be a regulatory idiotype.

3. Sherr *et al.* (31) have investigated the fine specificity of anti-Id suppressor T cells induced by intravenous injection of syngeneic spleen cells covalently coupled with the 4-hydroxy-3-nitrophenylacetyl (NP) hapten. Interestingly, these cells bound to anti-NP antibodies that express different levels of serologically detected NP[b] idiotypic determinants. These results suggest that anti-Id T suppressor cells can recognize idiotypic determinants on different NP reactive clones and therefore could have a large suppressor effect. Similarly, in the ferredoxin system, it was shown that the elimination of T suppressor cells by anti-Id antibodies against antibody specific for the N epitope

led to an overall increase in the antibody response specific for both N and C epitopes of ferredoxin (J. Levy, personal communication). This observation would suggest that the suppressor cells can exert their effect through a regulatory idiotope shared by both anti-N and -C antibodies.

Therefore, the regulatory idiotopes probably represent a category of idiotopes that function as immunogens in an autologous system and play an important role in idiotype-determined regulatory mechanisms.

References

1. Bluestone, J. A., Sharrow, S. O., Epstein, S. L., Ozato, K., and Sachs, D. H. (1981). *Nature (London)* **191**, 233.
2. Bona, C., and Paul, W. E. (1979). *J. Exp. Med.* **149**, 542.
3. Bona, C., Hooghe, R., Cazenave, P.-A., Le Guern, C., and Paul, W. E. (1979). *J. Exp. Med.* **149**, 815.
4. Bona, C., Mond, J., Stein, K. E., House, S., Lieberman, R., and Paul, W. E. (1979). *J. Immunol.* **123**, 1484.
5. Bona, C. *et al.* (1980). *J. Exp. Med.* **151**, 1334.
6. Bona, C. (1981). *In* "B Lymphocytes in the Immune Response: Functional Development and Interactive Properties" (N. Klinman, D. Mosier, I. Scher, and E. Vitetta, eds.), pp. 437–447.
7. Bona, C., Heber-Katz, E., and Paul, W. E. (1981). *J. Exp. Med.* **153**, 951.
8. Cazenave, P.-A. (1977). *Proc. Natl. Acad. Sci. U.S.A.* **74**, 5122.
9. Cerny, J., and Caulfield, M. J. (1981). *J. Immunol.* **126**, 2262.
10. Cosenza, H., Julius, M. H., and Augustin, A. A. (1977). *Immunol. Rev.* **34**, 3.
11. Dzierzak, E. A., and Janeway, C. A. (1981). *J. Exp. Med.* **154**, 1442.
12. Gleason, K., and Kohler, H. (1982). *J. Exp. Med.* **156**, 539.
13. Grey, H. M., Mannik, M., and Kunkel, H. G. (1965). *J. Exp. Med.* **121**, 561.
14. Hiernaux, J., Bona, C., and Baker, P. J. (1981). *J. Exp. Med.* **153**, 1004.
15. Hiernaux, J., and Bona, C. (1982). *Proc. Natl. Acad. Sci. U.S.A.* **79**, 1616.
16. Jerne, K. J., Roland, J., and Cazenave, P.-A. (1982). *EMBO J.* **1**, 243.
17. Jerne, N. (1974). *Ann. Immunol. (Paris)* **125C**, 373.
18. Ju, S.-T., Benecerraf, B., and Dorf, M. E. (1980). *J. Exp. Med.* **152**, 170.
19. Karol, ? (1978). *J. Exp. Med.* **148**, 1488.
20. Kunkel, H. G., Mannik, M., and Williams, R. C. (1963). *Science* **140**, 1218.
21. Kunkel, H. G. (1970). *Fed. Proc., Fed. Am. Soc. Exp. Biol.* **9**, 55.
22. Lieberman, R., Bona, C., Chien, C. C., Stein, K. E., and Paul, W. E. (1979). *Ann. Immunol. (Paris)* **130C**, 247.
23. Liu, Y. N., Bona, C., and Schulman, J. L. (1981). *J. Exp. Med.* **154**, 1525.
24. Lynch, R. G., Graft, R. J., Sirisinha, S., Simms, S. G., and Eisen, H. N. (1972). *Proc. Natl. Acad. Sci. U.S.A.* **69**, 1540.
25. Metzger, D. W., Miller, A., and Sercarz, E. (1980). *Nature (London)* **287**, 540.
26. Miller, G. G., Nadler, P. I., Hodes, R. J., and Sachs, D. H. (1982). *J. Exp. Med.* **155**, 190.

27. Oudin, J., and Michel, M., (1963). *C.R. Hebd. Seances Acad. Sci.* **257**, 805.
28. Oudin, J. (1971). *Proc. Natl. Acad. Sci. U.S.A.* **68**, 2616.
29. Pierce, S. K., Speck, N. A., Gleason, K., Gearhart, P. J., and Kohler, H. (1981). *J. Exp. Med.* **154**, 1178.
30. Rubinstein, L. J., Yeh, M., and Bona, C. A. (1982). *J. Exp. Med.* **156**, 506.
31. Sherr, D. H., Yu, S.-T., and Dorf, M. (1981). *J. Exp. Med.* **154**, 1382.
32. Trenkner, E., and Riblet, R. (1975). *J. Exp. Med.* **142**, 1121.
33. Urbain, J., Winkler, M., Franssen, J. P., and Collignon, C. (1977). *Proc. Natl. Acad. Sci. U.S.A.* **74**, 5126.
34. Victor, C., Bona, C., and Pernis, B. (1983). *J. Immunol.* **130**, 1819.
35. Winkler, M., Franssen, J. D., Collignon, C., Leo, D., Mariamé, B., Van de Walle, P., DeGroote, D., and Urbain, J. (1979). *J. Exp. Med.* **150**, 184.

Chapter 4

The Uniqueness and Boundaries of the Idiotypic Self

Nelson M. Vaz

Laboratory of Immunobiology
Biomedical Institute, UFF
Niteroi, Brasil

and

Carlos Martinez-A. and António Coutinho

Laboratory of Immunobiology
Pasteur Institute
Paris, France

I. A Change of Paradigm in the Immunological Theory

The publication of the network theory (1) marks the beginning of the end of nearly 100 years of "horror autotoxicus." Self–nonself discrimination is no longer the central question in immunology; it is no longer even a question (2). Positive recognition of self and autoreactivity are essential properties of the immune system, necessary for its development (3) and embodying its function.

Immunology is no longer part of microbiology, as the immune system is not a collection of thousands of independent clones of resting cells waiting to mount an "immune response" and eliminate bacteria or viruses. The immune system is turned inward rather than outward, and its inherent internal activity is quantitatively more important than the accidental disturbances resulting from introduction of "external antigens." A normal, conventionally bred and fed adult mouse contains $1–1.5 \times 10^6$ "background-activated" immunoglobulin-secreting cells in its lymphoid organs which account for the production of serum antibodies. The larger part of this activity, however, is truly independent of environmental stimulation, because germ-free mice, fed on chemically defined, low molecular weight diets, also contain $0.5–1 \times 10^6$ background secreting cells (4). Intentional immunization of such mice with complex antigens, such as heterologous erythrocytes or bacteria, and the quantitative comparisons of such immune responses with the ongoing internal activity, provide the best demonstration that immune responses are "accidents de parcours" in the life of an immune system.

Starting from simple postulates on the extent of paratopic and idiotypic diversity, network perspectives provide the immune system with self-determined internal complementarities necessary (and sufficient) to its evolutionary requirements, ontogenic development, and maintenance of dynamic steady states. These internal controls are implicit in the self-determined organization of the system (2) and to a large extent are autonomous (although not independent) of environmental driving pressures; they represent the key to the completeness of the system repertoire (5) and its prometheic characteristics (6).

As often happens when paradigms shift, the new perspectives are not easily perceived; the ideas are far from being completely explored, and their consequences are not suspected. We shall try to outline very briefly some of the implications of the network theory which, in our opinion, deserve critical consideration and a more thorough theoretical approach.

II. Are We Concerned with the Most Complex System in Biology?

A. THE NERVOUS AND IMMUNE SYSTEMS: A COMPARISON

The network theory is based on the extreme diversity of antibodies and clonal receptors of lymphocytes. The numbers are impressive, and they immediately suggest comparisons with other complex systems and important evolutionary implications. Jerne has calculated that the immune system of a man contains 2×10^{12} lymphocytes and 10^{20} antibody molecules (7), whereas the nervous system is made up of only 3×10^{10} cells (8). Complexity, however, is brought about by the specific interactions among these structural elements, so that the nervous system can contain 10^{14} synapses or more (8). On the other hand, we have at present little or no information on the corresponding numbers in the immune system; they could in fact be as high, if not higher. Thus, indications exist for a high degree of connectance within the B-cell and antibody repertoires (9; D. Holmberg, unpublished observations) and between antibodies and helper T-cell repertoires (10). Actually, the only reason for adopting a conservative position in this respect is the lack of available information on the functional relevance of such interactions.

The nervous system does appear to embody a network of interactions, set by positional diversity, mediated by substances that are biochemically active within precise ranges of concentration, and enriched by the structural diversity (differentiative types) of its cellular components. On the other hand, the immune system displays a similar degree of complexity in terms of its component cell types, their structural diversity, and their functional performance. The cellular interactions in this "elementary" network are also mediated by a variety of biochemically active "factors" with synergistic or antagonistic effects on the various target cells. The argument could even be made that positional diversity is also important in the immune system, and that the systemic circulation and mobility of antibodies and cells greatly multiply the possibilities at this level. In other words, a network structurally similar to that of the nervous system is provided by B cells, helper cells, cytotoxic T cells, macrophages, the various subclasses of antibodies, and all lymphocyte-specific growth and maturation factors *even in the absence of clonal diversity.* In addition, however, the immune system produces 10^7 or 10^8 different proteins, many orders of magnitude greater than all the rest of the vertebrate body, and this unique property brings about a complex network of variable regions that does appear to be placed at a different qualitative level of complexity in comparison with the elementary networks of cell types and mediators.

B. STRUCTURAL RENEWAL OF THE IMMUNE SYSTEM

If this were not sufficient, three other properties of lymphocytes help to vastly augment the levels of complexity in the immune system. First, let us consider the dynamics of the cellular components. As pointed out before (5), although the number of cells in the nervous system decreases from birth (8), new lymphocytes are produced from stem cells throughout life and at astonishing high rates: As many as 10 or 20% of the whole B-cell compartment and at least a few percent of all T cells are renewed every day (11–13), and many of these newly formed lymphocytes survive for a very short time (13–15). That is, throughout life, the immune system retains full potentiality for developing a whole new set of structural components precisely at the level of diversity embodying the complex network. It is our conviction that we must discover the rules and mechanisms selecting, for long life spans, a few rare elements from the pool of newly formed lymphocytes. An understanding of the reasons for such a turnover will constitute a major advance in our knowledge of the economy of the immune system.

C. LYMPHOCYTE EXPANSION AND MATURATION

Related to this property of structural renewal in the system is a second one, unique to lymphocytes, namely, the fact that differentiated lymphocytes divide and mature upon specific stimulation. Thus, a single lymphocyte can produce a progeny of 1000 in only 1 week of mitotic activity, providing the immune system with the enormous plasticity required by an adaptive system. Furthermore, activated lymphocytes mature to effector functions; a plasma cell, for example, produces 1000-fold more antibodies than a resting B lymphocyte. In summary, this unique property of clonal expansion and maturation allows the immune system to expand any given structural component (antibodies in particular) by increasing its concentration 1 million times in 1 week. When ontogenic development has been completed, there are few if any other body components that can so dramatically and in such a short time vary in concentration under physiologic conditions.

D. SOMATIC MUTATION

Finally, perhaps the most important component of structural innovation is brought into the system by the apparently unique rates of mutation (and possibly other mechanisms of somatic variation) of genes encoding variable regions. This property not only leaves the upper limits of diversity essentially open and introduces all the possibilities of mimicry so important to the very concept of networks but also brings about, in the short lifetime of a clone, possibilities of genetic variation that would take infinitely longer for germlines to achieve in evolutionary time. It is clear that the short life cycles of microorganisms, as compared to those of vertebrates, have imposed prometheic evolutionary strategies, such as the completeness of repertoires, in order to ensure an antiinfectious defense. It is not clear, however, how much of that completeness is in fact derived by somatic mutation or carried in germlines. Furthermore, if most (or all) somatic mutation takes place *after* initiation of clonal expansion on stimulation of competent precursor cells, antiinfectious immunologists could reframe that evolutionary race by equating bacterial with lymphocytic doubling times. The disadvantage of lymphocytes (30–60-fold longer doubling time) would perhaps be compensated for by the higher rates of mutation of antibody genes (probably at least 100-fold higher). Alternatively, if somatic mutation takes place before stimulation, along with the process of B-cell generation from precursors in bone marrow, B-cell repertoires are equally diverse at all levels, and virgin repertoires reaching the periphery are already complete. This, in turn, would impose strict requirements for the selection of available repertoires which would go far beyond the putative property of germline gene collections of being *dispersed* (16).

Also at this level lies the alternative between a Socratic or Jernean (17) perspective of the system which can never learn anything (new antibodies), but only recall and *select*, and those views which define the immune system as a learning machine and are, therefore, somewhat "informative." In fact, if we set aside the archaic postulates that contradict principles of protein synthesis, informative theories of antibody formation and current convictions of antigen-dependent somatic hypermutation and selection arrive at very similar conclusions. Both views propose that most of the antibodies produced by the individual in response to an antigen did not exist before immunization, nor did the structural genes needed to encode them. Obviously, learning from Jerne, we would like to consider as correct both of his basic postulates: selection from an extremely diverse population of antibodies generated (before immunization) by extensive somatic mutation.

It may be argued, however, that those two views are not at all mutually exclusive and that both pathways participate in generating a striking property of the immune system, which can properly be defined as
creativity. Thus, if creativity is the performance of a function not
specifically selected for in evolution, the high-affinity recognition of
(and responses to) any newly synthesized molecule must be accepted
as an example of that definition. In addition, common sense tells us
that creativity is highly individual, and we know very well how
greatly immune reactivities and antibody patterns vary between syngeneic individuals. The chances of DNA recombination and mutation
certainly participate in the establishment of such stringent individuality, but it would appear that variability arises not only from the low
probability of arriving at the same solutions but also from the individuality in choosing, from all those available, a given set of solutions
(paratopes and idiotopes) to the same problem (an integrated network).

In fact, to the *potential* and *available* repertoires defined by Jerne,
we could add another, constituted by the set of specificities that are
being used (the *actual* repertoire) to describe three sets of specificities: (1) what can be made; (2) what has been made and can be used
(precursor B-cell repertoire); and (3) what is actually being used (circulating antibody repertoire). The first is genetically determined, reflects the history of the species, and draws the limits of the others; the
second is derived ontogenically in a process which, through maternal
influences (18), implicates many generations and reflects the history
of the recent ancestors. The third and last set of specificities is ephemeral, determined at each moment by the present experiences which
define the history of the individual, but on the basis of the "recursive"
properties of the immune system, it will influence all future *actual*
(and *available*) repertoires. Thus, ephemeral as it may be, this last
system of contacts constitutes, at any moment, the immunological
(idiotypic) self.

III. An Organism-Centered Perspective of the
Immune System

Network perspectives, as opposed to clonal perspectives which are
antigen centered, are organism centered: The activity of the immune
system is seen as (self)-determined by the network organization itself,
rather than being driven by chance contacts with foreign materials
evoking immune responses. The heart of clonal concepts, and of the

question of self versus nonself discrimination, is the immune response paradigm, according to which the activity of the immune system is nothing but a collection of (essentially independent) immune
responses. According to this idea, each (specific) immune response
includes sets of effector cells and corresponding sets of regulator cells,
but there is no provision for self-determined (i.e., autonomous) activities of the system, which is therefore controlled externally. Thus, the
system would be antigen driven, a typical model of cause-and-effect,
(antigenic) stimulus–(immune) response relationships. As opposed to
these ideas, the heart of network perspectives is the autonomy of the
immune system, its ability to self-determine its actions. Self-determination, on the other hand, is essential to an understanding of three
important developments of the last 20 years, namely, cellular interactions, the genetic control of immune events, and the idiotypic network.

A. THE NATURE OF IMMUNE ACTIVITY

There is now abundant experimental evidence to demonstrate that
immune activity consists of complex interactions between different
types of lymphoid cells. From a clonal perspective, these interactions
serve the main purpose of controlling clonal expansion and differentiation and are essentially *intraclonal* events. From a network perspective, every clone and clonal product is at the same time recognizing
and being recognized by other clones and clonal products. These
interactions, therefore, are essentially *interclonal* activities, and antigen molecules serve as links between previously disconnected
clones. In clonal perspectives, these interactions control independently the activity of each clone. From a network perspective, the
activity of each clone is subordinate to the activity of the network.
These interactions are the network itself; without them, the system
could not operate as a system.

The notion of self-determination is also crucial to an understanding
of the genetic control of the (immune) events embodied in these cellular interactions. In a clonal perspective that is antigen centered, most
efforts to elucidate the nature and functions of immune response
genes have focused on the characterization of antigen-specific receptors. These efforts, however, led to the discovery of MHC-restriction
phenomena, the essence of which is the establishment of clonal activities as subordinate to the organization of the network from which the
clone originated, in the absence of the external "specific" antigen
(19, 20).

Finally, the notion of self-determination is also essential to envisage the circularity, that is, the organizational closure, of the idiotypic network. If it must (self)-determine its own actions and recognitions, the organization of the network must be closed on itself, even if open to interactions with external antigens. The notion of a system (self)-determining its own actions may be disturbing at first, but if the system is not in control of its own actions, what is? This notion of organizational closure is, of course, not necessary from a clonal perspective, because these views lack altogether the need for global plans of organization in the immune system.

B. RECURSION, EIGEN BEHAVIOR, AND
COGNITIVE DOMAINS

Three important notions may be introduced in immunology to help understand the self-determination of the immune system: recursive behavior, eigen states, and cognitive domains (2). The term *recursion* describes the idea that the immune system, like other important biological systems, operates through circular causality, and it suggests that the system tends to repeat itself, to have rhythms. Essentially, it means that a system is able to undergo state transitions which are determined by the previous state of that very same system, and that such states are arranged in circular chains.

The term *eigen behavior* was first used by Jerne (1) in his formulation of the idiotype network to designate the succession of stable states in the immune system. The prefix *eigen* denotes the fact that such stability crucially depends on the circularity of the system's construction. To ignore the self-referential structure of the system and its ability to change eigen states continuously and recursively amounts to disregarding altogether the mechanisms of operation of the system (2). This capacity to generate a variety of adaptive eigen behaviors is typical of large, interconnected natural systems (2, 21–23), a belief supported by a solid body of mathematical and systemic developments (24, 25).

The notion of *cognitive domain* was developed by students of the nervous system to denote the interdependence of the characteristics of the organism's nervous system and the domain of its possible interactions (25). It is an everyday experience that different organisms perceive their surroundings differently; what is relevant to an animal (and in which way it is relevant) depends on both the animal's genetic background and its individual history. This concept may be applied to the lymphoid system. The *actual* repertoire of paratopes expressed by the system at any moment will define its cognitive domain at that moment; that is, it will determine which contacts are relevant to the (immunological) self and which are not and therefore remain as non-sense. Whatever may be recognized as an epitope (idiotope) may be so recognized because it has a degree of resemblance to an already existing set of epitopes (internal images) in the network. Self-recognition and the recognition of novelty are one and the same process.

What is not present in the cognitive domain of the system and does not participate in the establishment of eigen states remains as nonsense (cybernetic noise) and does not participate in the immunological self. The continuous introduction of new materials into the internal environment, from both internal and external sources, brings about disturbances, waves of activity in the immune network, reflecting the continuous acquisition of new eigen states and consequently modifications of its cognitive domain. Through these compensatory changes in its clonal structure, the system incorporates, more often than not, new materials in the activity of the self. The ontogeny of an immune system is, therefore, never completed; it actually began generations earlier with the individual's ancestors. Thus, maternal influences, through the transmission of idiotypes across the placenta and/or in the milk, are prominent examples of natural incorporation of new materials in the activity of the self, providing the first wave of significant influences in the emergent lymphoid system, which profoundly affect the organization of its repertoires (18). Simultaneously, this process allows for a unique example in biology: the nongenetic transmission of experiences to progenies, that is, the eigen behavior is also a property of two independent but connected immune systems.

Other internally generated body components, such as emergent lymphoid cells and the antibodies they produce, as well as some externally derived materials, are continuously being transformed and assimilated without need of modifications in the pattern of changes that connect the components of the lymphoid system and the body as a whole. We should perhaps make a distinction between "foreign-familiar" materials, such as the usual components of the diet and the normal microbiota, and "foreign-foreign" materials. The former, in previous and sustained contacts, have already made their imprint, and the present eigen states consider them; they have been "assimilated." The latter, although able to connect with components of the system, thus penetrating its cognitive domain, are not assimilated by the network in its present eigen state. Thus, these foreign-foreign materials cause disturbances in the organization requiring compensatory

changes, until a new equilibrium is reached permitting the assimila-
tion of the new material into the self—turning it into foreign familiar.
These disturbances correspond to what immunologists call "immune
responses."

Interestingly, much of the relevant material generated by the system itself through the emergence of new lymphocyte clones is actually not incorporated by the self, as the *surviving* lymphocyte clones
are only a small proportion of all those continuously generated. The
vast majority of these cells disappear in a few days, perhaps from lack
of stimulatory connections with the present eigen state of the network.

Foreign materials that penetrate the organism by natural routes are
thought of as invariably inducing immune responses. Although this
might actually be the case, these "responses" often consist of adaptations that provide for *decreases* as well as increases in the ostensive
responsiveness of the system. When this happens, immunologists
speak of "tolerance." Evidently, therefore, natural tolerance is neither
the functional opposite of immunization nor is it restricted to immature animals.

C. BOUNDARIES OF THE COGNITIVE DOMAIN

A crucial issue in this perspective is the definition of the boundaries
of the cognitive domain of the lymphoid system. Being complete (5),
the paratopic universe can potentially recognize all body structures
and is not limited to the recognition of idiotopes on antibody molecules or external antigens. Thus, patterns of configuration in all body
molecules might be seen as playing a role in the generation of internal
complementarities which embody the eigen states of the lymphoid
system. Being also complete, the idiotypic universe can successfully
mimic all nominal antigens, including any other component of the
internal environment. It is quite clear, however, that although idiotypic "internal images" can be functionally relevant and actually substitute for the "original" in its absence, they do not annihilate that original (the nonidiotypic "antigen") when it is present. Consequently,
idiotypic diversity does not provide an ivory tower for the system, that
is, idiotypic internal images do not save the immune system from
having to deal with other antigens that are not its own. Most developments of the network theory fall short of considering the immune
system's universe as embedded in a larger universe of proteins and
other molecular patterns that makes up the body of a vertebrate. In
essence, as the immune system perceives nanogram amounts of a

given idiotype, we consider it likely that it also perceives nanogram amounts of any other protein of the internal environment.

In this immunosomatic perspective, let us first consider the implications for the immune system itself. Provided that there is no elimination of self-recognizing clones—the basic postulate in the network theory—the universe of patterns within the immune system and the internal complementarities they embody are the idiotypic and paratopic repertoires *plus* the patterns of all other molecules in the body. Although the system is self-determined, its eigen states, and consequently its very repertoires, are also influenced by all other body components and foreign-familiar materials that have previously been assimilated into self. In other words, the immune system of a rat that genetically lacks albumin cannot be the same as the immune system of an otherwise identical but normal rat. If idiotypes and paratopes compose an equilibrated network by mutual neutralization and stimulation, then the immune steady states of a diabetic individual cannot be the same as those of another individual with normal circulating levels of insulin, because the hormone will also participate in those complementarities and substitute for its internal image. The antibody repertoire of H-2^d mice must be different from that of congenic mice expressing on every cell of the body H-2^k molecules, which participate in a different circuit of network interactions.

In essence, we are here extending to all other components of the internal environment that have been incorporated into self the original postulates of the network theory. As Jerne said, even if the immune system did not start as a network, once a given level of diversity is reached, it cannot avoid internal recognition and regulation. We are simply including *all* self patterns that can be recognized by paratopes or mimicked by idiotopes *in the same universe* of interactions, where each structural component is important in the establishment of repertoires and their regulation. In this sense, all body components belong in the immune system, and the structure of the system is largely a consequence of the rest of the organism. It is probably misleading, therefore, to consider regulatory influences of idiotypes and paratopes in the development and maintenance of immune steady states while ignoring the roles of epitopes in other body proteins.[3]

---

[3] The question of the relative importance of each structural component in the internal environment is complex, as it relates to molar concentrations, to functional properties other than binding to paratopes or mimicking idiotopes, and even to topologic constraints. For example, MHC products or lymphocyte-specific growth factors cannot be dealt with in the same manner as actin.

A prime example of these perspectives is the determination by MHC products of the immune system cognitive domain. Furthermore, from the functional point of view, there is no logical reason why an antigen-sensitive B-cell precursor should recognize an idiotope on antibodies, or epitopes on hormone molecules, in qualitatively different ways, given their similar circulating concentrations and the exclusion of "clonal abortion." Previously, we believed that such a contradiction in the network theory required a solution for self–nonself discrimination. Here, in the framework of an organism-centered perspective, this is no longer a question, because all self components are treated the same way as participating in the immune network in eigen states that allow (and regulate) the effector function of each particular molecule. As in other historical examples of shifts in paradigms, there are no solutions for the previous problems and puzzles. The rupture with previous theoretical frameworks creates new perspectives in which old questions make no sense and need no answers.

It could appear misleading to blur so greatly the boundaries of the cognitive domain of the system, which amounts to blurring the boundaries of the self. The lymphoid system is largely a consequence of the previous states of the lymphoid system itself: *It is self-determined.* The present view, however, in no way questions the self-determination of the immune system. We maintain that only *self* counts, and what self is has previously been (self)-determined by the immune system.

IV. The Immune System Is More Than an Antiinfectious Machine

The consequences of this perspective of the immune system for other systems and functions of the organism are many. First, let us recall the extraordinary importance that evolution has conceded to the immune system: (a) probably more DNA is used to encode structural elements of the immune system than in any other system in the body; (b) the number of proteins produced by the immune system alone is several orders of magnitude greater than that of all other systems combined; (c) some of the loci at the MHC, precisely those which are immune components "par excellence," constitute the most polymorphic system known in biology; and (d) compared to antibodies, no other structural components of vertebrates can vary so dramatically in concentration and over time under physiologic conditions. It appears inescapable to us that the extent of this diversity (contributing mimicry and/or neutralization of any other body component), as well as this extraordinary plasticity, must have consequences in the normal physiology of other body functions. It is also obvious to us that a normal individual producing a set of immunoglobulin idiotopes mimicking the epitopic profile of insulin must produce less of the hormone than another normal individual who instead expresses a given concentration of antibody paratopes that neutralize insulin. That is, the eigen states of the immune system influence the physiologic equilibria in other molecular interactions.

We are far from being clear about the experimental and theoretical directions that follow from this perspective. Let us simply state that we consider autoimmune diseases as the best demonstration of these concepts. We consider such pathologic states as examples of disregulation of the physiologic interactions and control carried out by the immune system on all other body functions. In contrast to advocates of classical perspectives, therefore, we distinguish self-recognition and autoreactivity from what is usually designated as autoimmunity. Autoimmune diseases are, for the enlarged network concepts presented here, what pathology is for normal physiology. The existence of autoantibodies (not only to other antibodies but also to any other body structure), the stimulation by self-antigens of immunocompetent cells, need not lead to pathology, malfunction, or destruction of such components. Rather, all body components and the immune system itself exist in an equilibrium ontogenically established, but defined by eigen states within the same *self*, mutually adapted such that destructive immune mechanisms can be neutralized by other elements or even purposedly used, if necessary, in the economy of the organism. Most components in this steady state are renewed; some new ones appear and others disappear. At all times, from its self-determination and by its plasticity and diversity, *the immune system defines individuality and maintains the limits of self.*

A. EVOLUTION OF THE IMMUNE FUNCTION

As seen above, what has not been previously delineated as self and consequently did not participate in the establishment of the present eigen state, may or may not fall within the cognitive domain characteristic of the system. If it does, its introduction into the internal environment may lead to an immune response that results in tolerance, that is, in the incorporation of the foreign into self rather than its destruction or elimination.

In other situations, immune responses do appear to be definitely directed at the neutralization, destruction, and elimination of the foreign materials. We will distinguish two main categories of such immune responses which, for obvious quantitative and other reasons, have occupied immunologists for many years. Let us first consider the evolutionary origins of the immune function. The immune system of vertebrates appears to have evolved from two major primordial types of recognitional functions, carried by distinct sets of genes, molecules, and cells, and submitted to different evolutionary pressures. The T-cell branch of modern immune systems appears to have evolved from recognition systems which in primitive invertebrates already controlled cell-to-cell interactions, both in germline (sperm–egg interactions) and in somatic cells (histocompatibility reactions). The main characteristics of this T-cell branch are the positive recognition of self (particularly evident in primitive species in which nonself is actually ignored) and a repertoire directed to cell surface structures exhibiting polymorphism within species. Because the species reproduce sexually, such polymorphic patterns may well be self for any normal individual. The evolution of this recognition system has involved the differentiation of specialized cell types to carry out this function (and the corresponding loss of such performance by all other somatic cells), which then must learn ontogenetically what self is.

This, in turn, brought about the positive recognition of nonself and, in particular, the impossibility of the coexistence of two different (T-cell) immune systems in the same organism, that is, *the demarcation of individuality through the uniqueness of each immune system.* Thus, the polymorphic markers (MHC) can coexist in individuals (heterozygotes, polypoids or chimeras), but in every case only one immune system is allowed; that is, the individual immune system will always delineate the unique constellation of polymorphic markers in a unified perspective of self, thereby defining itself as a single (and also unique) immune system. This may have provided the evolutionary reasons for the maintenance of individuality in a much deeper and broader sense than the mere protection against microorganism invasion. In modern immune systems, these evolutionary principles are still apparent, as rejection is observed only when the foreign nonsense is part of another immune system, or when it impinges and modifies self to make it appear as if it came from another immune system. Thus, T-cell reactivity leading to destruction of tissues or cells does require the recognition of the most "immunological" products of MHC, namely, those selectively expressed by bone marrow-derived cells. The elimination of virus-infected cells also requires their mimicry of another immune system's cells. Here again, maintenance of individuality appears teleologically to be the most satisfying concept, and immune responses to be the remnants of evolutionary stages that imposed the present set of strategies.

B. PRIMITIVE RECOGNITION MECHANISMS

Another kind of immune reactivity, which is obviously directed outward, concerns nonsense materials that carry marks of an evolutionary past preceding the existence of immune systems. This other branch of primitive recognition mechanisms which evolved to make up vertebrate immune systems discriminates structures that do not exist in the species and, consequently, are nonself with certainty (26). The constancy of these differences allows for the use of stereotyped responses requiring relatively little adaptability from the lymphoid system. Such substances are primarily bacterial products, such as endotoxin, which readily evoke B-cell and macrophage responses but toward which T lymphocytes show no reactivity. Perhaps the most spectacular of these remnants of an antiinfectious evolutionary past is the ability of lipid A to stimulate 10–50% of all B lymphocytes in a mouse (27).

V. Conclusions

Obviously, the immune system is still competent and effective in providing protection against infection, but the present concepts imply that defense against invasion by microorganisms is not the only biological function of the system and not even the most relevant. Similarly, we do not speak of the skin as the major antiinfectious system, nor we consider defense to be the main function of that organ (although it might well be). Similarly, the human nervous system performs functions already apparent in primitive nervous systems, but the brain is also something with which we think. There is a higher level of organization in the nervous and immune systems which transcend the thresholds of internal complementarities and autonomous stimulation in cellular networks. Thus, the primitive biological function, evolutionarily controlled by environmental pressures, is no longer the only function selected for, and the systems are free to evolve to levels of exaptation (28) which largely exceed those original performances.[4]

The biological world, as we see it today, is only one of many possible results of evolution and not necessarily the best. Contemplating 1 million years of evolution of human societies, we realize part of the truth of this statement. By asking what the (immunological) self is, we are raising, from a new angle, cognitive issues which have troubled mankind from its origin. Time may be ripe for an answer: Self is *self-referential*. Knowing the world is knowing yourself, and knowing yourself is your only (and unique) way of knowing the world. To us, it is tantalizing to understand that fundamental issues pertaining to the definition of individuality may now be approached with the molecular, cellular, and organismic tools of experimental immunology. These material tools may permit us to answer questions that could not be approached from other perspectives. Let us hope that there will be enough time and wisdom.

References

1. Jerne, N. K. (1974). *Ann. Immunol. (Paris)* **125C**, 373.
2. Vaz, N. M., and Varela, F. J. (1978). *Med. Hypotheses* **4**, 231.
3. Adam, G., and Weiler, E. (1976). *In* "The Generation of Antibody Diversity: A New Look" (A. J. Cunningham, ed.), p. 1. Academic Press, New York.
4. Hooijkass, H., Benner, R., Pleasants, J. R., and Wostmann, B. S. (1983). Submitted for publication.
5. Coutinho, A. (1980). *Ann. Immunol. (Paris)* **131D**, 235.
6. Ohno, S. (1978). *Compr. Immunol.* **5**, 197.
7. Jerne, N. K. (1978). *In* "Basel Institute for Immunology Annual Report 1977," p. 1. Basel Institute for Immunology, Basel.
8. Changeux, J.-P. (1982). *In* "L'Homme Neuronal." Fayard, France.
9. Bernabé, R. R., Coutinho, A., Martinez-A., C., and Cazenave, P.-A. (1981). *J. Exp. Med.* **154**, 552.
10. Coutinho, A., Forni, L., Holmberg, D., and Ivars, F. (1983). *Nobel Symp.* **55**, 273.
11. Osmond, D. G., and Nossal, G. J. V. (1974). *Cell. Immunol.* **13**, 132.
12. Scollay, R. G., Butcher, E. C., and Weissman, I. L. (1980). *Eur. J. Immunol.* **10**, 210.
13. Freitas, A. A., Rocha, B., Forni, L., and Coutinho, A. (1982). *J. Immunol.* **128**, 54.
14. Freitas, A. A., and Coutinho, A. (1981). *J. Exp. Med.* **154**, 994.
15. Rocha, B., Freitas, A. A., and Coutinho, A. (1983). *J. Immunol.* (in press).

[4] As defined by Gould and Vrba (28), *exaptation* refers to "features that now enhance fitness but were not built by natural selection for their current role." Therefore, it does not include creativity of no survival value, in which part of the brain and lymphoid activity appears to engage.

16. Cohn, M. (1982). *Bull. Inst. Pasteur (Paris)* **80,** 300.
17. Jerne, N. K. (1966). *In* "Phage and the Origins of Molecular Biology" (J. Cairns, G. S. Stent, and J. Watson, eds.), p. 301. Cold Spring Harbor Lab., Cold Spring Harbor, New York.
18. Bernabé, R. R., Coutinho, A., Cazenave, P.-A., and Forni, L. (1981). *Proc. Natl. Acad. Sci. U.S.A.* **78,** 6416.
19. Bevan, M. J. (1977). *Nature (London)* **269,** 417.
20. Zinkernagel, R. M. (1978). *Immunol. Rev.* **42,** 224.
21. Walker, C. R., and Ashby, W. R. (1972). *Kybernetik* **6,** 387.
22. Lazlo, E. A. (1970). "An Introduction to System's Philosophy." Harper Torchbook, New York.
23. May, R. (1973). "Model Ecosystems." Princeton Univ. Press, Princeton, New Jersey.
24. Varela, F. J., and Goyrcer, J. (1977). *Prog. Cybernet. Syst. Res.* **3.**
25. Maturana, H. R., and Varela, I. J. (1980). "Antopoiesis and Cognition." Reidel Publ., Dordrecht, Netherlands.
26. Coutinho, A. (1975). *Transplant. Rev.* **23,** 49.
27. Andersson, J., Coutinho, A., Lernhardt, W., and Melchers, F. (1977). *Cell* **10,** 27.
28. Gould, S. J., and Vrba, E. S. (1982). *Paleobiology* **8,** 4.

Idiotypes in the Immune System

Chapter 5

Structural Properties and Genetic Control of an Idiotype Associated with Antibodies to the *p*-Azophenylarsonate Hapten[1,2]

Michael F. Gurish and Alfred Nisonoff

Department of Biology, Rosenstiel Research Center
Brandeis University, Waltham, Massachusetts

[1] Supported by grants AI-17751 and AI-12895 from the National Institutes of Health.
[2] Abbreviations: Ar, *p*-azophenylarsonate; BSA, bovine serum albumin; C or V, constant or variable region of immunoglobulin; CAF_1, (BALB/c × A/J)F_1; CRI, intrastrain cross-reactive idiotype; H or L chains, heavy or light chains; HIS, hyperimmune suppressed; HP, hybridoma product (monoclonal antibody); Id, idiotype; Igh, immunoglobulin heavy chain gene locus; Kb, kilobases; KLH, keyhole limpet hemocyanin.

I. Introduction

An intrastrain cross-reactive idiotype (CRI_A) is associated with a substantial proportion of the anti-p-azophenylarsonate (anti-Ar) antibodies of all A/J mice inoculated with the Ar derivative of keyhole limpet hemocyanin (KLH-Ar). Investigations of this system in several laboratories have provided information on a number of topics, including the relationship between molecular structure and idiotypy; genetic linkage of idiotype expression to loci controlling heavy (H) and light (L) chains; the role of germline genes and somatic mutation in the expression of the idiotype; the presence of major and minor cross-reactive idiotypes in the A/J strain; the relationship of the minor idiotype to a major idiotype of BALB/c mice; and the role of idiotypy in the regulation of humoral and cell-mediated immune responses. Much of this work has been reviewed recently (Greene *et al.*, 1982; Capra *et al.*, 1982). In this chapter, we will focus on the nature of the response to the Ar hapten and will not consider in any detail investigations on regulation. Besides attempting to bring the subject up to date, we will present interpretations of data relating to the genetic control of the idiotypic response.

II. Linkage of CRI_A Expression to Genes Controlling C_H Regions and Kappa Chains

A. LINKAGE TO C_H GENES

CRI_A is present in the anti-Ar antibodies of the A/J ($Igh-1^e$) and AL/N ($Igh-1^d$) strains. It is not, however, produced by NZB mice that are $Igh-1^e$ but differ from A/J at the $Igh-5$ (delta chain) locus, or by AKR mice which, like AL/N, are $Igh-1^d$ (Pawlak and Nisonoff, 1973). The possibility was considered that AKR or NZB might fail to produce CRI_A because of the absence of appropriate L chains. However, mice resulting from an F_1 cross of AKR or NZB with BALB/c mice failed to produce CRI_A on immunization with KLH-Ar (Laskin *et al.*, 1977). Because, as discussed later, BALB/c mice can synthesize the necessary L chains, this result suggests that the AKR and NZB strains fail to produce the requisite H chains. As indicated below, AKR is also one of a small number of strains that cannot provide the L chains needed for CRI_A expression.

Linkage to the *Igh* locus was shown by tests carried out with C.AL-9 and later with C.AL-20 congenic mice, bred by Dr. Michael Potter (Pawlak *et al.*, 1973a,b). C.AL mice carry the Igh-1^d allotype of the AL/N strain on a BALB/c background. The observation that such mice produce CRI_A demonstrated linkage of expression of the idiotype to the *Igh* locus. In our experience, virtually all immunized C.AL-20 mice produce CRI_A; however, the percentage of anti-Ar antibodies that express the idiotype is somewhat lower on the average than that associated with the A strain. Similarly, nearly all (A/J × BALB/c)F_1 or (A/J × C57BL)F_1 mice produce CRI_A (Pawlak and Nisonoff, 1973; Laskin *et al.*, 1977), but an occasional F_1 mouse expresses very low levels (per unit weight of anti-Ar antibodies). These findings, together with those of Blomberg *et al.* (1972), provided early evidence for the close linkage of V_H and C_H genes. The linkage of CRI_A expression to the *Igh* locus has been confirmed by backcross studies with C58, PL, AKR, C57BL/6, CBA, SJL, C3H, and strain 129 mice (Laskin *et al.*, 1977; Gottlieb *et al.*, 1979; Brown *et al.*, 1981b).

Congenic A.By mice, which have a strain A background but a different H-2 type, produce CRI_A in amounts quantitatively similar to those of strain A. Conversely, the presence of the H-2 genotype of strain A on an unrelated background was not associated with the formation of CRI_A (Pawlak and Nisonoff, 1973). The production of CRI_A by F_1 mice indicated that the failure of the other (non-A) parental strain to produce CRI_A is not attributable to the presence of genes controlling the synthesis of a suppressor of CRI_A (Pawlak and Nisonoff, 1973).

We have never been able to remove antibodies to the CRI_A idiotype by exhaustive adsorption onto large amounts of nonspecific A/J immunoglobulins bound to Sepharose. In addition, assays for CRI_A are carried out in the presence of added normal A/J serum to ensure removal of antibodies to nonspecific immunoglobulins. Subsequent to the appearance of a report suggesting the presence of low levels of CRI_A in normal A/J immunoglobulins (Wysocki and Sato, 1981), we carried out quantitative investigations in which the sensitivity of the assay for idiotype was maximized (Barrett and Nisonoff, 1982). Using thoroughly adsorbed anti-CRI_A, we were still unable to detect significant quantities of molecules bearing CRI_A in nonimmune A/J sera; the upper limit set by these experiments was 140 ng/ml, a value about 13 times lower than that reported by Wysocki and Sato. Possible reasons for this apparent discrepancy were discussed.

For use in structural studies, we prepared substantial quantities of antibodies, of which more than 90% expressed CRI_A. This was done by using ascitic fluids induced by immunization using a 9 : 1 ratio of complete Freund's adjuvant to antigen solution (Tung *et al.*, 1976). Ascitic fluids from individual mice were selected that contained a relatively high content of CRI_A. The anti-Ar antibodies were affinity purified and subjected to preparative isoelectric focusing, and the fraction with pI 6.7–6.9 was isolated (Tung and Nisonoff, 1975). More than 90% of these antibodies, which were essentially all IgG_1, expressed CRI_A. That CRI_A appears in other classes and subclasses of immunoglobulin was subsequently demonstrated when monoclonal CRI_A^+ antibodies were prepared (Lamoyi *et al.*, 1980a; Marshak-Rothstein *et al.*, 1980a,b).

Studies carried out in collaboration with Dr. Klaus Eichmann provided evidence for a crossover event involving V_H genes encoding two different idiotypes: One idiotype, designated A5A, is associated with antistreptococcal antibodies of strain A mice; the other is CRI_A (Eichmann *et al.*, 1974). The experiments were made possible by Eichmann's discovery of a mouse, obtained by backcrosses involving BALB/c and A/J mice, which was homozygous for the BALB/c heavy chain allotype (Igh-1^a) but nonetheless expressed the A/J A5A idiotype in its antistreptococcal antibodies. This mouse, BB♂7, was in turn backcrossed to BALB/c females. About half of the offspring were A5A$^+$, a finding consistent with the presence of an A5A gene in BB♂7. However, none of the offspring of this backcross expressed CRI_A. This finding is consistent with the possibility that the association of A5A with the Igh-1^a allotype in mouse BB♂7 had resulted from a crossover event occurring somewhere between the V_H genes encoding A5A and CRI_A. The result also implied that the gene encoding CRI_A resides closer to the C_H region of the genome in Igh-1^e mice than does the gene encoding A5A. These results demonstrated the presence of two distinct germline V_H genes controlling different antibody specificities. A discussion of subsequent experiments of this type is provided by Weigert and Potter (1977).

B. LINKAGE TO THE KAPPA CHAIN LOCUS

The observation of linkage of CRI_A expression to the *Igh* locus, in congenic F_1 and backcross mice, seemed somewhat paradoxical because the presence of the appropriate L chain is required for expression of the idiotype (Schroeder, 1974). The possibility was considered that the apparent absence of genetic linkage to a locus controlling L chains might be caused by the ability of each of the strains used in breeding studies to provide the necessary L chains; under these circumstances, CRI_A would appear to be linked only to the *Igh* locus. An opportunity to test this hypothesis was provided by the finding of Edelman and Gottlieb (1970) that a few strains of mice, including PL, C58, RF, and AKR, express a polymorphism in the V_K region characterized by the presence of an additional cysteine-containing peptide. The gene controlling expression of this phenotype is very closely linked to the *Lyt-2,3* locus on chromosome 6 (Gottlieb, 1974).

To test the possibility of linkage of CRI_A expression to the kappa chain locus, mice were obtained by backcrossing (A/J × PL/J) F_1 males to PL/J females (Laskin *et al.*, 1977). It was observed that the presence of the A/J allotype in the offspring was not sufficient to ensure the production of CRI_A. All mice that were homozygous for the *Lyt 3.1* genotype of PL/J, irrespective of their Igh allotype, failed to produce the idiotype, i.e., for production of the idiotype, it was necessary that a mouse possess genes controlling both Igh-1^e and Lyt-3.2, both characteristic of the A/J strain. When either of these genes was absent, the mouse failed to produce CRI_A. These findings were subsequently extended to other strains that express Lyt 3.1, namely, C58 (Gottlieb *et al.*, 1979) and AKR (Brown *et al.*, 1981b). Homozygosity for the *Lyt* genes of C58 and AKR resulted in failure to produce CRI_A, even in the presence of the appropriate, Igh-1^e heavy chain gene.

III. Preparation of Monoclonal Antibodies with Anti-Ar Activity

Many of the experiments to be discussed below made use of monoclonal hybridoma products (HP) with anti-Ar activity. These were obtained by fusion of A/J immune spleen cells with BALB/c myeloma tumor cells. HP 25, HP 42, HP 45, and HP 52 were obtained with the 45.6TG1.7 cell line of Matthew D. Scharff, which secretes L and H chains characteristic of the MPC 11 tumor (Gill-Pazaris *et al.*, 1979). All other HP were obtained by using the Sp2/0-Ag14 line of Shulman *et al.* (1978), which secretes no L or H chains before or after fusion.

IV. A Minor Intrastrain Cross-Reactive Idiotype (CRI_m) in A/J Anti-Ar Antibodies

The existence of an intrastrain cross-reactive idiotype distinct from CRI_A, present in A/J anti-Ar antibodies, was discovered during screening of monoclonal antibodies with anti-Ar activity (Gill-Pazaris *et al.*,

1979). It was found that about 20% of the wells contained antibodies with anti-Ar activity that were negative in the conventional assay for idiotype (i.e., caused minimal displacement of labeled anti-Ar antibodies from rabbit anti-Id) but nonetheless interacted with some of the rabbit anti-Id antibodies. This interaction was demonstrated by the capacity of rabbit anti-Id to prevent the adherence of such monoclonal anti-Ar antibodies to BSA-Ar-coated wells in polyvinyl chloride plates. This result can be explained on the basis that the inhibitory anti-Id antibodies are reactive with only a minor fraction of serum anti-Ar antibodies, and that the monoclonal antibodies we are discussing correspond to this minor fraction. This would account for the failure of such monoclonal antibodies to cause substantial inhibition in the conventional assay for idiotype. A large excess of anti-Id directed against minor serum components would, however, prevent the binding of monoclonal antibodies expressing the minor idiotype to a plate coated with BSA-Ar. Hereafter in this discussion, we will refer to molecules that react with conventional anti-Id, but differ from CRI_A, as bearing minor cross-reactive idiotypic determinants (CRI_m).

Experiments were next carried out in which radiolabeled HP expressing CRI_m were used as ligands in radioimmune assays (Gill-Pazaris *et al.*, 1979). It was found that A/J anti-Ar antisera or affinity-purified A/J serum anti-Ar antibodies were capable of displacing each labeled HP almost completely from anti-Id. In contrast, a monoclonal HP that expresses CRI_A failed to cause appreciable displacement of any of these HP. (This same CRI_A^+ HP was a strong inhibitor of the binding of labeled serum antibodies to rabbit anti-Id.) These results are consistent with the presence of a subpopulation of anti-Id antibodies that recognize HP or serum antibodies expressing CRI_m but do not recognize CRI_A, i.e., with the presence of two serologically distinct idiotypes in A/J anti-Ar sera.

Variability of expression of CRI_m was studied by testing anti-Ar sera from individual A/J mice as inhibitors of binding to anti-Id of three labeled HP that express CRI_m. Antisera from individual mice were found to vary enormously in their capacity to displace these labeled ligands. The data are shown in Table I. Although nearly all of the sera were capable of displacing each HP from anti-Id, there is obviously great variation in the degree of expression of the minor idiotype in individual sera. In contrast, nearly all of the antisera were roughly equivalent in their capacity to displace labeled pooled A/J anti-Ar antibodies from the same rabbit anti-Id preparation; this reflects the presence of a fairly constant concentration of CRI_A. (In all cases, data

TABLE I

Inhibition of Binding of Labeled CRI_m^+ HP or Labeled
A/J anti-Ar Antibodies to Anti-Id Antibodies: Inhibitors,
Anti-Ar Antisera from Individual Mice[a]

Inhibitor (Serum number)	Anti-Ar required (ng) for 50% inhibition using 4 labeled ligands[b]			
	A/J Anti-Ar	HP 42	NP 45	HP 52
1	9	710	900	230
2	7	250	160	130
3	6	380	70	70
4	9	3000	340	660
5	9	220	280	180
6	10	5700	1600	370
7	11	190	250	80
8	9	>9300	>9300	>9300
9	11	~7500	4600	4000
10	11	7100	2500	1800

[a] Data are from Gill-Pazaris et al. (1979).
[b] Ten ng of labeled ligand (specifically purified anti-Ar antibody from serum or HP) were used in each test. The rabbit anti-Id antibodies were prepared against specifically purified A/J anti-Ar. Control sera included nonimmune A/J serum, A/J anti-KLH-benzoate, A/J antitrinitrophenyl, and A/J antistreptococcus (group A). None of these caused 50% inhibition when 1 μl was employed in the assay.

are expressed as weights of anti-Ar antibodies required to cause 50% inhibition in the competitive radioimmunoassay.) The high concentrations of antibodies needed for displacement of the CRI_m^+ HP indicate that the concentrations of minor idiotypes in A/J antisera are quite low; further evidence on this point is discussed below. That the inhibition observed is caused by anti-Ar antibodies was demonstrated by adsorption experiments; passage through a column of BGG-Ar-Sepharose removed essentially all inhibitory activity. Antisera prepared against KLH-benzoate, the trinitrophenyl group, or group A streptococci were not inhibitory in assays for CRI_A or CRI_m (Gill-Pazaris et al., 1979).

These studies were extended to three additional HP (R8.2, R19.9, R21.10), each of which expresses CRI_m by the criteria discussed above (Gill-Pazaris et al., 1981). As indicated above, these HP were prepared by using the nonsecreting Sp2/0-Ag14 cell line as the fusion partner with A/J spleen cells. It was found that two of the three CRI_m^+ HP (R8.2 and R19.9) contain L chains that are closely related serologically to L chains present in CRI_A^+ molecules. This was demonstrated by chain recombination experiments; the L chains of R8.2 or R19.9, but not of R21.10, when allowed to recombine with H chains obtained from CRI_A^+ anti-Ar antibodies, yielded recombinant products that expressed CRI_A by the criterion of inhibition in the standard radioimmunoassay. The H chains of the CRI_m^+ HP did not yield CRI_A^+ products when recombined with L chains of CRI_A^+ molecules. Because all three HP express CRI_m, but only two have L chains serologically similar to those of CRI_A, these findings provided evidence for the heterogeneity of CRI_m. Further data on heterogeneity are discussed below.

A. QUANTITATION OF THE FRACTION OF SERUM ANTI-AR ANTIBODIES THAT EXPRESS CRI_m

This question was approached by using ^{125}I-labeled, affinity-purified serum anti-Ar antibodies (Gill-Pazaris *et al.*, 1981). The latter were passed over an adsorbent consisting of Sepharose 4B conjugated to rabbit anti-Id antibody prepared against a CRI_A^+ HP (R16.7). This was shown to result in removal of essentially all CRI_A^+ molecules. The properties of the ^{125}I-labeled antibodies that did not adhere to the column were then studied. It was found that a maximum of 18% of this preparation could be bound by an excess of anti-Id. This corresponds to the presence in the unfractionated anti-Ar of about 8–10% of molecules bearing CRI_m when one allows for the enrichment that occurred upon passage over the anti-CRI_A column. In addition, individual HP that bear CRI_m failed to displace these nonadherent molecules from rabbit anti-Id. This provides further evidence for the heterogeneity of the CRI_m population, i.e., individual CRI_m^+ HP express only a small fraction of the serological specificities comprising CRI_m.

Further evidence that passage over the anti-CRI_A column separates the minor and major idiotypic components was obtained by using unlabeled rather than labeled affinity-purified serum anti-Ar antibodies. After passage over the column, it was found that the nonadherent population had lost its capacity to displace ^{125}I-labeled serum anti-Ar antibodies from anti-Id but retained the capacity to displace ^{125}I-labeled HP 21.10, a CRI_m^+ HP.

The finding of L chains in CRI_m^+ molecules that are related to those in CRI_A raised the question of whether those anti-Id antibodies that react with CRI_m are actually specific for L chains. Arguing against this possibility was the observation that the ^{125}I-labeled recombinant molecule $H_N L_D$ (where N refers to normal Ig and D to CRI_A) is not bound to an appreciable extent by anti-Id. In addition, unlabeled $H_N L_D$ is a very poor inhibitor of the binding of CRI_m^+ HP to anti-Id. Clarification of the degree and nature of the heterogeneity of CRI_m will probably require extensive structural studies on HP that express this minor idiotype.

An interesting sidelight of these results is that they demonstrate the utilization of similar or identical L chains in combination with different H chains. Similar observations were made by Clevinger et al. (1980), who studied dextran-binding HP.

In a subsequent study, the presence of CRI_m in individual sera was further investigated by competition radioimmunoassays in which the labeled ligand was serum anti-Ar expressing CRI_m rather than CRI_m^+ HP (Nelles and Nisonoff, 1982). The ligand was prepared by labeling pooled, affinity-purified serum anti-Ar antibodies and passing the antibodies over a column of Sepharose to which anti-CRI_A was conjugated. (The anti-CRI_A was prepared by immunization of a rabbit with the CRI_A^+ HP R16.7.) Serological testing showed that the material which passed through the column expressed CRI_m but not CRI_A. Anti-Ar-containing ascitic fluids from 26 individual mice were then studied quantitatively for their capacity to displace this labeled CRI_m preparation from anti-Id; the same ascitic fluids were also tested for their level of CRI_A by the competition radioimmunoassay. Again, it was found that the concentration of CRI_A (per unit weight of anti-Ar) in individual anti-Ar ascites varied over a narrow range, whereas the concentration of CRI_m varied dramatically among individual sera.

The data in Table II (Nelles and Nisonoff, 1982) demonstrate once again that individual CRI_m^+ HP are deficient in the idiotypic determinants that characterize the CRI_m of serum anti-Ar antibody. Whereas 43 ng of unlabeled CRI_m were capable of causing 50% displacement of labeled serum CRI_m, 2000 ng of each of three of CRI_m^+ HP failed to cause 50% inhibition. In addition, unlabeled HP R8.2 and HP R19.9, both of which are CRI_m^+, failed to displace another labeled CRI_m^+ HP, R21.10, from rabbit anti-Id.

In the same study, the absence of serologic cross-reactivity between CRI_A and CRI_m was confirmed by using monoclonal antiidiotope antibodies specific for an epitope present in CRI_A^+ molecules. Serum CRI_m, isolated as described above, and two different CRI_m^+ HP failed to react with each of two monoclonal anti-CRI_A HP.

The presence of the minor cross-reactive idiotype in A/J anti-Ar antibodies has been confirmed by Marshak-Rothstein et al. (1981).

TABLE II

Anti-Ar HP That Carry Minor Idiotypic Determinants are
Deficient in the Minor Idiotypic Determinants of Serum
Anti-Ar Antibodies[a,b]

	^{125}I-Labeled ligand [Anti-Ar required for 50% inhibition (ng)]	
Unlabeled inhibitor	Serum CRI_m^c	HP R21.10 (CRI_m)
Serum CRI_m^c	43 (99)[d]	800 (74)
HP R21.10 (CRI_m)	>2000 (20)	6 (96)
HP R8.2 (CRI_m)	>2000 (13)	>2000 (0)
HP R19.9 (CRI_m)	>2000 (12)	>2000 (3)
Anti-Ar ascites (pool)	68 (99)	890 (72)
HP R16.7 (CRI_A)	>2000 (16)	>2000 (0)

[a] Data are from Nelles and Nisonoff (1982).

[b] Inhibition tests were carried out with rabbit anti-Id directed against
A/J anti-Ar antibodies and 10 ng of the specifically purified ^{125}I-labeled
ligand.

[c] Serum CRI_m was obtained by adsorption of A/J anti-Ar antibodies on
Sepharose 4B conjugated with anti-Id directed against a CRI_A^+ HP
(R16.7).

[d] Numbers in parentheses show the percentage of inhibition by 2000
ng of the unlabeled inhibitor.

B. REGULATION OF CRI_m BY ANTI-Id ANTIBODIES

Our early work had shown the feasibility of suppressing the appearance of CRI_A by administration of rabbit anti-Id antibodies prior to
immunization with KLH-Ar (Hart *et al.*, 1972). Because such rabbit
antisera contain antibodies specific for both CRI_A and CRI_m, it was of
interest to ascertain whether CRI_m was also suppressed by the pretreatment with anti-Id. It was found that anti-Ar sera from each of five
idiotypically suppressed, hyperimmunized (HIS) mice failed to displace each of three labeled CRI_m^+ HP from rabbit anti-Id antibodies
(Gill-Pazaris *et al.*, 1981). In nearly all instances, 5000 ng of anti-Ar
from HIS mice failed to cause 50% inhibition of binding of the labeled
ligand, whereas the same quantity of anti-Ar antibodies from a nonsuppressed serum pool caused 80–90% inhibition (40–500 ng of anti-
Ar were required for 50% inhibition). Thus, preinoculation of rabbit
anti-Id causes a profound suppression of CRI_m as well as CRI_A.

It was subsequently found that CRI_A and CRI_m can be regulated
independently (Nelles and Nisonoff, 1982). This was shown by using

monoclonal anti-CRI_A antibodies prepared in BALB/c mice. Preinoculation of each of two such anti-Id antibodies resulted in virtually complete suppression of the subsequent appearance of CRI_A but had no significant effect on the level of CRI_m. In control experiments, conventional rabbit anti-Id again suppressed CRI_m as well as CRI_A.

V. Relationship of the Idiotypes of Anti-Ar Antibodies of A/J and BALB/c Mice

In collaboration with Alan R. Brown, it was found that A/J CRI_m is related to a major idiotype of BALB/c anti-Ar antibodies, which we designated CRI_C (Brown and Nisonoff, 1981; Brown et al., 1981a). The unexpected observation was made that rabbit anti-Id specific for A/J CRI_m binds an average of 5–10% of A/J anti-Ar antibodies but an average of roughly 40% of BALB/c anti-Ar antibodies. This BALB/c population was found to correspond to a major BALB/c anti-Ar idiotype. The weights of A/J anti-Ar antibodies required to cause 50% inhibition in a radioimmunoassay for CRI_C varied from 420 ng to greater than 10,000 ng; two of nine sera tested caused less than 50% inhibition (40 and 44%, respectively) when 10,000 ng was tested for inhibitory capacity. In contrast, the weight of BALB/c anti-Ar antibodies required to cause 50% inhibition in the same assay varied from 80 to 105 ng; three pools of BALB/c anti-Ar were tested. Through appropriate adsorption experiments, it was found that only one-third of the A/J CRI_m^+ antibodies are actually related to the BALB/c idiotype. (This provides additional evidence for the heterogeneity of A/J CRI_m.) The expression of CRI_C was highly variable among individual A/J anti-Ar antisera.

Evidence that CRI_A and CRI_C are serologically unrelated was obtained by testing CRI_A^+ HP as inhibitors of the binding of CRI_C by rabbit anti-Id antibodies. Each of four such HP was noninhibitory in the assay; 5000 ng caused 0–28% inhibition. Furthermore, adsorption of anti-CRI_C on an insolubilized CRI_A^+ HP had no detectable effect on the capacity of the anti-CRI_C to bind ^{125}I-labeled BALB/c anti-Ar antibodies.

When anti-CRI_C was adsorbed on A/J serum anti-Ar antibodies conjugated to Sepharose, the plateau level of binding of ^{125}I-labeled pooled BALB/c anti-Ar antibodies by the anti-CRI_C decreased to 15% of the total labeled population, as compared to 44% bound by unadsorbed anti-CRI_C. This indicates that about two-thirds of CRI_C molecules share idiotypic determinants with the anti-Ar antibodies of A/J mice. These experiments define two subpopulations of CRI_C, of which the larger is serologically cross-reactive with a portion of A/J CRI_m.

Further evidence for the relatedness of CRI_m and CRI_C was the observation that anti-Id specific for A/J CRI_m suppressed the subsequent formation of the major anti-Ar idiotype (CRI_C) in BALB/c mice (Brown et al., 1981a).

INDEPENDENT REGULATION OF CRI_A AND CRI_C IN F_1 MICE

(BALB/c × A/J)F_1 (CAF_1) mice were used to determine whether CRI_A and CRI_C are regulated independently when anti-Id antibodies are inoculated prior to immunization (Kresina et al., 1983). Such hybrid mice were found to express both idiotypes when immunized against the Ar hapten group. The data in Table III demonstrate that the two idiotypes are regulated independently. The anti-Id reagents used to induce suppression include one that is specific for R16.7, a CRI_A^+ HP; a BALB/c-derived monoclonal anti-CRI_A (2F6.4); and rabbit anti-Id prepared against affinity-purified BALB/c anti-Ar antibodies. Anti-Id(R16.7) and 2F6.4 both suppressed CRI_A while having a minimal effect on the subsequent production of CRI_C. Conversely, the anti-Id(BALB/c) suppressed CRI_C and had no significant effect on CRI_A formation. An anti-Id reagent prepared against serum A/J anti-Ar antibodies suppressed both CRI_A and CRI_C, a result consistent with the presence of both anti-CRI_A and anti-CRI_C in the anti-Id.

VI. Strain Distribution of CRI_C and Concentrations of CRI_C in Individual BALB/c Mice

CRI_C was identified in each of 40 individual BALB/c anti-Ar sera or ascitic fluids tested, i.e., all samples caused more than 50% inhibition in the radioimmunoassay for CRI_C (Brown and Nisonoff, 1981). It was further shown that the idiotypic determinants are localized on Fab fragments and that removal of anti-Ar antibodies from hyperimmune BALB/c serum completely removes the capacity of the serum to cause inhibition in the standard radioimmunoassay for the idiotype.

To quantify CRI_C in the anti-Ar antibodies of BALB/c sera, direct binding studies were carried out with ^{125}I-labeled, affinity-purified antibodies. The plateau values for two separate pools of antibodies

TABLE III

Independent Regulation of CRI_A and CRI_C in (BALB/c × A/J) F_1 (CAF$_1$) Mice

Preinoculation[a]	Anti-Ar required for 50% inhibition (ng)	
	CRI_A[b]	CRI_C[c]
CAF$_1$ normal serum	6, 25, 34	260, 210, 430
	10, 23	300, 210
CAF$_1$ nonspecific IgG	200, 140, 19	110, 39, 440
	37, 62	130, 150
Anti-Id(R16.7)[d]	All >2000	48, 59, 43
(five mice)		260, 31
HP 2F6.4[e]	All >2000	86, 230
(eight mice)		86, 230
		19, 35
		69, 33
Anti-Id(BALB/c)[f]	91, 770, 100, 60	All >2000
(nine mice)	420, 90, 620, 30, 40	
Anti-Id(A/J)[g]	All >2000	All >2000
(six mice)		

[a] CAF$_1$ mice were inoculated with two ip injections of the reagent indicated, with a 3-day interval. Starting 2 weeks later, they were immunized ip twice, with a 2-week interval, with 250 μg of KLH-Ar in CFA. The mice were bled 2 weeks after the final antigen injection.

[b] With 10 ng purified A/J anti-Ar antibodies as labeled ligand.

[c] With 10 ng purified BALB/c anti-Ar antibodies as labeled ligand.

[d] Two inoculations of 100 μg idiotype-binding capacity (three mice) or 0.1 μg idiotype-binding capacity (two mice) before immunization.

[e] Two inoculations of 100 μg protein (six mice) or 0.1 μg protein (two mice) before immunization.

[f] Two inoculations of 30 μg idiotype-binding capacity.

[g] Two inoculations of 100 μg idiotype-binding capacity.

were 20% and 40% of the total labeled ligand, respectively. When antibodies isolated from four individual immunized BALB/c mice (other than those that had contributed to the two pools) were tested, the binding plateaus varied from 38 to 65% of the labeled anti-Ar population.

The distribution of CRI_C in various strains of mice is shown in Table IV (Brown and Nisonoff, 1981). Strain 129, which like BALB/c is Igh-1^a, is strongly CRI_C^+. Three strains that are Igh-1^j, which is closely related to Igh-1^a, expressed little or no CRI_C in their antibodies. The Igh-1^j strains were formerly designated Igh-1^a but were shown to be distinct by using an anti-AKR Fab antiserum that subdi-

TABLE IV

Expression of CRI_C in Anti-Ar Antibodies of Mice
of Various Strains[a]

| Strain[d] | Igh-1 allotype | Anti-Ar required for 50% inhibition (ng) | |
		CRI_C[b]	CRI_A[c]
BALB/c	a	55	>5000
129	a	107	>5000
PL	j	1800	>5000
C3H/AN	j	>5000	>5000
CBA	j	>5000	>5000
C.B-20	b	4100	>5000
C57BL/6	b	>5000	>5000
RF	c	88	>5000
DBA/1	c	230	2600
SWR	c	>5000	>5000
C.AL-20	d	770	87
A	e	1800	37
NZB/B1N	e	>5000	>5000
RIII/2	g	200	>5000
SEA/Gn	h	75	>5000

[a] Data are from Brown and Nisonoff (1981).
[b] Using 10 ng ^{125}I-labeled BALB/c anti-Ar antibodies as ligand.
[c] Using 10 ng ^{125}I-labeled A/J anti-Ar antibodies as ligand.
[d] Anti-Ar from strains BALB/c, PL, C57BL/6, RF, and A were affinity purified from the pooled sera or ascites of more than 10 mice. For the remaining strains, anti-Ar sera pooled from 2–6 mice immunized with KLH-Ar were tested.

vides the Igh-1[a] allotype group (Spring and Nisonoff, 1974). This anti-serum identifies an allotypic marker present in the $C_H 1$ domain of the IgG_{2b} subclass. The results just discussed show that the same sub-grouping of strains applies to the CRI_C idiotype.

As is evident from Table IV, the C.B-20 and C.AL-20 congenic strains failed to produce significant concentrations of CRI_C. Because these strains express the allotypes of C57BL and AL/N, respectively, on a BALB/c background, their failure to produce CRI_C demonstrates close linkage of expression of CRI_C to the *Igh* locus.

Anti-Ar antibodies from two of three strains tested of the Igh-1[c] allotype (RF and DBA/1) express high concentrations of CRI_C in their anti-Ar antibodies. Two other strains that are CRI_C^+ are RIII/2 and SEA/Gn, which are Igh-1[g] and Igh-1[h], respectively.

In summary, the low levels of CRI_C in anti-Ar antibodies of the two allotype-congenic strains demonstrate close linkage of inheritance of this idiotype to the *Igh* locus. The expression of CRI_C in substantial concentrations is not confined, however, to strains of the Igh-1ᵃ allotype.

VII. Hapten-Binding Specificities of CRI_A^+ Anti-Ar Antibodies

Our initial studies on the hapten-binding characteristics of A/J anti-Ar antibodies were prompted by the following considerations. On the average, about half of the anti-Ar antibodies produced by individual A/J mice bear CRI_A. The regular appearance of the idiotype might be accounted for on the basis that such molecules are of relatively high avidity; this could result in selective triggering of those lymphocytes which express the idiotype. To investigate this possibility, we compared binding affinities of A/J anti-Ar antibodies having either a high or a low content of CRI_A (Kapsalis *et al.*, 1976). This was done either by selecting appropriate mice, including idiotypically suppressed mice, or through fractionation of purified anti-Ar antibodies by isoelectric focusing. Comparisons were made, first by equilibrium dialysis using the radiolabeled hapten (*p*-azobenzenearsonic acid)-*N*-acetyl-L-tyrosine (Ar-acetyl-Tyr). Relative avidities were then investigated by determining the effect of dilution on the binding of ^{125}I-labeled KLH-Ar (the immunogen) to the antibodies. Both sets of measurements were consistent in indicating that the CRI_A^+ family is slightly lower in both affinity and avidity than the CRI_A^- population. This appears to rule out the possibility that the regular appearance of CRI_A is attributable to a high avidity of receptors on lymphocytes.

The fine specificities of A/J anti-Ar antibodies were further investigated by using monoclonal HP (Kresina *et al.*, 1982). For 10 CRI_A^+ HP, the binding affinities for Ar-acetyl-Tyr varied over a fairly narrow range, from 0.41×10^6 to $2.2 \times 10^6 \ M^{-1}$. The value for serum anti-Ar enriched for CRI_A^+ antibodies was 0.60×10^6 to $0.65 \times 10^6 \ M^{-1}$. The shapes of the binding curves for the monoclonal antibodies were consistent, as expected, with homogeneity with respect to binding affinity. For three CRI_A^- anti-Ar HP, the binding affinities for the same hapten varied from 0.5×10^6 to $3.4 \times 10^6 \ M^{-1}$.

Despite the relative uniformity of binding affinities of the CRI_A^+ HP for Ar-acetyl-Tyr, these monoclonal antibodies exhibit considerable microheterogeneity with respect to the fine specificities of their combining sites. This was best illustrated by a comparison of their relative affinities for other haptens, particularly o-aminobenzenearsonic acid (o-Ar) and (p-azobenzenearsonic acid)-N-L-histidine (Ar-HIS). With the binding affinity for p-aminobenzenearsonic acid arbitrarily set at 1.0, the relative binding affinities for Ar-HIS varied by a factor of 20 among the CRI_A^+ HP and the affinities for o-Ar varied by a maximum factor of approximately 4. Of the haptens tested, Ar-acetyl-Tyr probably resembles the effective haptenic structure in the immunogen most closely (Mäkelä et al., 1977). The data therefore suggest that the monoclonal antibodies tested all interact in a quite similar fashion with the hapten structure present on the immunogen, but that differences in fine specificity are clearly evident when other haptens, such as Ar-HIS, are investigated.

VIII. An Unrelated Major Idiotype Associated with Antibodies to the Phenylarsonate Hapten in A/J Mice

Studies by Mäkelä et al. (1976) showed that an inherited idiotype is induced in A/J mice by immunization with a hapten consisting of p-azobenzenearsonate coupled to p-hydroxyphenylacetic acid; this hapten, in turn, is conjugated to lysine side chains of the protein carrier used for immunization. The hapten is designated ABA-HOP. In effect, it corresponds very closely to the immunogen we employ, with the exception that there is an additional spacer,

$$-\overset{\overset{\displaystyle O}{\displaystyle \|}}{C}-NH-CH_2-CH_2-CH_2-CH_2-,$$

between the hapten and the immunizing protein. In collaboration with Mäkelä's laboratory, it was found that the major idiotype induced by ABA-HOP clearly differs from CRI_A (Mäkelä et al., 1977). The content of CRI_A in anti-ABA-HOP antisera is, on the average, more than 30 times lower than that present in our conventional anti-Ar antisera. Conversely, the concentration of the major idiotype associated with anti-ABA-HOP is at least 20 times lower in antibodies prepared against KLH-Ar than in anti-ABA-HOP antibodies. It is evident that the presence of the additional spacer in the ABA-HOP hapten selectively induces a population of anti-Ar antibodies that includes only very small numbers of molecules carrying CRI_A. In mice undergoing a secondary response to ABA-HOP, the proportion of antibody molecules carrying the ABA-HOP major idiotype was at least 75%.

The anti-ABA-HOP antibodies have a higher affinity for various phenylarsonate derivatives than do molecules carrying CRI_A, and the tightness of fit around the second benzene ring is much greater. This was shown by the deleterious effect on binding to anti-ABA-HOP of substitutions in this ring of the hapten molecule.

IX. Serological Properties of Monoclonal CRI$_A^+$ HP

Hybridomas secreting anti-Ar antibodies were prepared in several laboratories, including our own (Estess *et al.*, 1980; Marshak-Rothstein *et al.*, 1980a,b; Alkan *et al.*, 1980; Walker and Morahan, 1981). We carried out the work described below with hybridomas produced by using the nonsecreting Sp2/0-Ag14 myeloma cell line. It was found that approximately 25% of anti-Ar-secreting hybridomas produce CRI$_A^+$ antibodies. All subclasses of IgG and an IgM protein were represented among the CRI$_A^+$ HP (Lamoyi *et al.*, 1980a). An HP was designated as CRI$_A^+$ if it was capable of causing 50% inhibition of binding in the standard radioimmunoassay, which uses rabbit anti-Id with ^{125}I-labeled A/J serum anti-Ar antibodies as ligand. As shown in Table V, the CRI$_A^+$ HP vary greatly in their inhibitory capacity in this system. For the 14 HP studied, 9–3200 ng was required to cause 50% inhibition. CRI$_A^-$ HP failed to cause more than 20% inhibition when 2000 ng were tested. Thus, CRI$_A^+$ HP exhibit microheterogeneity with respect to their idiotypic determinants (Lamoyi *et al.*, 1980a).

In the same study, it was found that individual monoclonal HP possess "private" idiotypic determinants that are not present in other monoclonal CRI$_A^+$ HP. This was evidenced by the inability of nonautologous HP to cause complete displacement in radioimmunoassays that measure competition. In some instances, serum anti-Ar antibodies also failed to cause complete displacement at the maximum level of anti-Ar tested, although private determinants are generally present at low levels in serum antibodies.

It was of interest that several individual HP were able to displace 85–94% of ^{125}I-labeled serum anti-Ar from its anti-Id antibodies. On the assumption that monoclonal antibodies are representative of serum antibodies, one might expect that the serum antibodies would contain a large collection of private idiotypic determinants that are not present on most individual CRI$_A^+$ HP. Perhaps the most likely explanation is that most private idiotypic determinants are present at such low concentrations in serum antibodies that they do not induce the formation of significant amounts of anti-Id antibodies. This would account for the fact that most of the anti-Id is directed against shared or "public" idiotypic determinants in the serum antibodies. The data indicate, in addition, that CRI$_A^+$ serum antibodies that are bound by

TABLE V

Displacement of Labeled A/J Anti-Ar from Its Rabbit Anti-Id
Antibodies by Unlabeled A/J Anti-Ar Antibodies or HP with
Anti-Ar Activity[a,b]

Unlabeled inhibitors	Amount required for 50% Inhibition (ng)	Inhibition by 2000 ng (%)
A/J serum anti-Ar	11	97
HP R16.7 (IgG_1)	9	94
93G7 (IgG_1)	12	90
R20.4 (IgG_{2b})	14	86
R26.5 (IgG_3)	17	85
R13.4 (IgG_3)	21	87
R10.8 (IgG_{2a})	180	60
R23.2 (IgG_{2b})	200	66
R9.3 (IgG_{2b})	300	65
121D7 (IgG_1)	300	71
R17.5 (IgG_{2b})	460	63
R24.6 (IgG_{2a})	1800	52
123E6 (IgG_1)	1900	51
124E1 (IgG_1)	2900	47
R22.4 (IgG_{2a})	3200	49
R8.2 (IgG_{2b})[c]	>2000	9
R18.11 (IgG_3)[c]	>2000	20
R19.9 (IgG_{2b})[c]	>2000	15
R21.10 (IgG_1)[c]	>2000	6

[a] Data are from Lamoyi et al. (1980a).
[b] Each test utilized 10 ng ^{125}I-labeled, purified A/J anti-Ar antibodies
and slightly less than an equivalent amount of rabbit anti-Id.
[c] HP R8.2, R18.11, R19.9 and R21.10 lack the major CRI (CRI_A).

anti-Id possess at least one idiotope in common with such inhibitory
HP and therefore in common with one another. The presence of private idiotopes in monoclonal CRI_A^+ anti-Ar antibodies has also been
noted by others (Marshak-Rothstein et al., 1980b).

Further evidence for the presence of one or more conserved
idiotopes in the CRI_A^+ family was obtained through a variation of the
serological procedure (Lamoyi et al., 1980b). The radioimmunoassay
was set up by allowing anti-Id directed against one CRI_A^+ HP to bind a
different, ^{125}I-labeled CRI_A^+ HP. The assay was carried out in this way
so as to eliminate effects due to private idiotypic determinants. Two
such sets of "heterologous" systems were investigated (Table VI). In
both cases, 12 of 14 CRI_A^+ were strong inhibitors and were nearly
equivalent in terms of the weight of anti-Ar antibody required to cause

TABLE VI

Inhibition by Unlabeled CRI_A^+ HP of Binding of Anti-Id
Antibodies to Heterologous Labeled HP[a,b]

Unlabeled inhibitor	Amount required for 50% inhibition (ng)		
	R16.7 R10.8	93G7 121D7	Anti-Ar Anti-Ar
Serum anti-Ar	15 (100)[c]	11 (100)	11 (97)
R16.7 (IgG_1)	12 (100)	8 (97)	9 (94)
93G7 (IgG_1)	7 (100)	9 (99)	12 (90)
R20.4 (IgG_{2b})	10 (92)	8 (92)	14 (86)
R26.5 (IgG_3)	12 (88)	10 (99)	17 (85)
R13.4 (IgG_3)	13 (100)	14 (97)	21 (87)
R10.8 (IgG_{2a})	8 (100)	7 (90)	180 (60)
R23.2 (IgG_{2b})	5 (100)	7 (91)	200 (66)
R9.3 (IgG_{2b})	9 (100)	10 (90)	300 (65)
121D7 (IgG_1)	17 (88)	16 (100)	300 (71)
R17.5 (IgG_{2b})	7 (100)	7 (91)	460 (63)
R24.6 (IgG_{2a})	6 (100)	7 (93)	1800 (52)
123E6 (IgG_1)	>2000 (35)	>2000 (19)	1900 (52)
124E1 (IgG_1)	1900 (51)	>2000 (44)	2900 (47)
R22.4 (IgG_{2a})	6 (100)	7 (92)	3200 (49)

[a] Data are from Lamoyi et al. (1980b).
[b] Each test utilized 10 ng of ^{125}I-labeled ligand and slightly less than an equivalent amount of rabbit anti-Id.
[c] The percentage by inhibition by 2000 ng is in parentheses.

50% inhibition. (The same 12 HP vary greatly in their inhibitory capacity in the standard radioimmunoassay with ^{125}I-labeled serum anti-Ar antibodies as ligand.) These results are consistent with the presence of a highly conserved idiotope in the 12 CRI_A^+ HP that were tested.

Two of 14 CRI_A^+ HP that were tested were poor inhibitors in the "criss-cross" assay as well as in the standard radioimmunoassay using serum antibodies as ligand. Thus, microheterogeneity also extends to the public idiotopes; however, most of the HP that we tested possessed at least one conserved idiotope.

A phenylarsonate derivative possessing two benzene rings was found to be a strong inhibitor in each of three criss-cross assays. The degree of inhibition at a concentration of 10 mM was 84–91%. This strongly suggests that the conserved idiotope is associated with the hapten-binding region of the molecule (Lamoyi et al., 1980b).

Further evidence for the presence of at least one conserved idiotope on A/J serum anti-Ar antibodies was obtained by using monoclonal anti-Id reagents; the B cells used for fusion were from immunized BALB/c mice (Nelles *et al.*, 1981). It was found, first, that 8 of 10 CRI_A^+ monoclonal antibodies tested possess an idiotope reactive with each of three monoclonal anti-Id reagents. When serum anti-Ar antibodies were tested, it was found that one of the monoclonal anti-Id antibodies was able to bind about 60% of the CRI_A^+ population, thus establishing the presence of a cross-reactive idiotope in this fraction of the CRI_A^+ antibodies.

As mentioned above, certain CRI_A^+ HP are able to displace serum antibodies almost completely from anti-Id. To account for the fact that the monoclonal anti-Id reacted with only 60% of the CRI_A^+ population, we suggest that another 30–40% of the CRI_A^+ serum population possesses at least one idiotope that is modified but still serologically cross-reactive with the public determinant. CRI_A^+ HP would be able to displace such molecules when used at sufficiently high concentration, but the affinity of monoclonal anti-Id for these cross-reactive molecules could be insufficient to permit direct binding at the very low concentrations used in such assays (Nelles *et al.*, 1981).

X. Amino Acid Sequencing of CRI_A^+ Antibodies from Serum and Hybridomas

Methods used for isolating CRI_A-enriched populations from ascitic fluids of immunized A/J mice were discussed previously (Tung and Nisonoff, 1975). Amino acid sequencing was carried out in the laboratory of Dr. J. D. Capra on the NH_2-terminal regions of L and H chains isolated from such CRI_A-enriched antibodies. A single homogeneous sequence was obtained, in both the framework and hypervariable regions, for each type of polypeptide chain (Capra *et al.*, 1977; Capra and Nisonoff, 1979). When monoclonal antibodies expressing CRI_A were subsequently prepared and studied, their sequences, although exhibiting microheterogeneity, differed from those obtained with serum antibodies in about 20–30% of the positions in the sequence (Capra *et al.*, 1982; Slaughter *et al.*, 1982). The reason for these differences is not clear. However, because CRI_A^+ serum antibodies and HP express the same public idiotopes, and because some of the private idiotopes of HP are also found in serum antibodies, the HP appear to be representative of the serum antibody population.

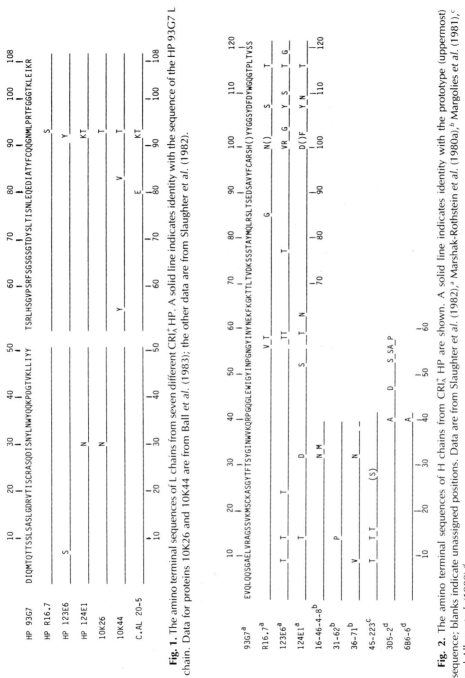

Fig. 1. The amino terminal sequences of L chains from seven different CRI$_A^+$ HP. A solid line indicates identity with the sequence of the HP 93G7 L chain. Data for proteins 10K26 and 10K44 are from Ball et al. (1983); the other data are from Slaughter et al. (1982).

Fig. 2. The amino terminal sequences of H chains from CRI$_A^+$ HP are shown. A solid line indicates identity with the prototype (uppermost) sequence; blanks indicate unassigned positions. Data are from Slaughter et al. (1982),[a] Marshak-Rothstein et al. (1980a),[b] Margolies et al. (1981),[c] and Alkan et al. (1980).[d]

Figures 1 and 2 are partial compilations of the NH_2-terminal amino acid sequences of L and H chains, respectively, of CRI_A^+ HP. If one compares the V_L sequences of pairs of CRI_A^+ HP (Fig. 1), the degree of homology averages about 96%. Substitutions, as compared to the prototype sequence, are seen in both framework and complementarity-determining (hypervariable) positions and are particularly frequent at positions 92 and 93 in the third hypervariable region. So far, no two complete V_L sequences have been found to be identical to one another.

A comparison of the sequences of V_H regions (Fig. 2) shows a similar pattern with, however, a somewhat higher frequency of substitutions; the average degree of homology between pairs of V_H regions nevertheless exceeds 90%. Although substitutions are again seen in both framework and hypervariable regions, they are much more concentrated in the hypervariable segments of V_H regions as compared to V_L. Substitutions are more prevalent in the second and third regions than in the first hypervariable region of the H chain.

XI. Investigations of Genes Controlling the Synthesis of H Chains of CRI_A^+ Molecules

Several studies of the control of CRI_A at the level of DNA have been reported (Estess *et al.*, 1982; Siekevitz *et al.*, 1982, 1983; Sims *et al.*, 1982) and are described below. The conclusions based on these studies may be summarized as follows.

1. There is a single germline gene for the V_H region of CRI_A^+ molecules and a single germline gene for V_L.
2. The presence of these two germline genes is necessary and sufficient for the production of CRI_A by a given strain of mouse. In all hybridomas studied so far that produce CRI_A^- anti-Ar HP, the germline V_H gene coding for CRI_A is not rearranged.
3. The V_H and V_L genes undergo somatic mutation in framework and hypervariable regions. As a consequence, CRI_A represents a family of molecules that is closely related but nonidentical in amino acid sequence. So far, no pair of CRI_A^+ molecules has proven to be identical with respect to either V_H or V_L sequence. The great similarity but nonidentity of amino acid sequences accounts for the existence of public and private idotopes in the CRI_A^+ family.

4. The V_H region of CRI_A^+ molecules makes use, almost exclusively, of the J_H2 sequence. Exceptions are two HP that utilize J_H4; one of these is only weakly CRI_A^+, as shown by serological assays.
5. The germline V_H gene that normally encodes CRI_A can undergo somatic mutations to such an extent that the gene product no longer expresses the idiotype.

The initial results obtained by Sims *et al.* (1982) utilized a complete V_H region cDNA probe in conjunction with the Southern blotting technique. The early results were difficult to interpret because of the large number of bands (approximately 20) obtained upon hybridization with an *Eco*R1 digest of mouse liver DNA. Subsequent studies were carried out with another probe, 1050 base pairs in length, that included the J_H region (Estess *et al.*, 1982). With A/J liver DNA (germline DNA), this probe hybridized with an *Eco*R1 fragment about 7 kb in length. With each of seven CRI_A^+ hybridomas, a new hybridizing restriction fragment of 5.8 kb was seen, that was not present in a digest of DNA of A/J liver or of the Sp2/0 parent myeloma line. It was concluded that the 5.8-kb band reflects a rearranged anti-Ar V_H gene and that in each CRI_A^+ hybridoma the same V_H gene is rearranged. These hybridization data do not exclude the possibility that more than one V_H gene is present in the 5.8-kb fragment. When a different restriction enzyme, *Sac*1, was used, all but one CRI_A^+ hybridoma exhibited a rearranged 7-kb band that was unique to the hybridomas. The one exception, hybridoma 124E1, yielded a 4-kb hybridizing band. Various explanations for the latter result, including the possible use of a different germline V_H gene in the 124E1 hybridoma, were discussed (Estess *et al.*, 1982). It should be noted that 124E1 inhibits relatively poorly in the radioimmunoassay for CRI_A.

The work of Siekevitz and colleagues (Siekevitz *et al.*, 1982, 1983) made use of a DNA probe that encompasses amino acid residues 15–90 of the V_H region. Although this probe hybridized with several restriction bands in the Southern blot of *Eco*R1-treated kidney DNA, the probe identified only a single strongly hybridizing band (6.4 kb). Of great interest was the observation that the presence of this band correlated with the Igh allotype of the strain of mouse under investigation; the studies included several CRI_A^+ as well as CRI_A^- strains. With one exception, only strains of mice that produce CRI_A, namely, A/J, C.AL-20, and AL/N, yielded the band. Negative strains included NZB, AKR, CBA, C57BL/10, CBA.Igh^b, and BALB/c. The DBA/2 strain is an exception in that it gave a moderately strong band at 6.4 kb, despite the fact that the strain is CRI_A^-.

Fairly extensive studies were carried out with Igh recombinant-inbred strains to test for linkage between expression of CRI_A and the presence of the strongly hybridizing 6.4-kb $EcoR1$ fragment. Each of several recombinant strains behaved either like the idiotype-positive parent (A/He) or like the idiotype-negative parent (BALB/c). Thus, each of six recombinant strains that are CRI_A^+ appeared to be identical to the A/He parent, i.e., the strongly hybridizing band was present. It was absent or expressed very weakly in the CRI_A^- strains.

The authors (Siekevitz $et\ al.$, 1982) considered the possibility that the 6.4-kb band might contain more than one gene that hybridizes with the incomplete V_H probe. When $EcoR1$ fragments of this size were cloned from embryonic DNA into bacteriophage, three different classes of gene were found. Only one of these, however, was identical in sequence to that of a V_H gene encoding a CRI_A^+ molecule. The other genes encoded polypeptides that would differ by at least eight amino acid residues. None of these eight residues were found in the protein sequences of 14 CRI_A^+ heavy chains. This led the authors to conclude that the other two germline genes are not utilized for the expression of CRI_A.

XII. Random Somatic Mutation versus Programmed Expression of Idiotypes

To explain the patterns of inheritance of CRI_A, we have proposed that genes controlling the idiotype are inherited in the germline or derived from a germline gene by a small number of somatic mutations (Kuettner $et\ al.$, 1972; Ju $et\ al.$, 1977). In examining the V_H and V_L amino acid sequences obtained thus far, no regular patterns of amino acid substitutions have emerged. On the basis of their observation that certain private idiotopes of three CRI_A^+ HP appear in the anti-Ar antibodies of most (but not all) immunized strain A mice, Marshak-Rothstein $et\ al.$ (1980b) have proposed that the somatic processes that operate on the germline V_H and V_L genes are programmed to appear regularly (cf. Klinman $et\ al.$, 1976). Arguing against this possibility is our earlier finding that idiotypes of anti-Ar antibodies appearing in some individual A/J mice suppressed for CRI_A are nonrecurrent. Using a sensitive radioimmunoassay, we could not detect three of four such idiotypes in significant concentrations in a panel of 181 A/J mice that had been hyperimmunized with KLH-Ar. This panel included mice that were suppressed or nonsuppressed with respect to CRI_A. The latter data, of course, do not bear directly on the question of variation within the CRI_A family, but they do indicate that idiotypes can be nonrecurrent. This would argue against their programmed appearance.

The fact that private idiotopes of some HP can be detected in immune sera does not necessarily prove identity of amino acid sequences. We consider it possible, and more consistent with the available data on amino acid sequences, that the somatic processes operating on the germline genes are variable rather than programmed. This does not imply that no restrictions on somatic variation exist, but only that it does not appear to occur in a regular sequence in individual mice.

References

Alkan, S. S., Knecht, R., and Braun, D. G. (1980). *Hoppe-Seyler's Z. Physiol. Chem.* **361**, 191–195.

Ball, R. K., Chang, J.-Y., Alkan, S. S., and Braun, D. G. (1983). *Mol. Immunol.* **20**, 203–212.

Barrett, M. C., and Nisonoff, A. (1982). *Eur. J. Immunol.* **11**, 977–978.

Blomberg, B., Geckeler, W. R., and Weigert, M. (1972). *Science* **177**, 178–180.

Brown, A. R., and Nisonoff, A. (1981). *J. Immunol.* **126**, 1263–1267.

Brown, A. R., Lamoyi, E., and Nisonoff, A. (1981a). *J. Immunol.* **126**, 1268–1273.

Brown, A. R., Gottlieb, P. D., and Nisonoff, A. (1981b). *Immunogenetics* **14**, 85–99.

Capra, J. D., and Nisonoff, A. (1979). *J. Immunol.* **123**, 279–284.

Capra, J. D., Tung, A. S., and Nisonoff, A. (1977). *J. Immunol.* **119**, 993–999.

Capra, J. D., Slaughter, C., Milner, E. C. B., Estess, P., and Tucker, R. W. (1982). *Immunol. Today* **3**, 332–339.

Clevinger, B., Schilling, J., Hood, L., and Davie, J. M. (1980). *J. Exp. Med.* **151**, 1059–1070.

Edelman, G. M., and Gottlieb, P. D. (1970). *Proc. Natl. Acad. Sci. U.S.A.* **67**, 1192–1199.

Eichmann, K., Tung, A., and Nisonoff, A. (1974). *Nature (London)* **250**, 509–511.

Estess, P., Lamoyi, E., Nisonoff, A., and Capra, J. D. (1980). *J. Exp. Med.* **151**, 863–875.

Estess, P., Otami, F., Milner, E. C. B., Capra, J. D., and Tucker, P. W. (1982). *J. Immunol.* **129**, 2319–2322.

Gill-Pazaris, L. A., Brown, A. R., and Nisonoff, A. (1979). *Ann. Immunol. (Paris)* **130C**, 199–213.

Gill-Pazaris, L. A., Lamoyi, E., Brown, A. R., and Nisonoff, A. (1981). *J. Immunol.* **126**, 75–79.

Gottlieb, P. D. (1974). *J. Exp. Med.* **140**, 1432–1437.

Gottlieb, P. D., Wan, H. C.-W., Brown, A. R., and Nisonoff, A. (1979). *Proc. Int. Leuko-cyte Cult. Conf.* **12**, 317–329.

Greene, M. I., Nelles, M. J., Sy, M.-S., and Nisonoff, A. (1982). *Adv. Immunol.* **32**, 253–300.

Hart, D. A., Wang, A. L., Pawlak, L. L., and Nisonoff, A. (1972). *J. Exp. Med.* **135**, 1293–1300.

Ju, S.-T., Gray, A., and Nisonoff, A. (1977). *J. Exp. Med.* **145**, 540–556.

Kapsalis, A. A., Tung, A. S., and Nisonoff, A. (1976). *Immunochemistry* **13**, 783–787.

Klinman, N. R., Press, J., Sigal, N. H., and Gearhart, P. (1976). *In* "The Generation of Antibody Diversity: A New Look" (A. J. Cunningham, ed.), pp. 127–149. Academic Press, New York.

Kresina, T. F., Rosen, S. M., and Nisonoff, A. (1982). *Mol. Immunol.* **19**, 1433–1439.

Kresina, T. F., Nelles, M. J., Brown, A. R., and Nisonoff, A. (1983). In preparation.

Kuettner, M. G., Wang, A. L., and Nisonoff, A. (1972). *J. Exp. Med.* **135**, 579–595.

Lamoyi, E., Estess, P., Capra, J. D., and Nisonoff, A. (1980a). *J. Immunol.* **124**, 2834–2840.

Lamoyi, E., Estess, P., Capra, J. D., and Nisonoff, A. (1980b). *J. Exp. Med.* **152**, 703–711.

Laskin, J. A., Gray, A., Nisonoff, A., Klinman, N. R., and Gottlieb, P. D. (1977). *Proc. Natl. Acad. Sci. U.S.A.* **74**, 4600–4604.

Mäkelä, O., Julin, M., and Becker, M. (1976). *J. Exp. Med.* **143**, 316–328.

Mäkelä, O., Karajalainen, K., Ju, S.-T., and Nisonoff, A. (1977). *Eur. J. Immunol.* **7**, 831–835.

Margolies, M. N., Marshak-Rothstein, A., and Gefter, M. L. (1981). *Mol. Immunol.* **18**, 1065–1077.

Marshak-Rothstein, A., Siekevitz, M., Margolies, M. N., Mudgett-Hunter, M., and Gefter, M. (1980a). *Proc. Natl. Acad. Sci. U.S.A.* **77**, 1120–1124.

Marshak-Rothstein, A., Benedetto, J. D., Kirsch, R. L., and Gefter, M. L. (1980b). *J. Immunol.* **125**, 1987–1992.

Marshak-Rothstein, A., Margolies, M. N., Benedetto, J. D., and Gefter, M. L. (1981). *Eur. J. Immunol.* **11**, 565–572.

Nelles, M. J., and Nisonoff, A. (1982). *J. Immunol.* **128**, 2773–2778.

Nelles, M. J., Gill-Pazaris, L. A., and Nisonoff, A. (1981). *J. Exp. Med.* **154**, 1752–1763.

Pawlak, L. L., and Nisonoff, A. (1973). *J. Exp. Med.* **137**, 855–869.

Pawlak, L. L., Hart, D. A., Nisonoff, A., Mushinski, E. B., and Potter, M. (1973a). *Specific Recept., Antibodies, Antigens, Cells, Int. Convocation Immunol.*, [*Proc.*], *3rd, 1972*, pp. 259–269.

Pawlak, L. L., Mushinski, E. B., Nisonoff, A., and Potter, M. (1973b). *J. Exp. Med.* **137**, 22–31.

Schroeder, K. W. (1974). Ph.D. Thesis, University of Illinois College of Medicine, Urbana.

Shulman, M., Wilde, C. D., and Köhler, G. (1978). *Nature (London)* **276**, 269–272.

Siekevitz, M., Gefter, M. L., Brodeur, P., Riblet, R., and Marshak-Rothstein, A. (1982). *Eur. J. Immunol.* **12**, 1023–1032.

Siekevitz, M., Huang, S. Y., and Gefter, M. L. (1983). *Eur. J. Immunol.* **13**, 123–132.

Sims, J., Rabbitts, T. H., Estess, P., Slaughter, C., Tucker, P. W., and Capra, J. D. (1982). *Science* **216**, 309–311.

Slaughter, C. A., Siegelman, M., Estess, P., Barasoain, I., Nisonoff, A., and Capra., J. D. (1982). *In* "Developmental Immunology: Clinical Problems and Aging" (E. L. Cooper and M. A. B. Brazier, eds.), pp. 45–68. Academic Press, New York.

Spring, S. B., and Nisonoff, A. (1974). *J. Immunol.* **113**, 470–478.

Tung, A., and Nisonoff, A. (1975). *J. Exp. Med.* **141**, 112–126.

Tung, A., Ju, S.-T., Sato, S., and Nisonoff, A. (1976). *J. Immunol.* **116**, 676–681.

Walker, I. D., and Morahan, G. (1981). *Scand. J. Immunol.* **13**, 433–440.

Weigert, M., and Potter, M. (1977). *Immunogenetics* **5**, 491–524.

Wysocki, L. J., and Sato, V. L. (1981). *Eur. J. Immunol.* **11**, 832–839.

Chapter 6

Idiotype-Specific T Helper Cells

M. McNamara and H. Köhler

Department of Molecular Immunology
Roswell Park Memorial Institute
Buffalo, New York

I. The Role of T Cells in Idiotype Networks

Complementary idiotypic interactions (1, 2) are the basis of a network theory on the immune system first proposed by Jerne (3). Originally, this theory had dealt with the specific interactions of B-cell idiotypes and antiidiotypes; it was later extended to T cells and T-cell factors (4–6) because of the emerging evidence that T cells and their factors also interact through idiotype-antiidiotype recognition. Furthermore, both the B- and T-cell compartments interact and exert controlling effects upon each other via idiotypic specificities (7, 8). Thus, the immune system could be viewed as a delicate balance of complementary cells and their products; this status quo can be altered by the addition of antigen, idiotype, or antiidiotype. Perturbation of the system by antigen causes activation of B cells and production of antibody. Subsequently, antiidiotypic antibody responses are generated (9, 10). This idiotypic cycling has been reported in many systems (11, 12). Similar responses are generated by the introduction of idiotype or antiidiotype into the immune system. However, the exact role and specificity of idiotype-recognizing T cells which are stimulated and their regulatory function on B cells needs to be better understood.

According to the network theory of complementary idiotypy, the regulation is being carried out by idiotypically defined B and T cells.

There are considerable data to support this concept. Idiotype-specific suppressor T cells (13, 14) have been induced by idiotype immunization. Similarly, priming with antiidiotype has been shown to stimulate idiotypic suppressor T cells (15, 16). Much less is known, however, about the network involvement of helper T cells which may be activated by antigen, idiotype, or antiidiotype. Although the role and specificity of idiotype-defined suppressor cells have been fairly well described (13, 17, 18), there is much uncertainty and even controversy about the function of idiotype-specific T helper cells: Are they required for maintenance of B-cell clonal dominance (19)? Are they needed to induce memory B cells to secrete antibody (20)? Or are they responsible for helping idiotype-specific T suppressor cells (21) or antiidiotypic B cells (22)?

One of the reasons for this uncertainty surrounding idiotype-specific T cells is that the nature of the T-cell receptor is unknown. B-cell idiotypic receptors are specialized immunoglobulins; however, the chemical nature of idiotype or antiidiotype receptors on T cells is controversial (23). Although T-cell idiotypes behave serologically and functionally as immunoglobulins (24, 25), it has not been possible to detect rearranged Ig gene segments in T-cell lines (26, 27). The observed cross-reactivity between T-cell and B-cell idiotypes could be explained by suggesting that T-cell receptors and their factors mimic idiotypic structures. Thus, the T-cell receptors could be assumed to be chemically different from immunoglobulins and encoded by a set of separate genes that are not used for immunoglobulin expression.

We would like to discuss our examination of the effect of network perturbation on regulatory T helper cells. We have analyzed the fine specificity and induction pathway of T helper cells, which are stimulated either with a hapten-carrier antigen complex, with idiotype, or with serum or monoclonal antiidiotypes. The comparison of the idiotype specificities that are expressed by B and T cells has produced some new and unexpected findings.

The system we used for these studies is the response of BALB/c mice to phosphorylcholine (PC), which is dominated by the TEPC15 (T15) myeloma idiotype (28, 29). We used a modification of the Klinman splenic fragment culture technique (30) and examined the interaction of idiotype-recognizing T helper cells with hapten-specific B cells under limiting T-cell dose conditions, which allowed us to study individual T cells and their interactions. The data we obtained demonstrate that antigen, idiotype, or antiidiotype immunization can induce T-cell recognition of both T15-positive and T15-negative, PC-binding antibodies. There is further evidence that one T helper cell population is recognizing a shared idiotopic determinant between the idiotypically distinct antibodies. These data suggest that complementary idiotypic–antiidiotypic interactions in the T-cell compartment are less specific than those in the B-cell compartment; in other words, T cells "see" idiotypes differently than do B cells. T cells recognize a cross-reactive determinant shared by two idiotypes which can be distinguished by antiidiotypic antibodies.

II. Induction of Idiotype-Specific T Helper Cells

T helper cells specific for immunoglobulin idiotypes have been described in various reports (31, 32) and implicated in the cellular regulation of B-cell activation (19, 20, 22) and expansion. The methods by which these cells can be stimulated in a normal immune response are important when considering the role that these cells play in network regulation.

We were interested in studying various manipulations of the immune network, which might occur naturally in the course of an immune response and which are involved in the generation of idiotype-specific T-cell help. In our experimental system, the idiotype-recognizing T helper cells must be stimulated to be detected. Unprimed T cells, or T cells primed with an unrelated antigen, are not scored as idiotype-recognizing T cells. We found that priming with PC-Hy antigen, idiotypically distinct anti-PC idiotypes (T15 or MOPC167), anti-T15 antiserum, or monoclonal anti-T15 antibodies can induce T-cell help for both T15 and M167 idiotypes. Transfer of PC-Hy primed T helper cells to athymic recipients results in a T-cell dose-dependent response to the T-dependent antigens TNP-T15 and TNP-M167 (Table I). Priming with PC-Hy specifically induces idiotype-recognizing help because Hy-primed cells are not able to help in the anti-TNP response. Similarly, idiotype-recognizing T helper cells were also seen when priming with idiotype was performed (Table I). Donor T cells from mice immunized with either T15 or M167 can provide help for both trinitrophylated T15 and M167. In other words, we found that a T15-positive idiotype can induce T-cell recognition of both T15-positive and -negative antibodies.

Finally, we examined the stimulatory effect of low-dose priming of donor mice with anti-T15 antiserum or monoclonal anti-T15 antibodies. Interestingly, as summarized in Table I, we found that whereas

TABLE I

Comparison of Different Priming Modes of Idiotype-Specific T Help
Induced by T-Cell Priming.

T-Cell Priming with[a]	Idiotype Recognition of[b]
Serum anti-T15 idiotype	$M460^-$, $T15^{++}$, $M167^+$
Monoclonal anti-T15 idiotype	$T15^{+++}$, $M167^{+++}$
PC-Hy priming	$M460^-$, $MPC11^-$, $T15^{+++}$, $M167^{+++}$
T15 or M167-idiotype priming	$T15^{+++}$, $M167^{+++}$

[a] Serum antiidiotype-primed BALB/c donors were prepared by either neonatally suppressing mice with 5 ng A/He anti-T15 antiserum iv at birth or treating adult mice with 0.1 μg anti-T15 antiserum iv. The mice were used 6–8 weeks after priming. Monoclonal antiidiotype-primed mice were prepared by immunizing NBF1 male mice with 0.1 μg 4C11 or 10 ng F6-3 iv. These mice were used 8 weeks later. PC-Hy-primed NBF1 male mice were given 100 μg Hy in CFA 8 weeks before use and 100 μg PC-Hy in IFA 4 weeks before use. M167 or T-15-primed NBF1 males were given 100 μg T15 or M167 in CFA 8 weeks before use and 100 μg T15 or M167 4 weeks before use. Then 5×10^5 donor Ly2$^-$ T cells were transferred into athymic, nu/nu BALB/c recipients.

[b] Splenic fragment cultures were immunized with either TNP-T15, TNP-M167, TNP-M460, or TNP-MPC11 at 10^{-8} M TNP. From 48 to 96 culture supernatants were assayed for anti-TNP activity (and thus idiotype recognition) on days 9 and 12 by ELISA. − (negative) indicates that no help was detected (for TNP-conjugated myelomas). +, + +, and + + + (positive) indicate relative differences in the number of positive foci responding to TNP-conjugated myelomas.

immunization with the two monoclonal antiidiotypes, F6-3 and 4C11, generated T cells which recognize T15 and M167 equally well, anti-T15 antiserum immunization stimulated T help which preferentially recognized the T15 idiotype over the M167 idiotype. This is surprising when one considers that F6-3 and 4C11 are capable of distinguishing serologically between T15 and M167. One would expect priming with the monoclonal antibodies to generate more specific help than priming with an antiidiotype serum. Idiotypes F6-3 and 4C11 are specific for two different idiotypic determinants; one is on the PC site and the other is near the PC site (33). These idiotopes may be more frequent than the idiotopes recognized by anti-T-15 antiserum. Therefore, they may represent regulatory idiotopes (34). We also noted that intravenous low-dose priming of donor mice with 100 μg F6-3 induces a suppressive effect on T-cell help, whereas 1 μg 4C11 antiidiotype generates help for T15 and M167.

Viewed collectively, these four priming modes demonstrate both indirect network and direct priming of idiotype-recognizing T helper

TABLE II

B or T Cells as Inducers of Idiotype-Recognizing T Help

Cells transferred from PC-primed BALB/c mice[a]	Mice used as T-Cell donors[b]	Anti-TNP response[c]
—	PC-primed BALB/c	++
—	Hy-primed BALB/c	—
—	PC-primed NBF1 male	++
—	Hy-primed NBF1 male	—
Spleen cells	Normal NBF1	++
B cells	Normal NBF1	—
—	Normal NBF1	—

[a] Mice used as PC-primed donors were prepared as in Table I. PC-primed whole spleen cells or B cells were transferred into irradiated NBF1 male recipients.

[b] Hy-primed or PC-primed T cell donors were prepared as in Table I. Primed Ly2− T cells were transferred into athymic B/C recipients. Naive NBF1 Ly2− T cells were cotransferred with the PC-primed B cells into irradiated NBF1 male recipients. Splenic fragment cultures, prepared from either the nu/nu B/C recipients or the irradiated NBF1 recipients, were immunized with TNP-T15 at 10^{-8} M TNP.

[c] Anti-TNP activity as assayed by ELISA on days 9 and 12.

cells. Receptors of cells that recognized idiotype can be defined as "antiidiotype-like" according to network theory. PC-Hy or anti-idiotype priming cannot activate the idiotype-recognizing T cell directly; the priming must occur via an indirect circuit. Idiotype, on the other hand, can stimulate the T15- and M167-recognizing cells directly.

The direct and indirect methods of stimulating T cells which recognize idiotype provide some insight into the T-cell network. The fact that antigen stimulation, a common occurrence in nature, can activate the T helper network and, more specifically, can trigger an idiotype-specific T cell, attests to the biological significance of these cells. The concomitant stimulation of idiotope-recognizing T help along with B cells indicates a regulatory role for these T cells. The fact that both antiidiotype and idiotype can induce T cells that recognize two similar but idiotypically distinct antibodies demonstrates that, like B cells, these T helper cells are regulated via an idiotypic–antiidiotypic immunoregulatory circuit. However, unlike B cells, these helper cells appear to be nonidiotype specific by the criterion of B-cell recognition.

III. Cells Involved in the Induction Circuit of Idiotype-Specific T Helper Cells

T cells which recognize idiotype may play an important role in the regulation of the B-cell (antibody) network (2, 8). The elucidation of the cellular induction circuit which leads to activation of these anti-idiotype-like T cells by antigens may provide a clue to the nature of the T-cell receptor and, subsequently, address the question of the regulatory role these T cells play for B cells and antibody production.

In our system, the question arises whether indirect priming induces a T-T or a B-T circuit. To exclude the B-T circuit, we tried to induce T15 idiotype-recognizing T cells in defective NBF1 male mice, whose B cells are unable to respond to PC (35). Therefore, in these mice, PC-Hy priming, which we know induces the generation of T cells specific for T15 and M167, would be able to affect only the T-cell compartment. As can be seen in Table II, PC-Hy-primed NBF1 males can provide help for T15, indicating a TH1-TH2 cellular loop of induction. The evidence for the existence of a T-cell circuit is strengthened by the finding (Table II) that PC-primed B cells fail to induce T helper cells from a normal donor to recognize T15.

The TH1-TH2 induction circuit proposed here imitates the T-suppressor cell circuits that have been documented (6, 7, 36). The specificity of the TH1 cell, induced by antigen or, alternatively, anti-idiotype would be "T15-like." The finer specificity of this TH1 is not known. Whether there are many TH1 cells, each specific for a distinct idiotope, or whether there is a small number of these intermediate cells expressing conserved recurrent idiotopes, remains to be seen. Network stability could be provided for by assuming that for all of the inducing antigens or antiidiotypes there is a limited number of idiotypically defined inducing cells. The target specificity of these T-cell loops would resemble determinants that were named "regulatory idiotopes" (34).

IV. Specificity of Idiotype-Recognizing T Helper Cells

B cells and their products are defined as specific for a particular idiotype. Antigen stimulation of B cells results in the expression of clones of cells specific for idiotype and antiidiotype (6, 9). The fine specificity of T cells and their products remains unknown, however, mainly because the nature of the T-cell receptor is unknown (23). It is uncertain whether the T-cell receptor is as specific as the B-cell antibody receptor or is less specific. If T cells are "idiotype specific," it is possible that two kinds of idiotype-recognizing T cells exist, one which recognizes common regulatory idiotopes and another which is specific for unique idiotopes. It seems that a network based on equal tendencies for both B and T cells to recognize specific idiotypes and their somatic variants would be unstable. However, if the T cells involved in the regulation of the immune network were somehow restricted in their recognition of B-cell idiotypes, a greater degree of stability could be achieved.

In the work discussed here, we describe the fine specificity of the idiotype-recognizing T helper cells. By doing this, we learn more about the nature of the T-cell receptors and their function in immunoregulatory networks. We have already demonstrated that immunization with antigen, idiotype, or antiidiotype can generate an auto-antiidiotypic response in the form of idiotype-recognizing T cells. Furthermore, we have shown that these T cells can recognize two similar but idiotypically distinct myeloma proteins. This dual recognition raises the question of whether the priming scheme is inducing two distinct populations of T helper cells, each specific for either T15

TABLE III

Idiotype-Recognizing T Cells Responding to Different
Trinitrophenylated Idiotypes

In vitro antigens[a]	Idiotype characterization	Induction of idiotype T help (priming)[b]	Foci/10^6 transferred cells[c]
TNP-T15	T15$^+$, anti-PC	PC-Hy	0.30
		F6-3	0.42
		4C11	0.36
TNP-M167	T15$^-$, anti-PC	PC-Hy	0.33
		F6-3	0.48
		4C11	0.34
TNP-HPCG11	T15$^+$, anti-PC	PC-Hy	0.51
TNP-HPCG15	T15$^-$, anti-PC	PC-Hy	0.70
TNP-HPC104	T15$^-$, anti-PC	PC-Hy	0.07
TNP-M460	T15$^-$, anti-TNP	PC-Hy	0.07
TNP-MPC11	T15$^-$, unknown	PC-Hy	<0.11

[a] In vitro antigens were used at a concentration of 5×10^{-7} to 10^{-8} M TNP.
[b] The BALB/c and NBF1 male T-cell donors were primed as in Table I. Recipients were either *nu/nu* BALB/c mice or PC-primed BALB/c mice.
[c] Frequency indicates the number of TNP-specific foci detected per 10^6 cells transferred.

TABLE IV

Inhibition of Idiotype-Specific Recognition *in Vitro* by Idiotypes or Hapten

NBF1 T cell donor treatment[a]	In vitro antigen[b]	In vitro inhibitor[c]	Anti-TNP positive wells[d]	Percentage inhibition[e]
PC-Hy	TNP-T15	—	30	—
	TNP-T15	T15	4	87
		M167	2	93
		T15 + M167	4	87
		PC	2	93
	TNP-M167	—	33	—
		M167	2	90
		T15	12	64
		T15 + M167	7	79
		PC	4	88

[a] Donor NBF1 male mice were primed with PC-Hy and Ly2⁻ T cells prepared as described in Table I. Then 10^6 Ly2⁻ T cells were injected into athymic *nu/nu* BALB/c recipients.

[b] The splenic fragment cultures were immunized *in vitro* with TNP_7-T15 or TNP_{12}-M167 at 10^{-8} M TNP.

[c] Affinity-purified myeloma proteins T15 and M167 were used at 10^{-9} M protein. PC was used as an inhibitor at 10^{-7} M PC.

[d] From 48 to 96 fragments were cultured and assayed by ELISA for anti-TNP activity on days 9 and 12.

[e] Percentage inhibition was calculated by the following formula: [1 − (percentage positive with inhibitor/percentage positive without inhibitor)] × 100.

or M167, or one population of T helper cells specific for an idiotypic determinant shared between the two idiotypes. To resolve this question, we compared the T-cell responses to T15, M167, and other T15⁺ and T15⁻ hybridomas (Table III). Then we measured the precursor frequency for PC-primed T cells responding to TNP-T15 and TNP-M167 by limiting dilution analysis, and found that the frequencies of the two populations were indistinguishable within the limits of experimental variation. These data supported the notion that one T-cell population is induced by PC priming and that this population recognizes both T15 and M167 idiotypes as well as other anti-PC, T15-like antibodies. To substantiate further this idea of a "non-idiotype-specific" T helper cell, we performed various inhibition experiments on the responses to the two idiotypes. Using PC, unconjugated T15 or M167, or free T15 and M167 heavy and light chains, as in the *in vitro* inhibitors, we attempted to block the help for the T15 and M167 carriers. As is seen from Table IV, PC hapten inhibited the response to the two antigens completely. Titration of the PC inhibitor produced identical PC inhibition curves for TNP-T15 and TNP-M167. When unconjugated T15 and M167 were used as the inhibitors, both idiotypes blocked the help for both antigens equally well, further demonstrating that a shared determinant on the T15 and M167 molecules is being recognized by PC-primed T cells. The shared determinant on the two idiotypes seems to be mainly restricted to the heavy chain, as only T15 and M167 heavy chains could inhibit the anti-TNP response (32). Collectively, these data indicate that the PC-binding site on the T15 and M167 molecules, a highly conserved structure, is the target of recognition by the T helper cells, and that one population of T cells recognizes the shared determinant between the two idiotypes.

These specificity data indicate the idiotype nonspecificity of the idiotype-recognizing T-cell population. Antigen priming stimulates a population of helper T cells that recognizes a cross-reactive idiotope between T15 and M167 that is associated with the binding site. This non-idiotype-specific nature of the T-cell population should restrict the number of interactions with individual B cells. A model could be proposed for network stability in which T cells would see B cells as families of idiotypes. They could exert control over a mutating B cell repertoire by recognizing public, nonvarying idiotopes shared by idiotype families.

V. Conclusions

The immune system can be described as a network of interacting cells. Because of the importance of the T and B cells in the immune network, the elucidation of the nature of the interaction between these two populations of cells is essential for a complete understanding of the immune system. Various lines of evidence (1, 8) lead to the conclusion that these interactions are achieved through idiotypic complementarity. To explore this idea, one must study the cellular receptors involved. B-cell idiotypic specificities are clearly defined. Antisera produced against a particular antibody are specific for the respective idiotype. T-cell receptor specificity, however, is less well known. Whether T cells see idiotypes as individual determinants or as groups of related determinants remains a question.

In the present work, we addressed the question of idiotypic receptors on T cells. In our experimental model, we used two similar but idiotypically distinct myeloma proteins, T15 and M167, as carriers to study directly T helper cells specific for idiotype. We can prime these

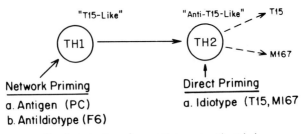

Fig. 1. Induction of non-idiotype-specific T help.

idiotype-recognizing T cells either directly, using T15 or M167 idiotypes, or indirectly, using anti-T15 antisera, monoclonal anti-T15 idiotype, or antigen. The induction of these antiidiotype T cells by PC antigen is evidence of their biological significance, and their induction by antiidiotype is further evidence of the existence of idiotype interactions between B and T cells. Priming of idiotype-recognizing T cells with antigen or antiidiotype cannot occur directly; a cellular induction loop must be involved. We have presented evidence for the existence of a TH1-TH2 circuit. The receptor specificity of the TH1 cell would be T15-like (Fig. 1), and that of the TH2 would be anti-T15-like.

The question of the fine specificity of these T cells is addressed by doing various inhibitions of T15 and M167 T-cell recognition. The data indicate that the antigen priming is inducing a single population of T cells which recognizes a shared determinant on the heavy chains of T15 and M167 that is involved in the PC-binding site. In other words, these T cells are heavy chain idiotope specific, as opposed to idiotype specific.

Viewed as a whole, these data provide evidence for a T-cell receptor that is functionally and biochemically different from a B-cell receptor. T cells could exert regulatory control over B cells by idiotopic recognition. The repertoire of constantly mutating B-cell idiotypes could be regulated by assuming that T cells recognize only a certain number of nonvariant idiotopes. Both T and B cells may have an equal tendency to produce variants of idiotypes, but the number of idiotopes involved in complementary network interactions would be limited. In the model, a hierarchy of idiotopes would exist in which certain functionally important idiotopes would be involved in T-B cell interactions, whereas others would remain unrecognized and unstimulated. This model describes the function of a balanced and regulated immune system.

References

1. Köhler, H., Rowley, D. A., Duclos, T., and Richardson, B. (1977). Complementary idiotypy in the regulation of the immune response. *Fed. Proc., Fed. Am. Soc. Exp. Biol.* **36**, 221.
2. Rowley, D. A., Köhler, H., and Cowan, J. D. (1980). An immunologic network. *Contemp. Top. Immnol.* **9**, 205.
3. Jerne, N. K. (1974). Towards a network theory of the immune response. *Ann. Immunol. (Paris)* **125C**, 373.
4. Julius, M. H., Cosenza, H., and Augustin, A. A. (1978). Evidence for autogenous production of T cell receptor bearing idiotypic determinants. *Eur. J. Immunol.* **8**, 484.
5. Eichmann, K., and Rajewsky, K. (1975). Production of T and B cell immunity by anti-idiotypic antibodies. *Eur. J. Immunol.* **5**, 661.
6. Owen, F. L., Ju, S.-T., and Nisonoff, A. (1977). Presence on idiotype-specific suppressor T cells of receptors that interact with molecules bearing the idiotype. *J. Exp. Med.* **145**, 1559.
7. Eichmann, K. (1974). Idiotype suppression. II. Amplification of a suppressor T cell with anti-idiotypic activity. *Eur. J. Immunol.* **5**, 511.
8. Kohler, H. (1980). Idiotypic network interactions. *Immun. Today* **1**, 18.
9. Kluskens, L., and Köhler, H. (1974). Regulation of immune response by autogenous antibody against receptor. *Proc. Natl. Acad. Sci. U.S.A.* **71**, 5083.
10. Rodkey, L. S. (1974). Studies of idiotypic antibodies. Production and characterization of auto-anti-idiotypic antisera. *J. Exp. Med.* **712**, 770.
11. Kelsoe, G., and Cerny, J. (1979). Reciprocal expansions of idiotypic and anti-idiotypic clones following antigen stimulation. *Nature (London)* **279**, 333.
12. Goidl, E. A., Schrater, A. F., Siskind, G. W., and Thorbecke, G. J. (1979). Production of auto-anti-idiotypic antibody during the normal immune response to TNP-Ficoll. I. Occurrence and AKR/J and BALB/c mice of hapten-augmentable, anti-TNP plaque-forming cells and their accelerated appearance in recipients of immune spleen cells. *J. Exp. Med.* **150**, 38.
13. Dohi, Y., and Nisonoff, A. (1979). Suppression of idiotype and generation of suppressor T cells with idiotype-conjugated thymocytes. *J. Exp. Med.* **150**, 909.
14. McKearn, J. P., and Quintans, J. (1980). Induction of idiotype-specific suppressor cells with soluble idiotype. *Fed. Proc., Fed. Am. Soc. Exp. Biol.* **39**, Suppl. 3, 1607.
15. Strayer, D. S., Lee, W. M. F., Rowley, D. A., and Köhler, H. (1975). Anti-receptor antibody. II. Induction of long-term unresponsiveness in neonatal mice. *J. Immunol.* **114**, 728.
16. Hart, D. A., Wang, A. L., Pawlak, L. L., and Nisonoff, A. (1972). Suppression of idiotypic specificities in adult mice by administration of anti-idiotypic antibody. *J. Exp. Med.* **135**, 1293.
17. Yamamoto, H., Nonaka, M., and Katz, D. H. (1979). Suppression of hapten-specific delayed-type hypersensitivity responses in mice by idiotype-specific suppressor T cells after administration of anti-idiotypic antibodies. *J. Exp. Med.* **150**, 818.
18. Bona, C., and Paul, W. E. (1979). Cellular basis of regulation of expression of idiotype. I. T-suppressor cells specific for MOPC 460 ID regulate the expression of cells secreting anti-TNP antibodies bearing 460 ID. *J. Exp. Med.* **149**, 592.
19. Bottomly, K., and Jones, F., III (1981). Idiotypic dominance manifested during a T-dependent anti-phosphorylcholine response requires a distinct helper T cell. *In* "B Lymphocytes in the Immune Respone: Functional, Developmental and Interactive Properties," p. 415. Elsevier/North-Holland, Amsterdam.

20. Woodland, R., and Cantor, H. (1978). Idiotype-specific T helper cells are required to induce idiotype-positive B memory cells to secrete antibody. *Eur. J. Immunol.* **8**, 600.

21. Cantor, H., Hugenberger, J., McVay-Boudreau, L., Eardley, D. D., Kemp, J., Shen, F. W., and Gershon, R. K. (1978). Immunoregulatory circuits among T cell sets. Identification of a subpopulation of T helper cells that induces feedback inhibition. *J. Exp. Med.* **148**, 871.

22. Cazenave, P.-A. (1977). Idiotypic-anti-idiotypic regulation of antibody synthesis in rabbits. *Proc. Natl. Acad. Sci. U.S.A.* **74**, 5122.

23. Jensenius, J. C., and Williams, A. F. (1982). The T lymphocyte antigen receptor-paradigm lost. *Nature (London)* **300**, 583.

24. Binz, H., and Wigzell, H. (1975). Shared idiotypic determinants on B and T lymphocytes reactive against the same antigenic determinant. I. Demonstration of similar or identical idiotypes on IgG molecules and T-cell receptors with specificity for the same alloantigen. *J. Exp. Med.* **142**, 197.

25. Szenberg, A., Marchalonis, J. J., and Warner, M. L. (1977). Direct demonstration of murine thymus-dependent cell surface endogeneous immunoglobulin. *Proc. Natl. Acad. Sci. U.S.A.* **74**, 2113.

26. Kronenberg, M., Davis, M. M., Early, P. W., Hood, L. E., and Watson, J. D. (1980). Helper and killer T cells do not express B cell immunoglobulin joining and constant region gene segments. *J. Exp. Med.* **152**, 1745.

27. Cayre, Y., Pallidino, M., Marcu, K., and Stavnezer, J. (1981). Expression of an antigen receptor on T cells does not require recombination at the immunoglobulin J_H-$C\mu$ locus. *Proc. Natl. Acad. Sci. U.S.A.* **78**, 3814.

28. Lee, W., Cosenza, H., and Kohler, H. (1974). Clonal restriction of the immune response to phosphorylcholine. *Nature (London)* **247**, 55.

29. Potter, M., and Lieberman, R. (1970). Common individual antigenic determinants in five of eight BALB/c IgA myeloma proteins that bind phosphorylcholine. *J. Exp. Med.* **132**, 737.

30. Pierce, S. K., Cancro, M., and Klinman, N. R. (1978). Individual antigen-specific T lymphocytes: Helper function in enabling the expression of multiple antibody expression. *J. Exp. Med.* **142**, 1165.

31. Gleason, K., Pierce, S. K., and Kohler, H. (1981). Generation of idiotype-specific T cell help through network perturbation. *J. Exp. Med.* **153**, 924.

32. Gleason, K., and Köhler, H. (1982). Regulatory idiotypes. T helper cells recognize a shared V_H idiotype on phosphorylcholine-specific antibodies. *J. Exp. Med.* **156**, 539.

33. Wittner, M. K., Bach, M. A., and Köhler, H. (1982). Immune response to phosphorylcholine. IX. Characterization of hybridoma anti-TEPC15 antibodies. *J. Exp. Med.* **128**, 595.

34. Bona, C. A., Heber-Katz, E., and Paul, W. (1981). Idiotype-anti-idiotype regulation. I. Immunization with a levan-binding myeloma protein leads to the appearance of auto-anti (anti-idiotype) antibodies to the activation of silent clones. *J. Exp. Med.* **153**, 951.

35. Mond, J. J., Lieberman, R. L., Inman, J. K., Mosier, D. E., and Paul, S. W. (1977). Inability of mice with a defect in B-lymphocyte maturation to respond to phosphorylcholine on immunogenic carriers. *J. Exp. Med.* **146**, 1138.

36. Sy, M. S., Bach, B. A., Dohi, Y., Nisonoff, A., Benacerraf, B., and Greene, M. I. (1979). Antigen- and receptor-driven regulatory mechanisms. I. Induction of suppressor T cells with anti-idiotypic antibodies. *J. Exp. Med.* **150**, 1216.

Chapter 7

Manipulating an Idiotypic System with Asymmetric Circuitry: Antiidiotypic Antibodies versus Idiotype-Recognizing T Cells[1]

Eli E. Sercarz and Christopher D. Benjamin

Department of Microbiology, University of California, Los Angeles
Los Angeles, California

I. The B Cell Predominant Idiotype and the T Helper Cell Idiotypes: Occupants of Separate Universes[2]

Previous work in studying the cellular interactions controlling the production of antilysozyme antibodies has indicated that the antigen-specific/MHC-restricted T helper cell (AgTh) occupies a detached regulatory niche (1). The predominant idiotype in the antibody system, IdXL, is expressed on more than 90% of secondary response antibodies and is also found on antigen-specific T suppressor cells (Ts). Furthermore, as in Fig. 1, one of the two Th cells depicted (IdXTh) is preoccupied with IdXL in that it recognizes the predominant idiotype on the surface of activated B cells. However, the AgTh is

[1] Supported in part by NIH Training Grant AI-07126 (C. D. Benjamin) and by American Cancer Society grant IM-263 and NIH grants AI-11183 and CA-24442.

[2] Abbreviations: Ag, antigen; BRC, burro erythrocytes; CFA, complete Freund's adjuvant; HEL, chicken eggwhite lysozyme; HUL, human lysozyme; IdXL, the predominant idiotype in the 2° antilysozyme response; MHC, major histocompatibility complex; NRIg, normal rabbit immunoglobulin; Th, T helper cell; and Ts, T suppressor cell.

101

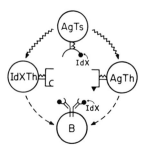

Fig. 1. Four cell types involved in the production of antibody to hen eggwhite lysozyme. The predominant idiotypic determinant on the secondary-response B cells is designated by a small solid circle on the receptor structure. This IdX determinant is also found on the Ag-specific T suppressor cell (AgTs). The MHC-restricted, Ag-specific T helper cell is shown to bear an idiotypic receptor different from IdXL. On the left is an IdXL-recognizing T helper cell. ⤳, suppression; ---→, help.

distinct from the IdXL regulatory universe in neither displaying IdXL$^+$ receptors nor recognizing IdXL, as assessed by a variety of techniques (1–3). Up to now, we have not looked for a predominant idiotypic species (Id2) among AgTh and other cells within this second idiotypic universe. Amplifying, augmenting, and contrasuppressor cells (4, 5) interacting with the AgTh family might belong to the IdXL or the alternative Id2 universe.

The evidence for T-cell recognition of Ig determinants is extremely strong and has been reviewed in several places (6–9). In the lysozyme system, it has been shown elsewhere (10) that at least two types of Th cells are employed in responses to HEL (hen eggwhite lysozyme), one specific for Ag in the context of MHC (AgTh) and another recognizing the predominant B-cell idiotype IdXL. It has been postulated that the AgTh might drive B cells to expand to a stage at which they favorably display an Ig epitope, such as the IdX idiotope. The IdXTh cells can be imagined to direct the further expansion of those B cells bearing this predominant idiotope and to provide a positive selective force which maintains this idiotype.

II. Driving B-Cell Maturation with T Cells and Other Agents

Studies of B-cell stimulation have involved several types of reagents: anti-heavy immunoglobulin variable and constant region antisera, antigens, mitogens, and growth differentiation factors. Recent work (11) has indicated that in order for the B cell to be activated sufficiently to produce antibody (PFC), a sequential series of interactions with a variety of nonspecific inducer molecules is necessary after the initiating contact with one of these agents. The generalized paradigm indicates that a stimulus from one of these ligands will induce the display of a receptor specific for the next ligand in the series. Presumably, T cells serve as a source of the inducer ligands, such as BCGF (B cell growth factor). BCGF acts quite early in the life of the activated B cell, thus requiring an "early" Th cell to produce this inducer. This terminology makes the implicit suggestion that a *series* of T cells may provide the inducer factors required for continued further progress toward the final goal of antibody production. Thus, it is possible that a single T cell is *not* able to drive the B cell to produce antibodies of multiple classes in the complete absence of any residual proliferation or differentiation factors. On the contrary, a single Th cell's function may be just to drive the B cell part of the way to the next "pit stop," where a new T-cell driver takes over (12).

This requirement for coordination of T help is only one implication that can be derived from the information that a multiplicity of T-cell factors is utilized by the B cell. Another interesting implication is that the "memory B cell" is really a set of B cells trapped at one of the diverse transition states along the pathway to an end-cell stage.

No doubt, the Ig receptor can be perturbed by Ag or idiotype-recognizing molecules to perform an essential first step in the transformation of the B cell in the absence of other factors. Subsequently, each future step would require the correct entity to be displayed on the cell surface for recognition by a T cell. For example, the succession of T cells may be activated by (a) Ag + MHC; (b) idiotype + X; (c) isotype + Y; or (d) allotype + Z, where X, Y, and Z stand for restricting molecules on the B-cell surface.

The interaction of anti-IdXL with the virgin B cell can be thought of as initiating the proliferation and temporary display of the BCGF receptor. It is also conceivable that memory B cells at other stages of differentiation can also be addressed, and this possibility should be experimentally examined. In this chapter, we compare the possible role of serum anti-IdX and IdX-recognizing Th in regulating different lymphocyte functions in response to the protein Ag lysozyme.

III. Modulation of IdXL-Bearing B Cells in Responder Strain Mice

Experiments will be described in the antiidiotypic manipulation of lysozyme responder A/J mice and nonresponder B10 mice. In this

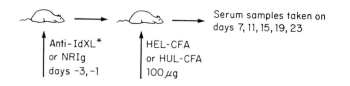

* 200 ng IBC, each injection

Fig. 2. Protocol for the antiidiotype manipulation experiments. Further details appear in the text.

"asymmetric" regulatory system, we have assumed that in the A/J mouse the predominant target of action is the B cell. Figure 2 describes the basic protocol of the experiments in the A/J mouse. Two injections of anti-IdXL seem to be necessary. The amount of antiidiotype used is in the low range of idiotype-binding capacity, and from the dictum of Rajewsky and his colleagues, it should stimulate its target B cells (13; K. Rajewsky, personal communication; 14).

The probe we utilized as a focus in these studies was the "koinotype" (15) of HEL-HUL (human lysozyme) cross-reactive clones. (*Koinotype,* a term chosen by Greek immunologist friends, refers to the entire set of clones with cross-reactive specificity.) HUL is a very distantly related lysozyme, with 52 of 129 amino acid residues changed.

The treatment of A/J mice with anti-IdXL has several consequences. First, it induces a "prememory" heightened state of reactivity. The subsequent response to HEL-CFA, provoked 3 days after the initial treatment, is extremely rapid in onset and may remain elevated compared to that of the untreated control for a prolonged time. Second, the antilysozyme that is produced is *all* IdXL-bearing, in comparison with the usual primary response to HEL, which has only a minor IdXL involvement. Third, the specificity of the response with respect to HEL-HUL reactive antibodies is typical. Thus, only about 1% of the HEL-induced antibody is cross-reactive with HUL.

Finally, and quite surprisingly, the affinity of the initial anti-HEL has the high secondary response characteristics. It is not at all clear why the IdXL⁺ B cells would have higher affinity for the Ag, but it introduces an unexpected factor into considerations of affinity maturation. In most systems examined, molecules with a predominant idiotype have been shown to be of average, nonremarkable affinity for Ag. This may not be true in all cases.

Even more striking sequelae are worth noting following anti-IdXL pretreatment with regard to specificity if HUL-CFA is the immuno-

TABLE I

Initial Production of Antibodies Highly Heteroclitic for
HEL in Anti-IdXL Pretreated, HUL-CFA Immunized
A/J Mice

Days after HUL-CFA immunization[a]	Average heteroclicity index[b]
7	0.06
11	0.48
15	0.61
19	0.83
23	1.50

[a] The average index for five mice is shown.
[b] Heteroclicity index of serum from anti-IdXL pretreated mice after HUL-CFA immunization. The index represents the binding of HUL divided by the binding of HEL.

gen. In this case, the initial composition of the antibody response is quite unusual. Thus, the early anti-HUL is strongly heteroclitic for HEL, as indicated by the heteroclicity indexes shown in Table I. Furthermore, in the typical response to HUL, HUL-HEL cross-reactive and IdXL$^+$ antibodies appear only at about the 5% level; however, after anti-IdXL pretreatment, the response during the first 11 days is shifted in the direction of overwhelming HEL-HUL cross-reactivity and IdXL positivity. Subsequently, an increasing amount of HUL-specific antibody is made, and the HUL-HEL cross-reactive antibody becomes a minority population by day 23. Nevertheless, the total amount of IdXL$^+$ anti-HUL remains close to 100–200 μg/ml between 11 and 23 days after antigenic challenge, a level 100 times greater than the one that appears in the absence of an initial antiidiotypic stimulus. The data are presented in greater detail in a forthcoming publication (16).

Two points should be stressed: (a) Following the two antiidiotypic injections, if no Ag was given, no IdXL$^+$ Ag-specific or Ag-nonspecific antibodies were ever detected. The antibody response is strictly dependent on antigen administration. (b) The effect of antiidiotype administration was transitory. Within 12 days, the prememory state had largely dissipated, and by 1 month the animals had apparently reverted to the unprimed level. This type of experiment will be repeated in the future in greater detail and with monoclonal antiidiotope antibodies.

It may be of interest to explore the diversity of types of silent clones represented in these experiments. Let us consider especially the HEL-HUL koinotype. First, it would have been expected that the members of this koinotype might have been equally well activated by HEL and HUL. It can be remembered, however, that immunization with HEL leads to only 1% representation of the HEL-HUL koinotype. HUL activates more of this koinotype to a level of 5% of the anti-HUL response. Previous work has shown that immunizing with keyhole limpet hemocyanin coupled to HUL increases the clonal diversity of the koinotypic antibodies detected by isoelectric focusing analysis (14). Second, while anti-IdXL pretreatment increases the HEL-HUL koinotype dramatically following HUL immunization to nearly 100%, ordinarily much of this population is silent. Third, the heteroclitic clones must represent another population which remains quiescent.

Although complicated T-cell-linked factors leading to clonal dominance may steer the response in one direction or another (15, 17, 18), it is also true that if dominance were stochastic, the HUL-HEL koinotype would occasionally be dominant in at least some individuals. This is never the case. Clearly, anti-IdXL treatment can strongly influence the specificity as well as the idiotypy of the antibody response. Priming with anti-IdXL not only provokes the IdXL$^+$ cells selectively but concomitantly also selects out members of the HEL-HUL koinotype because of the accidental association of IdXL with one or more of the specificities within this koinotype.

IV. Effect of Anti-IdXL on Ts in Nonresponder H-2^b Mice

The only other predictable target for anti-IdXL is the idiotype-bearing, Ag-specific Ts cell (see Fig. 1), which is most easily studied in nonresponder H-2^b strains. In these experiments, the induction of AgTs by the first HEL-CFA injection was assessed by challenge with HEL coupled to erythrocytes (HEL-RBC) 4 weeks later.

If low doses of anti-IdXL served to *activate* Ts, it would have been difficult to detect *in situ* upon subsequent challenge, because HEL-CFA itself induces suppression. Apparently, the AgTs were inactivated even at the dose level of antiidiotype (200 µg idiotype-binding capacity) used in each injection, so that subsequent injection of HEL-CFA primed for a vigorous PFC response to HEL-RBC challenge 4 weeks later. Table II shows the two experiments of this type; the level

TABLE II

Anti-IdXL Manipulation that Allows an Anti-HEL Response
in Nonresponder Mice

Serum Treatment[a]	Ag Priming	Ag Challenge[b]	Experiments	
			1	2
None	CFA	HEL-BRC	977[c]	1253
None	HEL-CFA	HEL-BRC	120	54
NRIg	HEL-CFA	HEL-BRC	195	122
αIdX-HEL	HEL-CFA	HEL-BRC	1047	824

[a] According to the protocol in Fig. 2.
[b] In this Ag challenge, 10^8 HEL-BRC were injected iv 4 weeks after priming into B10 mice.
[c] HEL-specific plaque-forming cells per 10^6 nucleated spleen cells.

of response obtained is equivalent to that in a congenic responder, B10.A. Unfortunately, the idiotypy of the response in these anti-IdXL-treated mice has not yet been studied. Given the principle that lower doses of antiidiotype promote and high doses inhibit cellular responsiveness (13), it would be expected that in addition to affecting the Ts precursor, the IdXL-bearing B cells might also be activated, making the response quite IdXL positive. The proportion of the response that is $IdXL^+$ should be a faithful index of the effect on the B-cell population.

The evidence is consistent with the hypothesis that there is a single avenue leading to suppression in the response to HEL: An N-terminal epitope on HEL is the single suppressor cell-inducing entity on the molecule. After HEL administration, the IdXL-bearing Ts is induced and is then responsible for down-regulating the anti-HEL response. Disturbance of this process, either by "amputating" the suppressor-inducing determinant from HEL (19) or by anti-IdXL treatment of the mouse which targets the Ts, abrogates the suppression.

It remains to be established whether Ts truly can be activated at some very low level of anti-IdXL. If so, there would be two very important corollaries to be examined with essential implications for antiidiotype therapy.

1. If a desirable T-cell suppression is difficult to induce or detect (as in an HEL-responsive strain whose Ts bear IdXL), treatment with low doses of antiidiotype could be employed to initiate the

suppression. The suppression might even dominate the expected simultaneous induction of the B-cell idiotypic response.
2. The existence of independent Ts and Th idiotypic universes, the conjunction with dosage differences in cell activation, should permit *in vivo* manipulation in any desired direction.

V. Conclusions: The Relative Roles of Antiidiotype Antibodies and Idiotype-Recognizing T Cells

The transitory effect of low doses of anti-IdXL administered in these experiments may conceivably mimic the physiological role of antiidiotypic antibody molecules in regulating the anti-HEL response. In previous articles, we have focused on the IdXL-promoting role of IdXL-recognizing T-helper cells (IdXTh), which seem to be responsible for the positive selection of IdXL-bearing B cells in the secondary anti-HEL response (1, 12). The major selective force eventuating in the particular relationship among IdXL-bearing and IdXL-recognizing lymphocytes was postulated to be the need for regulatory simplicity (1). A multiplicity of idiotypes would lead to a less easily coordinated system of regulation.

Low levels of antiidiotypic antibodies directed against the predominant idiotype could reinforce and abet the dominance first instituted by IdXTh. High levels of anti-IdX, in accord with the work of Rajewsky and his colleagues, would finally down-regulate the B-cell response, and also prevent antibody secretion by developed plasma cells (20). Of course, IdX-specific suppressor cells would share this regulatory function.

Granted that the modulation by antiidiotypic antibodies that we have described is short lived, the resultant cell population produces a vigorous response that is high in affinity and IdXL positive. As an activator of "immune memory," anti-IdXL is efficient and very rapid: A 3-day period is sufficient to produce a nearly maximal effect. It may very well be, however, that establishment of a permanent state of B-cell memory is a role reserved to the IdXTh, whose interaction may serve as an irreversible signal for a vital genetic switching event.

We can assume that the first interaction of antiidiotype or Ag with the receptors on the virgin B cell will have similar and immediate effects. However, after this, when the Ag in the receptor is internalized and processed within the B cell (21), display of the Ag in conjunction with Ia molecules will differentiate the sequelae. In the case of the antigenic stimulus, the AgTh will be able to continue to stimulate the activated B cell further. However, after antiidiotypic antibody induction, propagation of the response would probably require IdX-recognizing T helper cells.

An interesting question is whether anti-IdX antibody molecules should be regarded as having a singular function. Together with the IdXL-specific T helper and T suppressor cells, this assemblage could comprise a potent regulatory force for the modulation of IdXL-bearing cells. The immune system probably utilizes a variety of not quite parallel systems to accomplish similar but distinguishable ends. This is a clever sort of redundancy; in fact, it can be expected that the function of a specified task. For example, a particular cell, factor, or antibody may have the identical target cell but function at a different optimal time.

The basis for positive selection of the $IdXL^+$ B cells would still appear to reside in the existence of the IdXTh. How this cell type is triggered remains a question, although presumably IdXL on the B-cell surface together with a restriction element might be a suitable signal. Surely anti-IdXL antibody formation must be a later event, whose production probably requires an Ig-recognizing Th to collaborate with an anti-IdXL-synthesizing B cell. Anti-IdX formation should occur only when enough immunogenic IdXL arises: From the results cited, the first anti-IdXL might then be expected to act to induce *more* IdXL. This positive feedback loop could be part of an integrated system favoring the existence of predominant idiotypes such as IdXL.

Suppressive signals could most probably be derived from IdXL-recognizing Ts, conceivably arising directly via B-cell stimulation. High levels of anti-IdXL may represent a last bastion of defense against overactive idiotype production. Preliminary experiments on the augmentation of antilysozyme PFC with low levels of lysozyme (S. Eaton, M. Benveniste, H. Hosseinzadeh, and D. Duong, unpublished) indicate that during a typical secondary response, some anti-HEL PFC are intrinsically inhibited from secretion, presumably by anti-IdXL [20]. Thus, not much time is required to produce the inhibitory anti-IdXL. Alternatively, it is conceivable that the augmentation could be caused by displacement of suppressor T-cell products rather than anti-IdXL in the HEL-induced augmentation of PFC.

Another viewpoint is one that gives greater primacy to the preexistent network of intercellular interactions established from birth. With all cell types in predominant idiotypic circuits already activated and/or suppressed into metastable balance, new ligands supplied during immunization would assume the role of perturbation agents rather than agents inducing new cell types. Although the many differences between the primary and secondary responses to lysozymes tend to suggest less of a well-established marriage than a new affair, it may be hoped that a way will be found to settle this issue conclusively.

VI. Summary

The regulatory system controlling the response to lysozyme in the mouse is asymmetric in that certain regulatory cells belong to the predominant idiotypic universe and others to alternative universe(s). This situation allows the modulation of B-cell and Ts-cell responses by the provision of antiidiotype antibodies directed against the predominant idiotype without affecting the T helper cells. This modulation affects the affinity, specificity, and kinetics of the subsequent response to lysozyme in a dramatic manner. The relative role of antiidiotypic antibodies and idiotype-recognizing T cells was considered.

References

1. Sercarz, E. E., Araneo, B., Benjamin, C., Harvey, M., Metzger, D., Miller, A., Wicker, L., and Yowell, R. (1983). In "Immune Networks," Ann. N.Y. Acad. Sci. (in press).
2. Araneo, B., Metzger, D., Yowell, R., and Sercarz, E. (1981). Proc. Natl. Acad. Sci. U.S.A. 78, 499–503.
3. Harvey, M., Adorini, L., Miller, A., and Sercarz, E. (1979). Nature (London) 281, 594–596.
4. Gershon, R. K., Eardley, D. D., Durum, S., Green, D. R., Shen, F. W., Yamauchi, K., Cantor, H., and Murphy, D. B. (1981). J. Exp. Med. 153, 1533–1546.
5. Tada, T., Ochi, A., Miyatani, S., Abe, R., Yagi, J., and Yamauchi, K. (1983). In "Ir Genes: Past, Present and Future" (C. Pierce, J. Kapp, B. Schwartz, S. Cullen, and D. Shreffler, eds.). Humana Press, Clifford, New Jersey (in press).
6. Eichmann, K. (1978). Adv. Immunol. 26,195–254.
7. Janeway, C. (1980). In "Strategies of Immune Regulation" (E. E. Sercarz and A. J. Cunningham, eds.), pp. 179–198. Academic Press, New York.
8. Janeway, C., Sercarz, E. E., Wigzell, H., and Fox, C. F., eds. (1981). "Immunoglobulin Idiotypes." Academic Press, New York.
9. Urbain, J., Wuilmart, C., and Cazenave, P.-A. (1981). Contemp. Top. Mol. Immunol. 8, 113–148.
10. Adorini, L., Harvey, M. A., and Sercarz, E. E. (1979). Eur. J. Immunol. 9, 906–909.
11. Howard, M., and Paul, W. E. (1983). Annu. Rev. Immunol. 1, 307–33.
12. Sercarz, E. E., and Metzger, D. (1980). Springer Semin. Immunolpathol. 3, 145–170.
13. Kelsoe, G., Reth, M. and Rajewsky, K. (1980). Immunol. Rev. 52, 75–78.
14. Rajewsky, K., and Takemori, T. (1983). Annu. Rev. Immunol. 1, 569–607.

15. Sercarz, E., Cecka, J. M., Kipp, D., and Miller, A. (1977). *Ann. Immunol. (Paris)* **128C**, 599–609.
16. Benjamin, C. D., and Sercarz, E. E. (1983). In preparation.
17. Herzenberg, L., Hayakawa, K., Hardy, R., Tokuhisa, T., Oi, V., and Herzenberg, L. A. (1982). *Immunol. Rev.* **67**, 5–32.
18. Rosenberg, Y. (1982). *Immunol. Rev.* **67**, 33–58.
19. Yowell, R., Araneo, B., Miller, A., and Sercarz, E. (1979). *Nature (London)* **279**, 70–71.
20. Goidl, E. A., Schrater, A. F., Siskind, G. W., and Thorbecke, G. J. (1979). *J. Exp. Med.* **150**, 154–165.
21. Chesnut, R., and Grey, H. (1981). *J. Immunol.* **126**, 1075–1079.

Chapter 8

Biochemical, Functional, and Genetic Aspects of T-Cell Idiotypes

Bent Rubin

Centre d'Immunologie INSERM-CNRS de Marseille-Luminy
Marseille, France

I. Introduction[1]

In this volume, the term *idiotypes* is mostly used to mean antigenic determinants on the variable portions of immunoglobulin (Ig) mole-

[1] *Abbreviations:* AEF, allogeneic effector factor; CCG, chicken gamma globulin; C_H, constant region of heavy chain; DTH, delayed-type hypersensitivity; GA, polymer of glutamic acid and alanine; GAT, copolymer of glutamic acid, alanine, and tyrosine; Id, idiotype; Ig, immunoglobulin (M = mouse; R = rabbit); LDH, lactate dehydrogenase; KLH, keyhole limpet hemocyanin; mAb, monoclonal antibody; MHC, major histocompatibility complex; MLC, mixed lymphocyte culture; MW, molecular weight; NP, (4-hydroxy-3-nitrophenyl)acetyl; pA, protein A; PC, phosphorylcholine; SRBC, sheep red blood cells; Tcr, T-cell receptors; TGAL, poly(L-tyrosine, L-glutamic acid)poly(DL-alanine)poly(L-lysine); TNP, trinitrophenyl; V_H, V_L, variable regions on heavy or light chains.

cules. Two types of idiotypic determinants (idiotopes) are distinguished functionally: (1) combing site-related idiotopes [also called *paratopes* (Jerne *et al.*, 1982)] and (2) framework-related idiotopes. Antibodies against paratopes inhibit the interaction between antigen (hapten) and the specific antibody molecule, whereas antibodies against framework idiotopes do not necessarily inhibit such interactions. Although exceptions exist, most paratopes and idiotopes studied are conformational determinants dependent on elements from both heavy and light chain variable regions (V_H, V_L) (Imanishi-Kari *et al.*, 1979; Laskin *et al.*, 1977; Mäkelä and Karjalainen, 1977; Schiff *et al.*, 1979).

The subject of this chapter is idiotypes on T lymphocytes. The obvious question is whether T lymphocytes really express idiotypes in the strict sense of the term, that is, Ig idiotypes; in other words, whether or not T lymphocytes use the same variable region genes (V_H and V_L) as do B lymphocytes to produce their antigen-specific receptors. So far, this question has been addressed only by studies using anti-Id antisera or monoclonal antibodies (mAb) to detect the idiotype-like structures on specific T cells. The answers obtained are that in many but not all idiotypes, anti-Id systems, Id-like structures are found on both specific T-cell membrane molecules and their released, immunologically active molecules, such as helper factors and suppressor factors.

However, it should be emphasized that all these studies do not prove that T cells produce and secrete receptor molecules with immunoglobulin idiotypes (Id-Ig); it can only be concluded that T-cell receptor molecules bear determinants that cross-react serologically with Ig-Id. Sufficient amounts of data have been published showing that anti-Id antibodies can react with cell membrane molecules other than putative T-cell receptors (Tcr) (Sege and Peterson, 1978; Schreiber *et al.*, 1980; Volanakis and Kearney, 1981) and that mAb against T-cell antigens other than Tcr can react with Ig-Id (Pillemer and Weissman, 1981). Therefore, the definite answer to the question of whether or not T lymphocytes produce Tcr with Ig-Id must await the isolation and characterization of the Tcr structural genes.

In this chapter, we attempt to summarize studies using anti-Id antisera or mAb (1) to isolate and characterize putative Tcr molecules, (2) to locate the genes responsible for the synthesis of T-cell idiotypes, and briefly (3) to evaluate the function of T-cell idiotypes (see also other chapters in this volume). Despite the reservations mentioned above, such studies have already indicated that Tcr idiotypes are produced by genes linked to Ig V_H and C_H genes and that the Tcr heavy chain may have a structural buildup in domains similar to Ig heavy chains (Rubin *et al.*, 1980a).

II. The Concept of Antigen–Antibody Interactions and the Use of Anti-Id Antibodies

When injected with antigen, the experimental animal synthesizes specific Ig molecules (Ab1) with the capacity to react with the different antigenic determinants on the antigen. However, the specific Ig molecules produced possess variable region determinants which can act as immunogenic determinants (= idiotopes). Such determinants can elicit anti-Id antibodies (Ab2), which in turn can react with the Ab1 molecules. The production of Ab2 antibodies and their regulation of Ab1 synthesis during an immune response has been described (McKearn *et al.*, 1974). The two types of idiotopes, paratopes and framework idiotopes, may both induce anti-Id antibodies, and such anti-Id antibodies (Ab2) have been called Ab2a (antiframework: idiotope antibodies) and Ab2b (antiparatope antibodies) (Jerne *et al.*, 1982). Normally, one imagines that the antibody molecule reacts with antigen, although this interaction is a thermodynamic equilibrium between the two ligands. However, when it comes to the interaction between Ab1 molecules and their corresponding Ab2a and Ab2b molecules, it becomes almost a matter of definition whether Ab1 molecules react with Ab2 or Ab2 react with Ab1. Ab2b molecules may, in principle, contain structures similar to the antigen, so Ab1 may be assumed to react with both antigen and Ab2b; Ab2a molecules react with framework idiotopes, and these may be present on Ab1 molecules which display reactivity against different antigeneic determinants. Thus, Ab2a antibodies may be defined as molecules reacting with Ab1 molecules.

The network hypothesis states that Ab2 antibodies again can serve as immunogens and thereby induce the synthesis of Ab3 antibodies (Jerne, 1974; Cazenave, 1977; Urbain *et al.*, 1977). Such Ab3 anti-Ab2b may act as Ab1 antibodies. Because most idiotypes (Ab1) are produced by hyperimmunization and affinity chromatography on antigen columns (which may absorb Ab1 and Ab3 and possibly Ab2a in conjunction with Ab1 or Ab3), xenogeneic anti-Id antisera for example, may contain antibodies reacting against both Ab1 paratopes and framework idiotopes, and Ab2a and Ab3 antibodies (Suzan *et al.*, 1981).

It appears evident that if anti-Id antisera are used for the purification of Ab1 molecules, such affinity-purified Ab1 antibody molecules are contaminated with all types of molecules bearing determinants, which cross-react specifically with Ab1, Ab2, and Ab3 paratopes and idiotopes [e.g., Thy-1 (Pillemer and Weissman, 1981), C-reactive protein (Volanakis and Kearney, 1981), and hormone receptors (Schreiber *et al.*, 1980)]. Furthermore, molecules that react with Ig molecules "nonspecifically," such as complement components, Fc receptors, etc., will be "copurified." Therefore, after initial affinity fractionation, Ab1-like molecules have to be further characterized by antigen binding and reactivity with antisera against constant regions of Id-bearing Ig molecules, that is, antiallotype and/or isotype antisera.

This is exactly the strategy employed by many investigators using anti-Id antisera to isolate Tcr molecules (Rubin *et al.*, 1980a). However, care should be manifested when putative Tcr molecules have biochemical characteristics of the "contaminating" molecules mentioned.

III. Model Systems for the Study of T-Cell Idiotypes

Both T and B lymphocytes can recognize antigenic determinants via antigen-specific, membrane-bound receptors (Brondz, 1968; Golstein *et al.*, 1971; Miller and Mitchell, 1969; Mitchison, 1971; Rubin and Wigzell, 1973a,b; Rubin, 1976). Such receptors on mouse B lymphocytes are believed to be conventional Ig, coded for by genes located on chromosomes 12 (heavy chain), 6 (κ chain), and 16 (λ chain) (Valbuena *et al.*, 1978; Hengartner *et al.*, 1978; D'Eustachio *et al.*, 1981). The basic question is whether nature has created two different recognition systems: one, Ig expressed by B cells and another, as yet unidentified, expressed by T cells. The key finding which began the elucidation of this question was the pioneering work by Ramseier and Lindenmann (Ramseier *et al.*, 1977), followed by the studies of McKearn (1974), Binz and Wigzell (1975a,b,c), and Eichmann and Rajewsky (1975): Anti-Id antisera against Ig-Id reacted with T cells displaying the same specificity as the corresponding Id-bearing Ig molecules; and anti-Tcr antibodies raised in (A × B)F$_1$ animals against parental (A) T cells reacted with Ig molecules of A anti-B reactivity. These studies were later confirmed by other investigators using different systems, for example, the arsanyl-hapten system (Bach *et al.*, 1979; Hirai and Nisonoff, 1980), the NP-hapten system (Krawinkel *et al.*, 1976; Cramer *et al.*, 1981; Okada *et al.*, 1981), the phosphorylcholine (PC) system (Cosenza *et al.*, 1977; Köhler, this volume), the GAT system (Germain *et al.*, 1979; Theze *et al.*, 1982; Kapp *et al.*, 1981), the Henn lysozyme system (Sercarz and Metzger, 1980), and the TGAL system (Mozes and Haimovitch, 1979). Generally, three different approaches were used: (1) anti-Id antibodies were used to enumerate, fractionate, and isolate specific T cells and their products (Binz and Wigzell, 1977a,b); (2) anti-Id antibodies were employed to sensitize or elicit specific T- and B-cell responses (Rajewsky and Eichmann, 1977); and (3) antigen-specific T-cell proteins were isolated by interaction with antigen coupled to Sepharose and anti-Id antibodies were employed to demonstrate the presence of Ig-Id cross-reactive determinants on such T-cell products (Bach *et al.*, 1979; Hirai and Nisonoff, 1980; Cramer *et al.*, 1981; Mozes and Haimovitch, 1979; Krupen *et al.*, 1982). Basically, these studies have demonstrated that T and B cells (or Ig molecules) may share cross-reactive idiotypic determinants. According to recent concepts of network interactions, it is expected that one would find T and B cells displaying similar cross-reactive idiotypes in some but not all cases (Jerne, 1974; Jerne *et al.*, 1982). Experimentally, it has been found that variable region markers of putative Tcr vary less during an ongoing immune response than the B cell-Ig counterpart (Krawinkel *et al.*, 1978). Such concepts and experimental findings may explain in particular the experiments showing an absence of Ig-Id in T cells.

We have employed xenogeneic anti-Id antibodies against B6 anti-CBA Ig molecules as probes for the study of idiotypes on mouse alloantigen (B6 anti-CBA)-specific T cells (Rubin *et al.*, 1979). Thus, our studies have combined the approaches used by the group of Eichmann and Rajewsky (1975) (the production of anti-Id antibodies in Ig-tolerant xenogeneic animals) and the group of Binz and Wigzell (1975a,b,c), that is, the use of alloantigen-reactive T cells, which are present in an unusually high frequency in normal mice and are relatively easily enriched by various *in vivo* and *in vitro* manipulations (Nisbeth *et al.*, 1969; Wilson *et al.*, 1968; Lindahl and Wilson, 1977; Binz and Wigzell, 1975b,c; Dennert, 1979; Rubin *et al.*, 1980a). Our anti-Id antibodies (antiserum 5936) were used to isolate and characterize T-lymphocyte proteins bearing 5936-Id and to produce xenogeneic antisera against such 5936-Id-bearing T-cell protein. We will summarize our own results and compare these with the results of other investigators.

IV. Idiotypes on Normal and *in Vivo/in Vitro* Immunized T Cells

The anti-Id antisera 5936 was raised in a mouse-Ig tolerant rabbit (5936) immunized with B6 anti-CBA IgG (Rubin and Hertel-Wulff, 1978). This antiserum was shown to be a "true" anti-Id antiserum (Rubin *et al.*, 1979, 1980a), and the 5936 Ig-Id were produced by genes linked to the Igh-1^b allotype (C_H) genes of the B6 mouse (Suzan *et al.*, 1981). The quantitative expression of 5936-Id in anti-H-2^k antisera was regulated by *Ir* genes in the H-2 complex (Nordfang and Rubin, 1981; Suzan *et al.*, 1981). This antiserum was used to demonstrate Ig cross-reactive idiotypes on T cells by three different methods: indirect immunofluorescence, antibody- and complement-mediated cytotoxicity, and antibody binding revealed by ^{125}I-labeled protein A (pA). Table I summarizes the results of our experiments: Normal B6 T-cell populations contain 3–5% 5936-Id$^+$ cells; B6 T cells

TABLE I

5936-Id on Normal and Immune B6 T Cells

T-cell source[a]	5936-Id$^+$ cells[b] (%)	5936 + ^{125}I-pA[c] (cpm fixed)
B6-Spl.T	3 (0–10)	1.897
CBA-Spl.T	0 (0–0.3)	539
B6 anti-B10.BR LN T	4 (0–9)	1.928
B6 anti-B10.BR Spl.T	5 (0–6)	1.417
B6 anti-B10.BR PE T	3 (0–7)	1.457
B6 anti-B10.BR T-cell lines	32 (25–42)	5.620
B6.14a anti-B10.BR T-cell lines	8 (3–13)	806
CBA anti-B6 T-cell lines	4 (1–9)	1.023
B6 anti-B10.G T-cell lines	5 (1–8)	1.571
B6 anti-B10.BR T-cell clone 62c-7	57 (48–63)	7.842

[a] T cells were obtained by passage through Ig anti-Ig columns of: Spl, spleen cells; LN, lymph node cells; PE, peritoneal exudate cells. T-cell lines were produced as described elsewhere (Rubin *et al.*, 1980b). Clones were obtained from these lines by limited dilution in secondary MLC culture supernatants (Samuel *et al.*, 1982). B6.14a mice are CBA-allotype congenic B6 mice (Bourgois *et al.*, 1981).

[b] Percentage of cells labeled with fluorescein isothiocyanate (FITC)-labeled F(ab)$_2$ sheep anti-RIg (rabbit Ig) after preincubation of the cells with antiserum 5936. Preimmune 5936 serum of 5936 antiserum adsorbed on B6 anti-AKR IgG-Sepharose columns served as a control. In the different experiments, the control mixtures contained 1–6% of labeled cells.

[c] Cells were incubated with antiserum 5936, washed, and further incubated with ^{125}I-labeled pA. The amount of ^{125}I bound to the cells was determined by γ counting.

from mice hyperimmunized by H-2^k spleen cells contain the same proportion of 5936-Id$^+$ cells, that is, 3–5% (thus, the expression of 5936-Id on T cells is strictly regulated *in vivo*); B6 anti-B10.BR T-cell lines contain about 30% 5936-Id$^+$ cells; and T-cell clones derived by limited dilutions from such T-cell lines contain about 50% 5936-Id$^+$ cells. So far, five cloning experiments have been performed, and a mean of 42% of isolated clones contained about 50% 5936-Id$^+$ cells. The other clones contained either no 5936-Id$^+$ cells or variable amounts of 5936-Id$^+$ cells (0–25%). One clone (Table I, 62c) was re-cloned, and among positive clones (80%), again only about 50% 5936-Id$^+$ cells were found. Thus, it appears that even a homogeneous clonal T-cell population does not contain 100% 5936-Id$^+$ cells, but, perhaps dependent on the cell cycle, expresses more or less of 5936-Id$^+$ mem-

TABLE II

Strain Distribution of MLC Blasts Bearing the 5936-Id

MLC combination[a]	Responder cell phenotype		Detection of the 5936-Id[b]		
	H-2	Ig-1	IIF	AbC	pA
B6 anti-CBA	b	b	38 (18–60)	29 (15–36)	++++
B10 anti-B10.BR	b	b	41 (25–58)	28 (13–33)	++++
B6.5a anti-CBA	b	j	25 (18–30)	ND	ND
B6.9a anti-CBA	b	j	ND	2 (0–2)	ND
C3H.SW anti-CBA	b	j	3 (0–8)	2 (0–5)	−
BALB/B anti-CBA	b	a	6 (1–10)	5 (0–8)	−
A.BY anti-CBA	b	e	20 (18–26)	13 (3–18)	++++
B10.D2 anti-CBA	d	b	11 (9–19)	16 (5–22)	++
BALB/c anti-CBA	d	a	3 (0–7)	3 (0–8)	−
C3H.OH anti-CBA	o2	j	1 (0–5)	2 (0–6)	−
B6 anti-DBA/1	b	b	6 (0–11)	5 (0–9)	−

[a] MLC were initiated by culturing 20 × 10^6 Ig anti-Ig column-passed T cells (>95% Thy-1.2^+, <0.5% Ig$^+$ or Fcr$^+$) with 20 × 10^6 2000 R-irradiated stimulator spleen cells in 20 ml 5% FCS (fetal calf serum) in RPMI-1640 (Rubin *et al.*, 1980a). MLC blasts were harvested on days 3–5, purified by centrifugation on ficoll-isopaque (FIP, density = 1.077), and then analyzed. For B6.5a and B6.9a mice, see Table V.

[b] IIF, indirect immunofluorescence; AbC, antiserum and complement-mediated cytotoxicity. Values in parentheses are the range of results; pA, binding of antiserum to the MLC blasts, was detected using ^{125}I-labeled protein A. Arbitrary values of the amount of ^{125}I-labeled pA bound to 10^6 T blasts incubated with 5936 antiserum: ++++, >10-fold; ++, >5-fold binding over background; −, no significant binding; ND, not done.

brane protein. If only half of the T cells that potentially can express a given idiotype do express such idiotypes at a given moment, this means that the real frequency of 5936-Id$^+$ T cells may be as high as 5–10%. This figure is in agreement with the frequency of T cells reactive against a given H-2 haplotype (Nisbeth *et al.*, 1969; Wilson *et al.*, 1968; Lindahl and Wilson, 1977; Binz and Wigzell, 1975b).

Table II contains data on the strain distribution of 5936-Id$^+$ T cells among different mixed lymphocyte culture (MLC) blasts. It can be seen that the expression of 5936-Id$^+$ on T cells is associated with the Igh-1^b (and Igh-1^e) allotypes of the T-cell donor mice and with a reactivity against the H-2^k haplotype (Table I). The specificity of induction of 5936-Id$^+$ T cells was further analyzed by using stimulator cells from recombinant mice. The data in Table III indicate that genes in the *I*-

TABLE III

Mapping of the Genes Responsible for Expression of the H-2^k
Alloantigens, Which Stimulate the Induction of 5936-Id
on B6 T Cells

Exp. number	MLC combination[a]	Stimulator genotype				Id$^+$ T cells (%)[b]	
		K	IA	IE	D	IIF	Ab + RC
1	B6 anti-CBA	k	k	k	k	43	ND
	B6 anti-B10.A	k	k	k	d	21	ND
	B6 anti-C3H.OH	d	d	d	k	8	ND
	B6 anti-DBA/1	q	q	q	q	9	ND
	CBA anti-B6	b	b	b	b	1	ND
2	B6 anti-B10.BR	k	k	k	k	37	31
	B6 anti-B10.A(4R)	k	k	b	b	32	27
	B6 anti-B10.MBR	b	k	k	q	34	25
	B6 anti-B10.A(5R)	b	b	k	d	5	<5
	B6 anti-B10.AQR	q	k	k	d	29	28
	B6 anti-C3H.OH	d	d	d	k	6	<5
	B6 anti-B10.G	q	q	q	q	3	<5
	B6 anti-B10.D2	d	d	d	d	11	8

[a] B6 spleen cells were passed through Ig anti-Ig columns and stimulated with 25 × 10^6 (2000 R) stimulator cells of the indicated genotypes. Exp. 1: MLC blast cells were harvested on day 5 (Rubin *et al.*, 1979). Exp. 2: Primary MLC were left for 14 days, and then 2.5 × 10^6 responder T cells were stimulated with 25 × 10^6 stimulator cells. MLC blasts were harvested after day 4 (Rubin *et al.*, 1980b).

[b] IIF, indirect immunofluorescence; Ab + RC, antibody and complement-mediated cytotoxicity (see Table II); ND = not done.

A^k region are responsible for the membrane antigen(s), which induce the synthesis of 5936-Id on B6 T cells.

V. Interaction of Anti-Id Antibodies and T Cells

The most direct evidence for Ig cross-reactive idiotypes on T cells using anti-Id antisera comes from absorption studies. Binz and Wigzell (1975a) have produced anti-Id antisera in $(A \times B)F_1$ hybrid rats against normal parental type A T cells or against A anti-B Ig molecules. A anti-B T cells absorb all activity in these two types of antisera against A anti-B T cells, while leaving some activity in anti-(A anti-B) antisera against A anti-B Ig molecules. However, A anti-B Ig molecules absorb all activity against A anti-B T cells from both types of antisera. Such results indicate that A anti-B T cells and A anti-B Ig share Id determinants. In addition, anti-(Ig A anti-B) antisera contain antibodies which react against idiotypes found on the A anti-B Ig molecules but which are absent on the A anti-B T cells. With their reagents, they found 2–10% Ig-Id$^+$ T cells among normal T cells (Binz and Wigzell, 1975a,b,c). The data summarized in Table IV show that B6 anti-CBA Ig preparations can absorb all activity from antiserum 5936 against B6 anti-CBA T cells, whereas absorption with B6 anti-CBA T cells leaves activity against B6 anti-CBA Ig molecules (Rubin et al., 1980a). Furthermore, we can show that antibodies in antiserum 5936 absorbed, and subsequently eluted from B6 anti-AKR IgG-Sepharose columns, precipitate [^{35}S]cysteine-labeled B6 anti-CBA T-cell protein that has a molecular weight (MW) of about 75,000 (Fig. 1). This experiment demonstrated that the antibodies in antiserum 5936 that react with internally labeled B6 anti-CBA T-cell protein react with B6 anti-AKR IgG molecules of MW 150,000 (Suzan et al., 1982) and having mouse IgG$_1$ characteristics as judged by fractionation on DEAE-Sephacel, protein A-Sepharose, and serological reaction with rabbit anti-IgG$_1$ antiserum (Nordfang and Rubin, 1981; Suzan et al., 1982). IgG$_1$ antibodies from B6 anti-B10.G or B6.9a anti-CBA antisera do not absorb the antibodies in antiserum 5936 which react with B6 anti-CBA T cells (Fig. 1).

Krammer and Eichmann (1977) produced antireceptor/Id antisera in $(B6 \times AKR)F_1$ mice against AKR anti-B6 MLC blasts. Such antisera stained about 35% of AKR anti-B6 T cells and only 5% of SJL anti-B6 or AKR anti-SJL T cells. The binding of soluble B6 alloantigen to AKR anti-B6 T cells (after trypsin treatment and overnight incubation) was

TABLE IV

Absorption of Antiserum 5936 with B6 Anti-CBA IgG or T Cells

		Activity of 5936 Antiserum On		
		B6 anti-CBA T cells[b]		B6 anti-CBA IgG[c]
		Id+ cells (%)	C (%)	Titer in RIA
Antiserum[a]	Absorption[a]			
5936	—	28	100	1 : 3200
5936-NA	B6 anti-CBA T cells	<1	<4	1 : 3450
5936-E	B6 anti-CBA T cells	19	68	1 : 1080
5936-NA	B6 anti-CBA IgG	<1	<4	<1 : 10
5936-E	B6 anti-CBA IgG	21	75	1 : 9600

[a] One milliliter of 5936 antiserum (1 : 5 dilution) was absorbed on either B6 anti-CBA T cells or B6 anti-CBA IgG-Sepharose. Nonabsorbed (NA) protein and absorbed and subsequently eluted material (E) were concentrated to 1 ml before assay. Elution from cells, isotonic glycine buffer pH 3; from Sepharose, 3 M NH_4SCN (Nordfang and Rubin, 1981).

[b] Measured by indirect immunofluorescence.

[c] Control, NA, or E preparations of 5936 antiserum were titrated in the radioimmunoassay (RIA) against ^{125}I-labeled B6 anti-CBA F(ab)$_2$ fragments. Titer = the dilution of 5936 which gives 50% of the maximal binding (Nordfang and Rubin, 1981).

inhibited by the F_1 anti-(AKR anti-B6) antisera; the inhibitory activity of these antisera could be partially absorbed by AKR anti-B6 antisera (Krammer, 1978; Krammer and Eichmann, 1977).

Thus, Ig-Id have been found to be present as markers of T-cell membrane proteins involved in the specific reactivity of T cells, that is, possible markers of variable regions of specific T-cell receptors. Although they are outside the scope of this chapter, two other types of Ig-variable region determinants have been tested as markers of Tcr molecules: (1) a1 allotypes in rabbits and (2) V_H determinants detected by a rabbit antimouse V_H antiserum. Some investigators found rabbit a1 allotypes on specific rabbit T cells (Krawinkel et al., 1977b; Cazenave et al., 1977), whereas others failed to demonstrate such determinants on rabbit T cells (Jensenius et al., 1977; Wilder et al., 1979); and (2) anti-V_H antisera have been used to detect V_H determinants on antigen-specific Tcr (Puri et al., 1980; Eichmann et al., 1980;

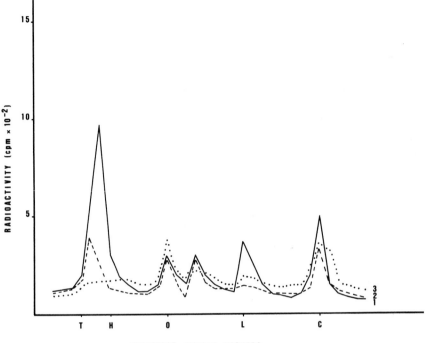

Fig. 1. Internal labeling of 5936-Id⁺ T-cell protein from T-cell line 62 (B6 anti-B10.A(4R)/B10.MBR). Three days after restimulation, the T cells were labeled for 6 h with [^{35}S]cysteine in 10% FCS/EHAA medium without essential amino acids (Suzan *et al.*, 1982). Labeled cells were lysed in 0.2% NP-40/0.01 M Tris, pH 8.0. The lysates were precleared four times with preformed rabbit Ig (RIg)-sheep anti-RIg complexes and then immunoprecipitated with preformed complexes of sheep anti-RIg and antiserum 5936 absorbed and eluted from (1) B6 anti-B10.A IgG-Sepharose, (2) B6 anti-B10.G IgG-Sepharose, or (3) B6.9a anti-B10.BR IgG-Sepharose. The precipitates [of similar size because of addition of normal RIg to (2) and (3)] were dissolved and subjected to SDS-PAGE under reducing conditions in a 10% gel. Molecular weight markers: T, transferrin (80,000); H, human serum albumin (67,000); O, ovalbumin (43,000); L, light chains (23,000); C, cytochrome C (12,500).

Ben-Neriah *et al.*, 1980), although others failed to repeat these results using their own reagents (Jensenius *et al.*, 1981).

VI. Induction of Specific T Cells by Anti-Id Antibodies

More indirect evidence for Ig-Id on T cells comes from studies using anti-Id antisera to sensitize or elicit specific T-cell immune responses. Eichmann and Rajewsky (1975) showed that guinea pig anti-(A5A) antibodies of class IgG_1 selectively induced group A streptococcal carbohydrate-specific T helper cells, whereas the same type of anti-Id antibodies of the IgG_2 class induced specific T suppressor cells in normal mice (Eichmann, 1975). Subsequently, the experiments have been repeated by several other groups (Frieschknecht *et al.*, 1978; Bluestone *et al.*, 1981; Miller *et al.*, 1981; see Rubin and Pierres, 1981), and the results were repeated using mAb anti-Id : DTH reactions in the Ars (Thomas *et al.*, 1981) or PC system (Arnold *et al.*, 1982), and help or suppression of *in vitro* antibody responses (Cerny *et al.*, 1982). J. Theze (personal communication, 1982) could induce GAT-specific T-cell lines *in vitro* by immunizing mice with either GAT or mAb anti-(anti-GAT) and challenging T cells from such mice with either GAT or mAb anti-Id, and vice versa. Thus, it appears certain that injection of anti-Id antibodies *in vivo* can induce and elicit specific T-cell responses. The mechanisms of these interactions are not understood, although one favorite hypothesis is that the anti-Id antibodies interact directly with and trigger T cells *in vivo*. However, antigen and anti-Id antibodies seem to trigger T cells in a different way, as the antigen-induced but not the anti-Id antibody-induced DTH response is H-2 restricted (Arnold *et al.*, 1982).

VII. Detection of Idiotypes on T-Cell Products
Isolated by Antigen-Specific Immunoadsorbents

The third approach was to use antigen-specific columns to isolate antigen-specific T-cell proteins and determine whether these T-cell molecules expressed Ig-Id cross-reactive determinants. Krawinkel *et al.* used NP-coupled nylon dishes to isolate anti-NP binding T-cell material. Such T-cell material could be shown to express the NP-heteroclitic marker (Krawinkel *et al.*, 1977a), an Ig-V_H region marker (Imanishi and Mäkelä, 1974), V_H markers (Cramer *et al.*, 1979), and Ig anti-NP idiotopes detected by mAb (Cramer *et al.*, 1981). Nisonoff *et al.* showed that Arsanyl-specific T-cell suppressor molecules could be isolated on Arsanyl-Sepharose columns, and such material expressed the cross-reactive anti-Ars idiotype(s) (Bach *et al.*, 1979; Hirai and Nisonoff, 1980). Kapp *et al.* demonstrated that anti-GAT suppressor molecules from T-cell populations and hybrids carried the cross-reactive anti-GAT idiotypes (Germain *et al.*, 1979; Kapp *et al.*, 1981). Thus, this approach also demonstrates Ig cross-reactive Ig-Id on antigen-binding T-cell molecules.

VIII. Studies on the Genes Responsible for the Synthesis of T-Cell Idiotypes

As mentioned above, the three approaches used for studying T-cell idiotypes have shown the same picture: T-cell idiotypes are associated with Ig allotypes. Binz et $al.$ (1976) showed that their T-cell idiotype genes segregated in backcross and F_2 analysis with the IgC_H genes, and Hämmerling et $al.$ (1976) showed that their anti-Id antibodies could induce Ig-Id T cells only in mice carrying the same IgC_H genes as the "parental" Id-bearing antibodies (i.e., A.J and BALB/c mice, respectively). Nisonoff et $al.$ showed that suppression induced by their Id-bearing suppressor molecules occurred only in mice carrying the same IgC_H genes as the mice that had produced the suppressor molecules (Dietz et $al.$, 1981). Thus, these studies demonstrated that the possible structural genes for T-cell idiotypes were linked to IgC_H genes. However, Krammer and Eichmann (1977), using their anti-Id antisera and backcross analysis, showed that both IgC_H genes and H-2 genes were necessary for the expression of their idiotypes on T cells. From these studies, it was not clear whether both types of genes acted as structural genes for T-cell idiotypes.

We studied the expression of the 5936-Id on T cells and B-cell products in three types of backcross animals: (1) (B6 × C3H.SW)F1 × C3H.SW, B6 (H-2^b, Igh-1^b) mice being high responders and C3H.SW (H-2^b, Igh-1^j) mice being nonresponders or low responders; (2) (B10. × B10.D2)F1 × B10.D2 mice, B10.D2 (H-2^d, Igh-1^b) being low or intermediary responders; and (3) (B6 × C3H.OH)F1 × C3H.OH mice, C3H.OH mice (H-2^{o2}, Igh-1^j) being nonresponders or low responders. The results of these experiments demonstrated that 5936-Ig idiotype genes were linked to Igh-1^b allotype genes and that genes within the H-2^b-gene complex regulated the quantitative expression of these idiotypes (Suzan et $al.$, 1981). 5936-Id on T cells from such backcross mice stimulated in $vitro$ MLC with B10.BR stimulator cells were present in high amounts on (1) H-2^b, Igh-1^b/Igh-1^j T cells, (2) H-2^b/H-2^d, Igh-1^b T cells, and (3) H-2^b/H-2^{o2}, Igh-1^b/Igh-1^j T cells (Figs. 2–4). Thus, our experimental results are in accordance with those of Krammer and Eichmann: T-cell idiotypes are closely linked to Igh-1 allotype genes, but their quantitative expression is linked to genes in the H-2 complex. However, the enormous spreading of results obtained with H-2^{o2}, Igh-1^b/Igh-1^j mice (Fig. 4, group III) indicates that a closer study of chromosome 12 markers of such individual mice is necessary in order to fully understand the regulation of T-cell idiotypes. Furthermore, these data call for attention when pooling cells from such backcross mice (Krammer and Eichmann, 1977).

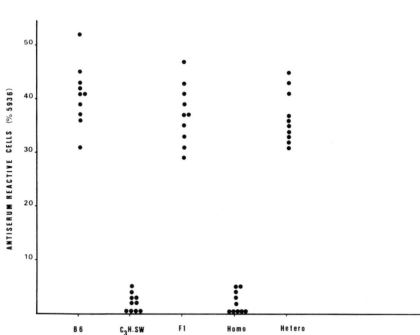

Fig. 2. Segregation of 5936-Id with Igh-1^b allotypes in H-2^b mice. Spleen and lymph node cells from individual B6, C$_3$H.SW, (B6 × C$_3$H.SW)F$_1$, and homozygous (homo) or heterozygous (hetero) Igh-1 backcross mice ((B6 × C$_3$H.SW) × C$_3$H.SW) were passed through Ig anti-Ig columns and stimulated *in vitro* with B10.BR spleen cells. After 5 days, anti-B10.BR responding T cells were treated with anti-Lyt2 antibody and complement, purified on FIP gradients (d = 1.090), and tested for expression of antiserum 5936 reactive cells by either indirect immunofluorescence or complement-mediated cytotoxicity (Suzan *et al.*, 1982, 1983). Results from two experiments were pooled in this graph.

We have produced antisera against isolated 5936-Id bearing T-cell molecules (Rubin and Bourgois, 1981). These antisera appear to detect allotypic determinants on membrane-associated T-cell molecules (Rubin *et al.*, 1980a; Rubin and Bourgois, 1981); they were also used in the backcross experiments mentioned above. These results were more clear-cut; T cells from Igh-1^b or Igh-1^b/Igh-1^j mice expressed the antiserum 6036-defined allotypes regardless of their H-2 types (Suzan *et al.*, 1982). Thus, both T-cell idiotypes (variable region?) and allotype (constant region?) genes were linked to Igh-1^b allotype genes; however, the expression of T-cell idiotypes but not T-cell allotypes was regulated by genes linked to the H-2 complex. Such data indicate that two different genes produce Tcr variable and constant regions.

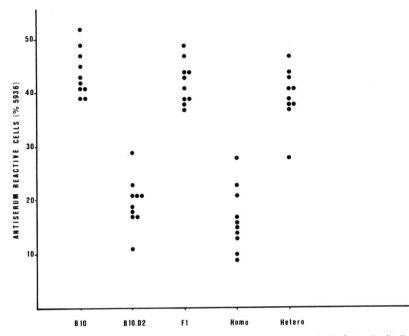

Fig. 3. Segregation of high reactivity against antiserum 5936 with H-2^b in Igh-1^b allotype mice. Spleen and lymph node cells from individual B10, B10.D2, (B10 × B10.D2)F$_1$, and H-2 homozygous (homo) or heterozygous (hetero) backcross [(B10 × B10.D2) × B10.D2] mice were treated as in Fig. 2. Each dot in the figure represents one mouse.

In addition to backcross analysis, we performed studies on the expression of T-cell idiotypes (and allotypes) on T cells from CBA-allotype congenic mice. The genotypes of the employed mice are given in Table V. An analysis of these results indicates that the 5936 T-cell idiotype genes are situated either within the V_H gene complex or centromeric to it (closely linked to the NP heteroclitic V_H marker). The 6036-allotype genes are situated either between the V_H and C_H genes or between the C_H genes and the crossing-over point of the B6.14a mice (i.e., between C_H and prealbumin genes) (Suzan *et al.*, 1982). Thus, it appears that T-cell idiotype genes and allotype genes are linked to *Igh-1* allotype genes and that such genes are the structural genes, at least for the Tcr heavy chain. However, the fact that genes linked to the H-2 complex can regulate the quantitative expression of T-cell idiotypes may indicate that such idiotypes are dependent on another polypeptide (the Tcr "light" chain), which is coded

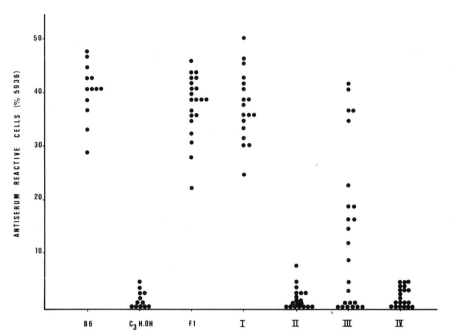

Fig. 4. Expression of 5936-Id on anti-B10.BR T cells is linked to Igh-1[b] allotypes. Spleen and lymph node cells from individual B6, C_3H.OH, (B6 × C_3H.OH)F_1, and (B6 × C_3H.OH)F_1 × C_3H.OH backcross mice (typed for serum Ig allotypes) were treated as in Fig. 2. The content of antiserum 5936 reactive cells and of anti-H-2[b]/anti-H-2[o2] reactive cells was analyzed by antiserum and complement-mediated cytotoxicity. The backcross animals were divided into four groups: I, H-2[b]/H-2[o2]; Igh-1[b]; II, H-2[b]/H-2[o2], Igh-1[j/j]; III, H-2[o2]/H-2[o2], Igh-1[b]/Igh-1[j]; IV, H-2[o2]/H-2[o2], Igh-1[j/j]. Results from two experiments are pooled. Each dot represent the results obtained with cells from one mouse.

for by genes in the H-2 complex. Such a model for Tcr is supported by the data of the Taniguishi/Tada groups, who have demonstrated that their antigen-specific suppressor factor is a molecule with two poly-peptides, one containing the antigen combining site and Igh-1 T-cell allotypes and another expressing I-J determinants (Tada *et al.*, 1980; Taniguishi *et al.*, 1981; Tokuhisa *et al.*, 1982). It also agrees with the finding that Ig idiotypes are dependent on both heavy and light chain elements (Imanishi-Kari *et al.*, 1979; Laskin *et al.*, 1977), but these studies (as have many others) have clearly shown that T-cell idiotypes are not dependent on the presence of "right" Ig light chain genes (Bach *et al.*, 1979; Hirai and Nisonoff, 1980; Krawinkel *et al.*, 1976; Cramer *et al.*, 1981).

TABLE V

Mapping of Genes Responsible for the Expression of 5936-Id and 6036 Allotypes on T Cells[a]

Mouse strain	Phenotype[b]			C_H Igh-1	Pre-albumin	Percentage of anti-B10.BR T cells[c] killed by RC and antisera		
	NP[H]	V_H S14	ABA-HOP			5936	6036	Anti-Thy
C57B1/6	+	−	−	b	0	25	37	98
CBA	−	+	+	j	a	1	3	97
B6.5a	+	−	+	j	NH	27	1	98
B6.9a	−	+	+	j	a	1	−1	96
B6.14a	ND	+	ND	j	0	1	−2	96
		V_H						
BALB/c		a		a	a	2	−2	98
11364		a		b	0	2	29	97

[a] Reproduced with permission from Suzan et al. (1982). Immunogenetics 16, 229–241.

[b] Mice were immunized with the respective antigens, and the resulting antisera were analyzed as described: NP[H], heteroclitic marker of NP-specific antibodies (Krawinkel et al., 1977a; S14 (Mäkelä et al., 1981); ABA-HOP (O. Mäkelä et al., 1976); Igh-1 (Rubin and Bourgois, 1981); prealbumin (Taylor et al., 1975). The presence of BALB/c V_H genes in 11364 mice was determined by the expression of the BALB/c Inulin idiotype by these mice (O. Mäkelä, personal communication).

[c] In the case of CBA T cells, these were stimulated with B6 spleen cells. Anti-Thy: AKR anti-C_3H hyperimmune antiserum (Rubin et al., 1979). RC, rabbit complement alone killed 5–10% of the cells. These values were subtracted from the experimental values.

IX. Function of T-Cell Idiotypes

In the present volume, several chapters are devoted to the function of T-cell idiotypes in helper or suppressor systems. Therefore, we will concentrate on the function of 5936 idiotypes in this chapter. 5936-Id are present on B6 T cells induced by I-A^k gene products (Table III). Such T cells express the Lyt-1$^+$,2.3$^-$ phenotype indicating that the 5936-Id$^+$ B6 T cells are helper cells (Suzan et al., 1983). It has not been possible so far to demonstrate 5936-Id on specific B6 helper factors or T cells. However, the helper factors of the CGG-specific helper T cell hybridoma T85-109-45/1 (Lonai et al., 1981a,b,c) express 6036 allotypes (P. Lonai and B. Rubin, unpublished). Because 5936-Id are always found on 6036 allotype-bearing molecules (Suzan et al., 1983), it may be assumed that 5936-Id-bearing molecules are also helper molecules. This was shown more directly by the experiments discussed below.

Helper T cells appear to recognize antigen in association with Ia gene products (Sprent, 1978; Zinkernagel, 1978). It is not known whether this joint recognition is caused by one or two T-cell receptors (Sprent, 1978; Zinkernagel, 1978; Matzinger, 1981; Kappler *et al.*, 1981; Nagy *et al.*, 1982). As mentioned before, a normal animal contains a very high frequency of alloantigen reactive T cells. This could be due to the possibility that T cells recognizing antigen in conjunction with self-MHC determinants cross-react with alloantigenic determinants (see Rubin *et al.*, 1980a). If this assumption is correct, one would assume that T cells reacting with antigen plus self-Ia may express the same idiotypes as T cells (with the same allotype genes) reacting with this self-Ia determinant as alloantigen. Therefore, we analyzed whether the 5936-Id expressed by B6 anti-I-A^k T cells were also expressed by B10.BR (H-2^k, Igh-1^b) T cells recognizing antigen in association with I-A^k gene products (Nagy *et al.*, 1982). Our experi-

TABLE VI

Inhibition of I-A but Not I-A/E Region Products Binding to TNP-Activated T Blasts with 5936 Antiserum[a]

Responder cells[b]	Preincubation[c] with	Incubation with soluble Ia[d]	Detection antibody[e]	I-subregion product detected	Antigen-binding blasts[f] (%)	Inhibition (%)
B10.BR anti-TNP (H-2^k, Igh-1^b)	—	B10.BR (Ia^k)	Ia-15	A^k	43.6	0
	5936	B10.BR (Ia^k)	Ia-15	A^k	3.0	93
	R anti-V$_H$	B10.BR (Ia^k)	Ia-15	A^k	4.0	91
	R anti-MIg	B10.BR (Ia^k)	Ia-15	A^k	41.3	5
	—	B10.BR (Ia^k)	Ia-7	A^k/E^k	42.3	0
	5936	B10.BR (Ia^k)	Ia-7	A^k/E^k	40.5	4
	R anti-V$_H$	B10.BR (Ia^k)	Ia-7	A^k/E^k	12.8	70
	R anti-MIg	B10.BR (Ia^k)	Ia-7	A^k/E^k	38.5	9
	—	—	Ia-15 + Ia-7	A^k + A^k/E^k	6.3	—
C3H anti-TNP (H-2^k, Igh-1^j)	—	B10.BR (Ia^k)	Ia-15	A^k	45.0	0
	5936	B10.BR (Ia^k)	Ia-15	A^k	41.7	7
	—	B10.BR (Ia^k)	Ia-7	A^k/E^k	24.3	0
	5936	B10.BR (Ia^k)	Ia-7	A^k/E^k	27.7	−14

[a] Reproduced with permission from Rubin *et al.* (1980). *Bull. Inst. Pasteur (Paris)* **78**, 305–348.
[b] Four-day primary anti-TNP cells were trypsin treated and incubated overnight at 37°C in TCGF-containing medium.
[c] Cells were preincubated for 15 min at 0°C and 30 min at 37°C with antisera at the following concentrations: 5936, 0.8 mg/ml; R anti-V$_H$, 13 mg/ml; and R anti-Ig, 0.3 mg/ml.
[d] Shed material from LPS activated B10.BR blasts (Nagy *et al.*, 1982).
[e] mAb (anti-Ia-15, clone 7/227.R7; anti-Ia-7, clone 13/18) were supplied by Dr. U Hämmerling. Final concentration was 1 : 15.
[f] Detected by indirect immunofluorescence. Background with anti-Ia-7 without antigen was 6.3%.

ments showed that B10.BR T cells recognizing TNP-I-A^k, LDH$_B$-I-A^k, or GA-I-A^k expressed 5936-Id and that the 5936-Id in these combinations were expressed on proliferating and/or helper T cells (Nagy *et al.*, 1982). The genes responsible for the synthesis of 5936-Id on B10.BR anti-TNP-I-A^k T cells were linked to Igh-1^b allotypes and, as shown in Table VI, the binding of I-A^k molecules to B10.BR anti-TNP-I-A^k cells was inhibited by antiserum 5936. The binding of CBA anti-TNP-I-A^k T cells was not inhibited, although the anti-V$_H$ antiserum inhibited the I-A^k binding to both types of cells. The results in Table VII show that B10.BR and B6 anti-I-a^k T cells can absorb all activity in antiserum 5936, demonstrating that it is the same antibodies in antiserum 5936 that react with the two types of cells.

Also, the binding of Ia^k antigen to B6 anti-B10.MBR T cells was inhibited by antiserum 5936, but the inhibition was less pronounced as compared with the self-Ia^k binding and was seen only when high concentrations of Ia^k antigen were used (Suzan *et al.*, 1983). These results may indicate that B6 anti-Ia^k T cells represent a heterogeneous cell population in regard to idiotype expression and antigen-binding avidity, the 5936-Id representing anti-Ia^k receptors of low avidity (Suzan *et al.*, 1983). The fine specificity of the inhibition of antigen bind-

TABLE VII

Absorption of Antiserum 5936 with B6 anti-IA^k and B10.BR
Anti-TNP/IA^k T Blast Cells

		Percentage of cells killed by antiserum 5936 and RC before or after absorption[b]		
Absorbing T blasts[a]	B6 anti-IA^k	B6.9a anti-IA^k	B10.BR anti-TNP	CBA anti-TNP
—	28	3	31	5
B6 anti-IA^k	3	1	−1	0
B6.9a anti-IA^k	27	0	33	4
B10.BR anti-TNP	5	−1	2	3
CBA-anti-TNP	29	2	27	1

[a] 200 μl antiserum diluted 1 : 5 was absorbed for 1 h at 37°C and 2 h at 4°C with 20 × 10^6 cells from T-cell lines 62 (B6 anti-4R/MBR), 71 (B6.9a anti-4R/MBR), or B10.BR (or CBA) T cells stimulated with TNP-coupled syngeneic spleen cells and harvested on day 5 after stimulation.

[b] Antiserum 5936 and rabbit complement-mediated cytotoxicity (see Table II).

ing was also determined using both antisera 5936 and 6036. The results in Table VIII show that antiserum 5936 inhibited only the binding of I-A^k molecules by B6 anti-B10.MBR T cells, whereas the binding of Ia^b or I-A^k/I-E^k molecules was not inhibited. By contrast, antiserum 6036 inhibited the binding of both Ia^b, I-A^k and I-A^k/I-E^k molecules by B6 anti-B10.MBR T cells. The binding of Ia^b, I-A^k and I-E^k molecules by C$_3$H anti-B10.MBR T cells was not inhibited by either antisera. These data indicate that 5936-Id and 6036 allotype-bearing T-cell protein are involved in the recognition of I-A^k gene products, whereas T-cell proteins carrying 6036 allotypes can also be involved in the recognition of Ia^b or I-E^k gene products. Thus, I-A^k gene products induce (Table III), keep proliferating in long-term cultures (Rubin *et al.*, 1980b; Suzan *et al.*, 1983), and bind to B6 5936-Id-bearing T cells with a possible helper function (Tables VI and VIII). As self-I-A^k recognizing B10.BR (or B10.A (4R)) T cells bear the 5936-Id regardless of their antigen specificity, our results are in favor of the

TABLE VIII

Inhibition of I-A^k but Not I-A^k/E^k Molecules Binding to Alloactivated B10 Anti-B10.MBR T Blasts with 5936 Antiserum

Responder cells[a]	Pre-incubation with [b]	Incubation with soluble Ia[c]	Detection antibodies[d]	I-subregion product detected A^k	Antigen-binding blasts[e] (%)	Inhibition (%)
B10 anti-B10.MBR	—	B10.MBR	anti-Ia-15 + Ia-19	A^k	47.5	0
	5936	B10.MBR	anti-Ia-15 + Ia-19	A^k	20.1	42
	6036	B10.MBR	anti-Ia-15 + Ia-19	A^k	4.6	90
	R anti-MIg	B10.MBR	anti-Ia-15 + Ia-19	A^k	43.5	8
	R anti-MIg	B10.MBR	anti-Ia-7	A^k/E^k	29.5	0
	5936	B10.MBR	anti-Ia-7	A^k/E^k	31.2	0 (−5)
	6036	B10.MBR	anti-Ia-7	A^k/E^k	7.1	76
	R anti-MIg	B10.MBR	anti-Ia-7	A^k/E^k	29.3	<1
	R anti-MIg	B10	anti-Ia-15 + Ia-8	A^b	31.3	0
	5936	B10	anti-Ia-15 + Ia-8	A^b	31.6	0
	6036	B10	anti-Ia-15 + Ia-8	A^b	5.2	83
	R anti-MIg	B10	anti-Ia-15 + Ia-8	A^b	33.0	0 (−5)

[a] See Table VI.
[b] See Table VI. R = rabbit.
[c] See Table VI.
[d] See Table VI. Anti-Ia-7 was derived from clone 13/18; anti-Ia-8 from clone B21-3.
[e] See Table VI. Background without antigen was <2.5%.

hypothesis that B10.BR T cells express two distinct paratopes, one specific for antigen (5936-Id$^-$) and one specific for self-I-A^k (5936-Id$^+$) (Nagy et al., 1982; see also Kappler et al., 1981; Lonai et al., 1981b).

X. Biochemical Analysis of 5936-Id-Bearing T-Cell Proteins

As was shown before (Rubin et al., 1980a; Rubin and Bourgois, 1981) and exemplified in Fig. 1, 5936-Id$^+$ T-cell proteins are produced by T cells, and the MW of membrane-bound molecules is about 75,000. We have used mostly B6 anti-H-2^k T-cell line supernatants for the isolation of 5936-Id$^+$ T-cell protein by antiserum 5936-Sepharose affinity chromatography, as described extensively elsewhere (Rubin et al., 1980a; Rubin and Bourgois, 1981; Bourgois et al., 1981). These molecules have also a MW of about 75,000, but they are easily degraded spontaneously into molecules with MWs of 62,000 and 50,000. The 50,000-MW molecule is relatively stable, and it appears to be a nonglycoprotein with an isoelectric point of about 4,8 (Rubin et al., 1980a). The amino acid composition of the 50,000-MW molecule is shown in Table IX, where it is compared with the amino acid composition of the heavy chain of MOPC 173 (Bourgois et al., 1981). This comparison shows that (1) the number of cysteyl residues is similar, suggesting that both molecules have a similar number of disulfide

TABLE IX

Comparison of the Amino Acid (A.A) Composition of Tcr-50 and the IgG$_{2a}$ MOPC 173 Heavy Chain

Amino acid	Tcr-50	Heavy chain	Δ[a]	Amino acid	Tcr-50	Heavy chain	Δ[a]
Asx	44.9	40.8	+4.1	Met	10.9	8.9	+2.4
Thr	24.0	35.0	−13.2	Ile	13.2	17.4	−4.2
Ser	30.0	49.9	−19.0	Leu	42.2	32.7	+9.5
Glx	56.8	36.9	+19.9	Tyr	13.3	17.7	−4.4
Pro	22.2	35.7	−13.5	Phe	18.7	12.8	+5.9
Gly	28.7	24.6	+4.1	Try	ND	11.2	—
Ala	35.8	18.4	+17.4	Lys	32.8	32.1	+0.7
Cys	10.7	10.9	−1.2	His	14.3	8.9	+5.4
Val	29.9	41.6	−11.9	Arg	16.2	12.8	+3.4

[a] For each residue, number of Tcr-50 minus number of heavy chain.

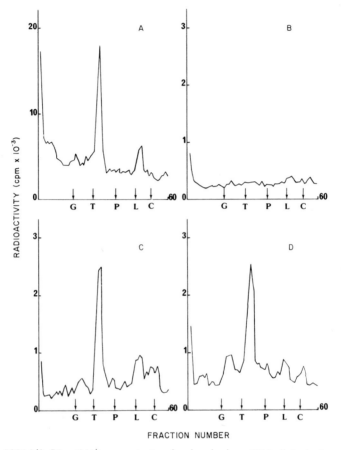

Fig. 5. 5936-Id[+], B6 anti-IA[k] supernatant molecules also bear 6036 allotypic determinants. B6 anti-IA[k] supernatants were passed through anti-Ig and antiserum 5936-Sepharose columns in series. Molecules adsorbed onto antiserum 5936-Sepharose were eluted with 3 M NH$_4$SCN, ^{125}I-labeled and (A) precipitated with *Staphylococcus aureus* coated with normal RIg (B), antiserum 5936 (C), or antiserum 6036 (D). Then they were subjected to SDS-PAGE under nonreducing conditions in a 6% gel. MW markers: G, IgG (150,000); T, transferrin (80,000); P, phosphocreatine kinase (40,000); L, light chain (23,000); C, cytochrome c (12,500). Reproduced with permission from Rubin et al. (1980a). *Bull. Inst. Pasteur (Paris)* **78**, 305–348.

bridges; (2) the number of prolyl residues is lower for the Tcr molecule, which could indicate that there is no hinge region at least in this part of the molecule; (3) the total number of neutral and aromatic residues is equivalent, although individual variations are observed; and (4) the number of hydroxyl residues is lower for the Tcr molecule, but the number of glutamyl residues is greater (57 instead of 37),

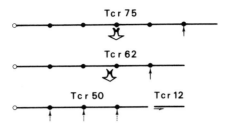

Fig. 6. Structure suggested for 5936-Id⁺ and 6036 allotype-bearing T-cell polypeptides. ●, regions susceptible to proteolysis; ○, blocked NH₂-terminal residue; →, region sequenced; ↑, site of spontaneous cleavage; ↑, site of possible cleavage by trypsin or chymotrypsin. For details, see text.

which is in agreement with the acidic isoelectric point observed (5 or below).

All the molecular forms of our Tcr molecules, 75,000-, 62,000-, and 50,000-MW molecules, bear 5936-Id and 6036 allotype (see Fig. 5 for the 75,000-MW molecule). However, none of them can be immuno-precipitated with anti-MIg antisera, antiallotype antisera, or anti-H-2/ mAb anti-Ia (B. Rubin, unpublished, and Rubin and Bourgois, 1981). The NH₂-terminal amino acid of the 50,000-MW molecule was blocked; this was also found for another T-cell protein with specificity for the TNP hapten (Cone *et al.*, 1981; Rosenstein *et al.*, 1981). We therefore undertook studies on the cleavage of the 50,000-MW molecule by different enzymes, and the results showed that treatment with trypsin resulted in two molecules with MWs of 37,000 and 12,000; treatment with chymotrypsin resulted in a single 25,000-MW molecular peak. As 5936-Id and 6036 allotypes have not yet been determined on these fragments, we can only suggest the following tentative model for the structure of our Tcr molecule (Fig. 6): a single polypeptide chain composed of six domains with an MW of 12,000.

In a few experiments, it was observed that the 62,000-MW molecule had degraded into two peaks with MWs of 50,000 and 12,000 (Tcr-50 and Tcr-12, respectively) in about similar proportions. Because we knew that the NH₂-terminal amino acid of the 50,000-MW molecule was blocked, the whole mixture was subjected to the amino acid se-quenator. A sequence of 11 amino acids was obtained, as shown in Table X (Bourgois *et al.*, in preparation). Comparison of the NH₂-terminal sequence of Tcr-12 with the region surrounding cysteine 29 in C_H domains was performed. All MR values are clearly below the AMV, indicating that stretch 1–11 of Tcr-12 presents some homology to stretch 20–30 of Cγ-1. A homology was also observed with stretch

TABLE X

Comparison of the NH$_2$-Terminal Sequence of Tcr-12 with the Region
Surrounding Cysteine 29 in Cγ1 Domains

Tcr-12[a]	Thr- Leu- Ser- Lys- Tyr- I/F[b]- Ala- Leu- I/F- Cys- I/F	MR[c]
M173-γ_{2a}	Thr- Thr- Gly- Ser- Ser- Val- Thr- Leu- Gly- Cys- Leu	1.10
M21	Ala- Ser- Gln- Ser- Met- Val- Thr- Leu- Gly- Cys- Leu	1.30
EU γ_1	Thr- Ser- Gly- Gly- Thr- Ala- Ala- Leu- Gly- Cys- Leu	1.10
SA γ_2	Thr- Ser- Glu- Ser- Thr- Ala- Ala- Leu- Gly- Cys- Leu	1.20
VIN γ_3	Thr- Ser- Glu- Ser- Thr- Ala- Ala- Leu- Gly- Cys- Leu	1.20
Rabbit γ	Thr- Pro- Ser- Ser- Thr- Val- Thr- Leu- Gly- Cys- Leu	1.00
Guinea pig γ_1	Thr- Ser- Gly- Ser- Met- Thr- Thr- Leu- Gly- Cys- Leu	1.15
Guinea pig γ_2	Thr- Ser- Gly- Ser- Met- Met- Thr- Leu- Gly- Cys- Leu	1.25

[a] Sequence of Tcr-12 (see Fig. 6) was undertaken with 4 nM of a mixture of fragments Tcr-12 and blocked Tcr-50 by using [^{3}H]phenylisothiocyanate and ^{14}C-carboxy methylation of reduced cysteyl residues. The other sequences are taken from Dayhoff (1976) and Kabat et al. (1979).

[b] In the analytic system used (HPLC), Ile (I), and Phe (F) migrated at the same position and were therefore not distinguished from one another.

[c] MR = minimum number of mutations required per codon. AMV = mean of average mutation values = 1.40 (Fitch, 1966). All MR values are clearly below the AMV, indicating that the stretch 1–11 of Tcr-12 presents some homology with stretch 20–30 of Cγ1. A homology was also observed with stretch 20–30 of Cγ3 and to a lesser extent with stretch 20–30 of the other C$_H$ domains of Ig heavy chains and stretch 79–89 of the hemoglobulin α chain. We thank Dr. Kabat, who helped us to find stretches representing matching residues.

20–30 of Cγ-3 and to a lesser extent with stretch 20–30 of the other C$_H$ domains of Ig and stretch 79–89 of the hemoglobulin α-chain. These data, together with the amino acid composition, the degradation profile, and the genetic linkage of Tcr V and C region genes to Ig heavy chain V and C region genes, suggest that antigen-binding T-cell receptor material (or its "heavy" chain) is related to the Ig family of molecules.

Our molecules look very much like the molecules described by others using similar systems (see Binz and Wigzell, 1981), the NP system (Krawinkel et al., 1976, 1977a; Cramer et al., 1979, 1981), the Arsanyl system (Bach et al., 1979; Hirai and Nisonoff, 1980), the KLH system (Tada et al., 1980; Taniguishi et al., 1981; Tokuhisa et al., 1982), the T$_{su}$ system (Spurll and Owen, 1981), the SRBC system (Fresno et al., 1981, 1982), the TNP system (Cone et al., 1981), and the AEF system (Delovitch et al., 1981). At present, we have found no structural evidence for a second Ia-bearing chain, as suggested by Tada and Taniguishi or Gershon et al. (Yamanshi et al.,

1982) and implicated by the genetic data (Krammer and Eichmann, 1977; the present article). However, because there might be differences in T-cell molecules recognizing antigen plus MHC and "only" MHC determinants, we are now studying 6036 allotype-bearing T-cell molecules from CGG-specific T-cell hybrids (Lonai et al., 1981a,b) and GAT-specific T-cell clones (Theze et al., 1982). Such cloned T cells do produce [^{3}H]leucine-labeled, Ia^k-bearing molecules, but whether they are involved in the specific antigen recognition is a question (Rubin, unpublished data). Another unsolved structural question is how many combining sites the native Tcr molecule expresses. The present guess seems to be two, but this is only considering either the "nominal" antigen combining site (Okuda et al., 1981; Cramer et al., 1980) or the MHC-specific combining site (Binz and Wigzell, 1977a,b).

XI. Molecular Biology of T-Cell Receptor Genes

Genetic mapping experiments in two different systems, the 5936-Id system (see preceding section), and the T_{su} system (Owen et al., 1981), suggested that the Tcr V genes are situated within or centromeric to the V_H genes, and the Tcr C region genes are situated either between V_H and C_H or between C_H and prealbumin genes. Two types of experiments were therefore carried out by many laboratories: (1) studies of rearranged Ig genes in T-cell clones or hybrids and (2) studies on cross-hybridization between Ig V or C region cDNA probes and mRNA from specific T cells. However, none of these experiments could show positive results, that is, T cells displayed no rearranged Ig genes, and no convincing cross-hybridization has been reported so far (Kronenberg et al., 1980, 1982; Kurosawa et al., 1981). The conclusions of these experiments were taken as absolute proof (by many investigators) of the nonidentity of Tcr and Ig heavy chain genes. This might well be true, but perhaps it is too early to state such rigorous conclusions. If (1) Tcr V and C region genes are duplicated Ig heavy chain V and C genes and (2) they are situated outside the Ig V_H and C_H genes, the distance between these V_T and C_T genes may be so large that mechanisms others than IgV$_H$/C$_H$ rearrangements are at play.

Recently, two groups of investigators isolated mRNA which in in vitro translation systems synthesize molecules with functional and serological properties similar to those produced in T cells: (1) KLH-specific suppressor factor (Taniguishi et al., 1982) and (2) GAT-specific suppressor factor (Wieder et al., 1982). The identification of these mRNA molecules and their corresponding DNA molecules will help us to understand the molecular mechanisms, at least for the construction of suppressor T-cell factors (receptors?).

XII. Conclusions

This chapter was written to summarize the experiments that strongly suggest that antibodies against certain inherited, public Ig-Id may cross-react with "idiotypes" on T cells. Evidence has been presented that such T-cell idiotypes were involved in antigen binding by and antigen-specific functions of their host T cells. Biochemical analysis of idiotype-bearing T-cell proteins and a comparison with T-cell proteins isolated by antigen binding or binding by antiallotype-isotype antibodies demonstrated that T-cell receptors may be constructed in a manner similar to that of Ig molecules by polypeptides which, at least in the case of the Tcr "heavy" chain, show structural analogies to Ig heavy chains. A reasonable candidate for Tcr "light" chains seems to be Ia-bearing polypeptides showing Ia specificities corresponding to the functional characteristics implicated for such subregion Ia gene products, for example, I-A = help; I-J(?) = suppression. However, in regards to the discussion in Section I of this chapter, we hope that we have drawn the limitations in the experiments and the interpretations of the presently available data on idiotypes on T cells.

Acknowledgments

The present work was supported by grants from CNRS (ATP 7071/72) and INSERM (CRL 81 1 0461). It is a pleasure to acknowledge the collaboration of Drs. A. Bourgois, B. E. Elliott, B. Hertel-Wulff, Z. Nagy, O. Nordfang, and M. Suzan. The skillful secretarial assistance by V. Bernay is gratefully acknowledged. The author thanks Dr. T. Delovitch for critically reading the manuscript and for many valuable discussions; Professor E. A. Kabat helped us to find stretches representing matching residues. I am most grateful for this kind assistance.

References

Arnold, B., Wallich, R., and Hämmerling, G. (1982). *J. Exp. Med.* **156**, 670–674.
Bach, B. A., Greene, M. I., Benacerraf, B., and Nisonoff, A. (1979). *J. Exp. Med.* **149**, 1084–1098.

Ben-Neriah, J., Givol, D., Lonai, P., Simon, M. M., and Eichmann, K. (1980). *Nature (London)* **285**, 257–259.

Binz, H., and Wigzell, H. (1975a). *J. Exp. Med.* **142**, 197–211.

Binz, H., and Wigzell, H. (1975b). *J. Exp. Med.* **142**, 1218–1230.

Binz, H., and Wigzell, H. (1975c). *J. Exp. Med.* **142**, 1231–1240.

Binz, H., and Wigzell, H. (1977a). *Contemp. Top. Immunobiol.* **7**, 113–167.

Binz, H., and Wigzell, H. (1977b). *Cold Spring Harbor Symp. Quant. Biol.* **41**, 275–284.

Binz, H., and Wigzell, H. (1981). *J. Exp. Med.* **154**, 1261–1278.

Binz, H., Wigzell, H., and Bazin, H. (1976). *Nature (London)* **264**, 639–641.

Bluestone, J. A., Sharrow, S. O., Epstein, S. L., Ozato, K., and Sachs, D. (1981). *Nature (London)* **291**, 233–235.

Bourgois, A., Kahn-Perles, B., and Rubin, B. (1981). *In* "Immunoglobulin Idiotypes" (C. Janeway, E. E. Sercarz, and H. Wigzell, eds.), pp. 449–458. Academic Press, New York.

Brondz, B. D. (1968). *Folia Biol. (Prague)* **14**, 115–126.

Cazenave, P.-A. (1977). *Proc. Natl. Acad. Sci. U.S.A.* **74**, 5122–5126.

Cazenave, P.-A., Cavaillon, J. M., and Bona, C. (1977). *Immunol. Rev.* **34**, 34–50.

Cerny, J., Heusser, C., Wallich, R., Hämmerling, G., and Eardly, D. D. (1982). *J. Exp. Med.* **156**, 719–730.

Cone, R. E., Rosenstein, R. W., Murray, J. H., Iverson, G. M., Ptak, W., and Gershon, R. K. (1981). *Proc. Natl. Acad. Sci. U.S.A.* **78**, 6411–6415.

Cosenza, H., Julius, M. H., and Augustin, A. A. (1977). *Immunol. Rev.* **34**, 3–33.

Cramer, M., Krawinkel, U., Melchers, I., Imanishi-Kari, T., Ben-Neriah, J., Givol, D., and Rajewsky, K. (1979). *Eur. J. Immunol.* **9**, 332–338.

Cramer, M., Krawinkel, U., and Mierau, R. (1980). *In* "Membranes, Receptors and the Immune Response" (E. P. Cohen and H. Köhler, eds.), pp. 345–358. Alan R. Liss, Inc., New York.

Cramer, M., Reth, M., and Grützmann, R. (1981). *In* "Immunoglobulin Idiotypes" (C. Janeway, E. E. Sercarz, and H. Wigzell, eds.), pp. 429–440. Academic Press, New York.

Dayhoff, M. O., ed. (1976). "Atlas of Protein Sequences and Structure," Vol. 6. Natl. Biomed. Res. Found., Washington, D.C.

Delovitch, T. L., Watson, J., Battistella, R., Harris, J. F., and Paetkan, V. (1981). *J. Exp. Med.* **153**, 107–128.

Dennert, G. (1979). *Nature (London)* **277**, 476–478.

D'Eustachio, P., Bothwell, A. L. M., Takaro, T. K., Baltimore, D., and Ruddle, F. H. (1981). *J. Exp. Med.* **153**, 793–800.

Dietz, M. H., Sy, M. S., Benacerraf, B., Nisonoff, A., Greene, M. I., and Germain, R. N. (1981). *J. Exp. Med.* **153**, 450–463.

Eichmann, K. (1975). *Eur. J. Immunol.* **5**, 511–517.

Eichmann, K., and Rajewsky, K. (1975). *Eur. J. Immunol.* **5**, 661–666.

Eichmann, K., Ben-Neriah, J., Hetzelberger, D., Polke, C., Givol, D., and Lonai, P. (1980). *Eur. J. Immunol.* **10**, 105–112.

Fitch, W. M. (1966). *J. Mol. Biol.* **16**, 9–28.

Fresno, M., McVay-Boudreau, L., Nabel, G., and Cantor, H. (1981). *J. Exp. Med.* **153**, 1260–1274.

Fresno, M., McVay-Boudreau, L., and Cantor, H. (1982). *J. Exp. Med.* **155**, 981–993.

Frieschknecht, H., Binz, H., and Wigzell, H. (1978). *J. Exp. Med.* **147**, 500–514.

Germain, R. N., Ju, S.-T., Kipps, T. J., Benacerraf, B., and Dorf, M. E. (1979). *J. Exp. Med.* **149**, 613–625.

Golstein, P., Svedmyr, E. A. J., and Wigzell, H. (1971). *J. Exp. Med.* **134**, 1385–1397.
Hämmerling, G. J., Blach, S. J., Berek, C., Eichmann, K., and Rajewsky, K. (1976). *J. Exp. Med.* **143**, 861–869.
Hengartner, H., Meo, T., and Müller, E. (1978). *Proc. Natl. Acad. Sci. U.S.A.* **76**, 4494–4499.
Hirai, Y., and Nisonoff, A. (1980). *J. Exp. Med.* **151**, 1213–1231.
Imanishi, T., and Mäkelä, O. (1974). *J. Exp. Med.* **140**, 1498–1511.
Imanishi-Kari, T., Rajnavolggi, E., Takemori, T., Jack, R. S., and Rajewsky, K. (1979). *Eur. J. Immunol.* **9**, 324–331.
Jensenius, J. C., Williams, A. F., and Mole, L. E. (1977). *Eur. J. Immunol.* **7**, 104–110.
Jensenius, J. C., Crone, M., and Kock, C. (1981). *Scand. J. Immunol.* **14**, 693–704.
Jerne, N. K. (1974). *Ann. Immunol. (Paris)* **125C**, 373–382.
Jerne, N. K., Roland, J., and Cazenave, P.-A. (1982). *EMBO J.* **1**, 243–247.
Kabat, E. A., Wu, T. T., and Bilowsky, H. (1979). "Sequences of Immunoglobulin Chains."
Kapp, J. A., Araneo, B. A., Ju, S.-T., and Dorf, M. E. (1981). *In* "Immunoglobulin Idiotypes" (C. Janeway, E. E. Sercarz, and H. Wigzell, eds.), pp. 387–396. Academic Press, New York.
Kappler, J. W., Skidmore, B., White, J., and Marrack, P. (1981). *J. Exp. Med.* **153**, 1198–1214.
Krammer, P. H. (1978). *J. Exp. Med.* **147**, 25–38.
Krammer, P. H., and Eichmann, K. (1977). *Nature (London)* **269**, 733–735.
Krawinkel, U., Cramer, M., Berek, C., Hämmerling, G., Black, S., Rajewsky, K., and Eichmann, K. (1976). *Cold Spring Harbor Symp. Quant. Biol.* **41**, 285–297.
Krawinkel, U., Cramer, M., Imanishi-Kari, T., Jack, S. R., Rajewsky, K., and Mäkelä, O. (1977a). *Eur. J. Immunol.* **7**, 566–573.
Krawinkel, U., Cramer, M., Mage, R. G., Kelus, A. S., and Rajewsky, K. (1977b). *J. Exp. Med.* **146**, 792–803.
Krawinkel, U., Cramer, M., Melchers, I., Imanishi-Kari, T., and Rajewsky, K. (1978). *J. Exp. Med.* **147**, 1341–1347.
Kronenberg, M., Davis, M. M., Early, P. W., Hood, L. E., and Watson, J. D. (1980). *J. Exp. Med.* **152**, 1745–1761.
Kronenberg, M., Kraig, E., Horvath, S. J., and Hood, L. E. (1982). *In* "Isolation, Characterization and Utilization of T Lymphocyte Clones" (C. G. Fathman and F. Fitch, eds.). Academic Press, New York.
Krupen, K., Araneo, B. A., Brink, L., Kapp, J. A., Stein, S., Wieder, K. J., and Webb, D. R. (1982). *Proc. Natl. Acad. Sci. U.S.A.* **79**, 1254–1258.
Kurosawa, Y., von Boehmer, H., Haas, W., Sakano, H., Traunerker, A., and Tonegawa, S. (1981). *Nature (London)* **290**, 565–570.
Laskin, J. A., Gray, A., Nisonoff, A., Klinman, N. R., and Gottlieb, P. D. (1977). *Proc. Natl. Acad. Sci. U.S.A.* **74**, 6000–6005.
Lindahl, K. F., and Wilson, D. B. (1977). *J. Exp. Med.* **145**, 500–518.
Lonai, P., Puri, J., Bitton, S., Ben-Neriah, Y., Givol, D., and Hämmerling, G. (1981a). *J. Exp. Med.* **154**, 942–951.
Lonai, P., Bitton, S., Savelkoul, J., Puri, J., and Hämmerling, G. (1981b). *J. Exp. Med.* **154**, 1910–1921.
Lonai, P., Puri, J., and Hämmerling, G. (1981c). *Proc. Natl. Acad. Sci. U.S.A.* **78**, 549–553.
McKearn, T. J. (1974). *Science* **183**, 94–98.
McKearn, T. J., Stuart, F. P., and Fitch, F. W. (1974). *J. Immunol.* **113**, 1876–1882.

Mäkelä, O., and Karjalainen, K. (1977). *Immunol. Rev.* **34**, 119–138.

Mäkelä, O., Julius, M., and Becker, M. (1976). *J. Exp. Med.* **143**, 316–331.

Mäkelä, O., Pasanen, V. S., Sawas, H., and Lehtonen, M. (1981). *Scand. J. Immunol.* **12**, 155–161.

Matzinger, P. (1981). *Nature (London)* **292**, 497–501.

Miller, G. G., Nadler, P. I., Asano, Y., Hodes, R. J., and Sachs, D. (1981). *J. Exp. Med.* **154**, 24–34.

Miller, J. F. A. P., and Mitchell, G. F. (1969). *Immunol. Rev.* **1**, 3–42.

Mitchison, N. A. (1971). *Eur. J. Immunol.* **1**, 18–24.

Mozes, E., and Haimovitch, J. (1979). *Nature (London)* **278**, 56–58.

Nagy, Z., Elliott, B. E., Carlow, D. A., and Rubin, B. (1982). *Eur. J. Immunol.* **12**, 393–400.

Nisbeth, N. W., Simonsen, M., and Zaleski, M. (1969). *J. Exp. Med.* **129**, 459–471.

Nordfang, O., and Rubin, B. (1981). *Immunogenetics* **12**, 497–509.

Okuda, K., Minami, M., Ju, S.-T., and Dorf, M. E. (1981). *Proc. Natl. Acad. Sci. U.S.A.* **78**, 4557–4561.

Owen, F. L., Riblet, R., and Taylor, B. A. (1981). *J. Exp. Med.* **153**, 801–810.

Pillemer, E., and Weissman, I. L. (1981). *J. Exp. Med.* **153**, 1068–1079.

Puri, J., Ben-Neriah, Y., Givol, D., and Lonai, P. (1980). *Eur. J. Immunol.* **10**, 281–284.

Rajewsky, K., and Eichmann, K. (1977). *Contemp. Top. Immunobiol.* **7**, 69–112.

Ramseier, H., Aguet, M., and Lindenmann, J. (1977). *Immunol. Rev.* **34**, 50–88.

Rosenstein, R. W., Murray, J. H., Cone, R. E., Ptak, W., Iverson, G. M., and Gershon, R. D. (1981). *Proc. Natl. Acad. Sci. U.S.A.* **78**, 5821–5825.

Rubin, B. (1976). *J. Immunol.* **116**, 80–85.

Rubin, B., and Bourgois, A. (1981). *Scand. J. Immunol.* **14**, 167–181.

Rubin, B., and Hertel-Wulff, B. (1978). *Scand. J. Immunol.* **7**, 523–527.

Rubin, B., and Pierres, M. (1981). *Immunol. Today* **2**, 208–209.

Rubin, B., and Wigzell, H. (1973a). *J. Exp. Med.* **137**, 911–931.

Rubin, B., and Wigzell, H. (1973b). *Nature (London)* **242**, 467–469.

Rubin, B., Hertel-Wulff, B., and Kimura, A. (1979). *J. Exp. Med.* **150**, 307–321.

Rubin, B., Suzan, M., Kahn-Perles, B., Boyer, C., Schiff, C., and Bourgois, A. (1980a). *Bull. Inst. Pasteur (Paris)* **78**, 305–346.

Rubin, B., Golstein, P., Nordfang, O., and Hertel-Wulff, B. (1980b). *J. Immunol.* **124**, 161–167.

Samuel, D., Denizot, F., Suzan, M., Rubin, B., and Golstein, P. (1982). *Cell. Immunol.* **71**, 139–147.

Schiff, C., Boyer, C., Millili, M., and Fourgereau, M. (1979). *Eur. J. Immunol.* **9**, 831–841.

Schreiber, A., Conrad, P. I., Andre, C., Vray, B., and Strosberg, A. D. (1980). *Proc. Natl. Acad. Sci. U.S.A.* **77**, 7385–7389.

Sege, K., and Peterson, P. A. (1978). *Proc. Natl. Acad. Sci. U.S.A.* **75**, 2443–2447.

Sercarz, E. E., and Metzger, D. W. (1980). *Springer Semin. Immunopathol.* **3**, 145–170.

Sprent, J. (1978). *Immunol. Rev.* **42**, 108–129.

Spurll, G. M., and Owen, F. L. (1981). *Immunol. Today* **2**, 75–77.

Suzan, M., Boned, A., Lieberkind, J., Valsted, F., and Rubin, B. (1981). *Scand. J. Immunol.* **14**, 673–685.

Suzan, M., Valsted, F., Boned, A., and Rubin, B. (1982). *Immunogenetics* **16**, 229–241.

Suzan, M., Elliott, B. E., and Rubin, B. (1983). *J. Immunol.* **130**, 1426–1431.

Tada, T., Hayakawa, K., Okumura, K., and Taniguishi, M. (1980). *Mol. Immunol.* **17**, 867–875.

Taniguishi, M., Scrito, T., Takei, I., and Tokuhisa, T. (1981). *J. Exp. Med.* **153**, 1672–1677.

Taniguishi, M., Tokuhisa, T., Kanno, M., Yaoita, Y., Shimizu, A., and Honjo, T. (1982). *Nature (London)* **298**, 172–174.

Taylor, B. A., Bailey, D. W., Cherry, M., Riblet, R., and Weigert, M. (1975). *Nature (London)* **256**, 644–646.

Theze, J., Kimoto, M., Gougeon, M. L., Moreau, J.-L., Sommé, G., Leclerq, L., and Fathman, C. G. (1982). *In* "Isolation, Characterization and Utilization of T Lymphocyte Clones" (C. G. Fathman and F. W. Fitch, eds.), pp. 399–406. Academic Press, New York.

Thomas, W. R., Morathan, G., Walker, I. D., and Miller, J. F. A. P. (1981). *J. Exp. Med.* **153**, 743–747.

Tokuhisa, T., Komatsu, Y., Uchida, Y., and Taniguishi, M. (1982). *J. Exp. Med.* **156**, 888–897.

Urbain, J., Wikler, M., Franssen, J. D., and Collignon, C. (1977). *Proc. Natl. Acad. Sci. U.S.A.* **74**, 5126–5131.

Valbuena, O., Marcu, K. B., Croce, C. M., Huebner, K., Weigert, M., and Perry, R. P. (1978). *Proc. Natl. Acad. Sci. U.S.A.* **75**, 2883–2888.

Volanakis, J. E., and Kearney, J. F. (1981). *J. Exp. Med.* **153**, 1604–1614.

Wieder, K. J., Araneo, B. A., Kapp, J. A., and Webb, D. R. (1982). *Proc. Natl. Acad. Sci. U.S.A.* **79**, 3599–3603.

Wilder, R. L., Yuen, C. C., Sher, I. I., and Mage, R. C. (1979). *Eur. J. Immunol.* **9**, 777–783.

Wilson, D. B., Blyth, J., and Nowell, P. C. (1968). *J. Exp. Med.* **128**, 1157–1174.

Yamanshi, K., Chao, N., Murphy, D. B., and Gershon, R. K. (1982). *J. Exp. Med.* **155**, 655–665.

Zinkernagel, R. M. (1978). *Immunol. Rev.* **42**, 224–241.

Chapter 9

Ontogeny of the HA-Responsive B-Cell Repertoire: Interaction of Heritable and Inducible Mechanisms in the Establishment of Phenotype

Michael P. Cancro, Mary Ann Thompson,
Syamal Raychaudhuri, and David Hilbert

Department of Pathology and Laboratory Medicine
University of Pennsylvania Medical School
Philadelphia, Pennsylvania

I. Introduction

It is well established that the potential antibody repertoire of a species is quite diverse, containing more than 10^7 unique specificities (Kreth and Williamson, 1973; Klinman and Press, 1975a; Köhler, 1976; Cancro et al., 1978b). Several molecular strategies which afford such great potential diversity have recently been inferred from analyses of immunoglobulin (Ig) variable region structural genes and their derived proteins (Mac et al., 1979; Weigert et al., 1980; Early et al., 1980; Kurosawa and Tonegawa, 1982; Shimizu et al., 1982; Gearhart et al., 1981). It is evident, however, that the antigen-responsive repertoire of an individual does not necessarily contain all members potentially afforded by genotype but may be a particular subset of these specificities (Hiernaux et al., 1981; Sigal, 1982; Cancro et al., 1981). The mechanisms responsible for determining which members from the library of potential specificities are phenotypically expressed remain poorly understood. Clearly, a knowledge of these mechanisms is essential to both understanding and effectively manipulating the humoral immune system.

A principal event in the establishment of repertoire phenotype is the appearance of an antigen-responsive B-cell pool during early life. We have recently studied the genetics and dynamics of repertoire phenotype during this formative period, and several aspects of the emerging repertoire's behavior have been established from this work. In addition, analyses of ligand-induced changes that occur during this period suggest that early events in repertoire formation may have profound consequences. First, particular specificities may be fixed and expanded by ligand challenge, resulting in a response which is dominated by these clonotypes in the adult. Second, clonotypes which would otherwise emerge are suppressed, resulting in their absence from responses in the adult. This chapter reviews the salient features of these studies, with attention to their implications for deliberate manipulations of repertoire phenotype.

II. Early Studies of Antibody Repertoire Ontogeny

In early ontogenetic studies, the concept of a controlled developmental appearance of specificities was introduced, based upon observations suggesting that the ability to mount humoral responses to particular antigens appeared at regular points in development

(Silverstein *et al.*, 1963; Sherwin and Rowlands, 1975; Rowlands *et al.*, 1974). More rigorous studies, using inbred mouse models, confirmed and extended this idea by demonstrating an ordered emergence of certain clonotypes within the 2,4-dinitrophenyl-(DNP), 2,4,6-trinitrophenyl-(TNP), and phosphorylcholine-(PC) specific responses of BALB/c mice (Klinman and Press, 1975b; Sigal *et al.*, 1976, 1977). Similar findings have also been reported for the murine responses to levan, dextran, and several additional haptenic compounds (Bona *et al.*, 1979; Fernandez and Möller, 1978; Sigal, 1977). This work is discussed extensively elsewhere (Sigal and Klinman, 1978; Klinman *et al.*, 1980). More recent studies (to be discussed here) using the murine response to influenza A hemagglutinin (HA) as a model have yielded data consistent with the idea that genetically identical individuals express similar patterns of repertoire acquisition (Cancro *et al.*, 1979; Cancro and Klinman, 1980; Cancro, 1982; Thompson and Cancro, 1982). Finally, data consistent with this concept have also been obtained in both avian and amphibian models (Huang and Dreyer, 1978; Du Pasquier and Wabl, 1978; Du Pasquier *et al.*, 1979).

The precise mechanisms which underlie this heritable pattern of repertoire phenotype formation are controversial. Such patterning reflects either intrinsic control over the activation and expression of *Ig* variable region genes (Klinman *et al.*, 1976) or selective clonal expansion and deletion mechanisms which act subsequent to *Ig* receptor expression. Because these mechanisms are clearly under genetic control regardless of which interpretation is correct, it appeared a reasonable first step to perform genetic studies of repertoire ontogeny in order to enumerate and identify the loci responsible.

III. Genetics of Antibody Repertoire Formation

A. THE MURINE INFLUENZA HA-SPECIFIC RESPONSE AS A MODEL

The genetics of repertoire formation have been approached primarily by limiting dilution analysis of murine B cells responsive to the HA molecule of the influenza strain PR8. The choice of this model is based upon its ability to resolve extensively the HA-responsive repertoire's clonal composition by reactivity pattern (RP) analysis of antibodies generated in limiting dilution culture (Bracialle *et al.*, 1976; Gerhard, 1976; Cancro *et al.*, 1978b). The general methodology is outlined in Fig. 1. The major advantage afforded by this model is that the behavior of the *entire* HA-responsive repertoire may be monitored, allowing changes or differences in repertoire composition to be detected which might be overlooked if only a few markers were followed. In addition, RP analysis can detect and positively characterize clonotypes not previously observed, providing an unbiased and comprehensive means of defining the repertoires of genetically disparate animals.

B. THE HA-SPECIFIC REPERTOIRES OF ADULT AND
   NEONATAL BALB/c MICE

As a preliminary to genetic studies, the HA-responsive primary repertoire of the adult BALB/c population was assessed by this technique and found to be very diverse (Cancro *et al.*, 1978b). Statistical treatment of this data suggested that the primary repertoire of adult BALB/c mice contains a minimum of 100–200 unique specificities (Wybrow and Berryman, 1973; Soper, 1980). It should be stressed that this great diversity is observed at the level of the entire adult *population*, because pools of adult B cells were employed in these estimates. It is difficult to establish whether a single adult mouse expresses more restricted heterogeneity among its B cells because of the small sample sizes obtained from any given individual. This point and its importance are discussed more extensively in Section VI. Diversity estimates of the secondary HA-specific repertoire among adult BALB/c mice have been performed by idiotype, RP, and amino acid sequence analyses of hybridoma antibodies. These estimates indicate over 1000 specificities (Staudt and Gerhard, 1982), some of which clearly result from somatic diversification mechanisms.

Similar analysis of the HA-responsive repertoire expressed by 12–14-day-old BALB/c mice showed the emerging HA-responsive compartment to be considerably less diverse than its adult counterpart (Cancro *et al.*, 1979). This conclusion was based on our finding that far fewer RPs are present in the neonatal population, coupled with the repeated observation of many clonotypes both within and between individual neonates. These results strengthened the concept that the phenotypically expressed repertoire emerges in a staged fashion among genetically identical individuals. More importantly, it demonstrated the feasibility of studying the genetics of repertoire formation by examining neonatal phenotypes in additional strains, F_1s, and congenics.

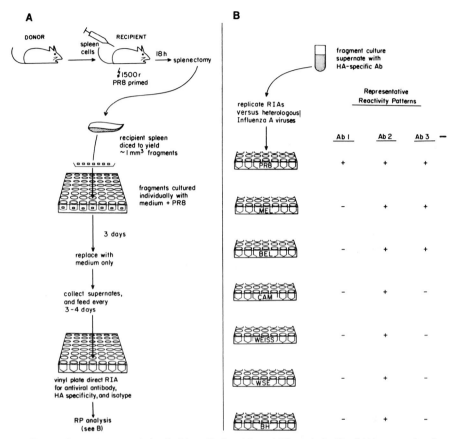

Fig. 1. General approach for limiting dilution (A) and RP analysis (B) of HA-responsive B cells. (A) shows the scheme used to generate monoclonal HA-specific antibodies by adoptive transfer and splenic fragment culture. Splenic cells from donor mice are passed to lethally irradiated primed recipients at doses which yield limiting dilution kinetics in the subsequent antigen-stimulated cultures. After 18 h, the recipient spleens are removed and diced to yield 1-mm³ fragments. These are cultured individually in the presence of antigen (PR8 virus). The medium is replaced with antigen-free medium 3 days later, and the cultures are then fed every 3–4 days. Culture supernates are harvested at each feeding, beginning on days 9–10 of culture. Typically, cultures will produce antibody until days 18–21 of culture. The collected supernates are assayed for antiviral antibody by radioimmunoassay and the supernates from a given positive fragment are pooled and then assayed for isotype and HA specificity. The monoclonal, HA-specific antibodies thus obtained are then assayed for RP. This type of analysis is schematized in (B). Because the antibodies are monoclonal, each one recognizes a single determinant on the immunizing (PR8) HA molecule. Depending on the distribution of the recognized determinant among the heterologous viral HAs, a characteristic array of positive and negative reactions is obtained for each antibody. Each potential pattern of reactions is termed a reactivity pattern (RP), and defines a clonotype or small set of clonotypes that is necessarily distinct from clonotypes yielding any other RP.

C. MULTIPLE LOCI MEDIATE REPERTOIRE FORMATION

1. Repertoire Formation in Heterozygotes

Characterization of a second strain, B10.D2, provided the basis for further genetic studies. Although these mice also showed a 12–14-day HA-responsive repertoire which was reproducible among individuals and smaller than its adult counterpart, the clonal composition differed considerably from that of BALB/c mice at the same age (Cancro and Klinman, 1980). This is evidenced by a similar frequency of HA-responsive B cells in the B10.D2 (Table I) but a considerable disparity in clonotype (RP) composition when compared to that of BALB/c (Fig. 2).

This observation provided the basis for genetic analysis of the heritable elements controlling emerging repertoire phenotype, because it demonstrated polymorphism(s) of these elements between B10.D2 and BALB/c mice. Accordingly, the HA-responsive repertoire of neonatal (BALB/c × B10.D2)F_1 mice was characterized. Because F_1s derived from inbred parents are genetically identical to one another (although heterozygous), the F_1s also show great similarity to one another at the same age. Comparison of the F_1s emerging repertoire phenotype to their parents' neonatal repertoires, however, reveals an intriguing phenomenon: The F_1's developmental pattern differs from

TABLE I

Frequencies of HA-Specific B Cells among Adult and Neonatal Mice[a]

Strain	Age	Total splenic cells transferred[b] $\times 10^{-7}$	HA-specific B cells per 10^6 splenic B cells[c]
BALB/c	8 weeks	152	13.0
B10.D2	8 weeks	103	8.0
(BALB/c × B10.D2)F_1	8 weeks	95	9.6
(C.B20 × B10.D2)F_1	8 weeks	40	11.0
C.B20	8 weeks	46	9.0
BALB/c	12–14 days	220	4.0
B10.D2	12–14 days	222	2.9
(BALB/c × B10.D2)F_1	12–14 days	212	2.5
(C.B20 × B10.D2)F_1	12–14 days	174	2.8
C.B20	12–14 days	188	2.6

[a] Splenic B cells from each strain and age shown were transferred to primed, irradiated recipients, and limiting dilution splenic fragment culture was performed.
[b] In each experiment, between 1 and 2 × 10^7 splenic cells were transferred to each recipient.
[c] Frequencies are given after correction for homing and cloning efficiency.

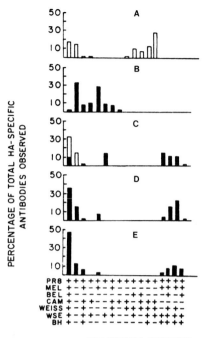

REACTIVITY PATTERN

Fig. 2. RP analysis and comparison of neonatal HA-specific repertoires among parental, congenic, and F_1 mice. The HA-specific antibodies derived from splenic fragment cultures were assayed for binding on six heterologous viruses by radioimmunoassay (RIA). Because they are monoclonal, each antibody recognizes a single determinant on the immunizing HA molecule. Depending on the distribution of the recognized determinant among these heterologous viral HA, a characteristic array of positive and negative reactions is obtained for each antibody. Each potential pattern of reactions defines a clonotype or a small set of clonotypes which is necessarily distinct from clonotypes yielding any other RP. The relative frequencies of all observed RP within the HA-specific repertoires of 12- to 14-day-old BALB/c (A), B10.D2 (B), (BALB/c × B10.D2)F_1 (C), (C.B20 × B10.D2)F_1 (D), and C.B20 (E) mice are shown. Also shown is an allotypic analysis of all antibodies derived from (BALB/c × B10.D2)F_1 neonates, which are heterozygous at the *Igh* locus (Igh^a/Igh^b). Each antibody derived from these F_1 was tested in a competitive RIA specific for IgM derived from the Igh^b haplotype. The shaded areas of each bar indicate the proportion of antibodies in each RP exhibiting reactivity in this assay. The histograms of the remaining strains, all of which are homozygous at the *Igh* locus, are shaded according to their appropriate allotype, but only several representative antibodies from these groups were actually tested in the assay.

that of both parents, because many parental clonotypes are absent and several novel clonotypes are expressed (Fig. 2). This compositional difference, coupled with the observation that neither the frequency of HA-responsive B cells (Table I) nor the overall degree of clonotype diversity differs from that of the parents, leads to several conclusions.

First, because F_1s derived from two inbred strains bear all the structural genetic information of both parents, the paucity of parental clonotypes cannot be caused by a lack of appropriate structural genes. Thus, some heritable regulatory phenomenon is required to explain this finding.

Second, the appearance of novel clonotypes (i.e., RPs seen in neither parent) can be explained by either of two mechanisms: (1) unique specificities are produced by combining V_H and V_L components from both parents in a single *Ig* molecule or (2) the clonotypes of parents and F_1s are similar but emerge in a different sequence, so that the F_1 repertoire at a given point in development may be different from that of the parents.

Finally, the degree of clonotype diversity observed in (BALB/c × B10.D2)F_1s is no greater than that seen among the parents at this age. Because it is known that BALB/c and B10.D2 differ at several V_H loci, this suggests that regardless of the *potential* diversity afforded by an expanded library of V-region genes, a subset of relatively fixed size is expressed at a given time within the primary pool. This concept and its implications are discussed further in Sections IV and VI.

2. Repertoire Formation in Allotype Congenics

The above experiments provided an opportunity to assess the role of allotype-linked loci versus remaining genetic background in controlling repertoire formation. Because BALB/c and B10.D2 are known to differ at the *Igh-1* locus, and because V_H structural genes are linked to *Igh-1*, it is reasonable to assume that these loci might play an important role in repertoire development. Specifically, C.B20 and (C.B20 × B10.D2)F_1 neonates were used to determine whether the novel pattern of clonotype appearance among (BALB/c × B10.D2)F_1s was caused by heterozygosity at *Igh-1* linked loci alone, or whether background loci were also instrumental in this process. Because (C.B20 × B10.D2)F_1s are identical to (BALB/c × B10.D2)F_1s except for homozygosity at *Igh-1*, the pattern of clonotype emergence in these mice should be like that of B10.D2s if allotype-linked loci alone were responsible. Inspection of Fig. 2 shows that this is not the case. Instead, 12–14-day-old (C.B20 × B10.D2)F_1s express an HA-responsive repertoire most similar to that of (BALB/c × B10.D2)F_1. The alternative hypothesis, that the developmental pattern is completely independent of *Igh-1*-linked loci, was critically tested by characterizing the repertoire of 12–14-day-old C.B20 mice. Because this repertoire also closely resembled the (BALB/c × B10.D2)F_1 and (C.B20 ×

B10.D2)F_1 repertoires, it appears that multiple loci are responsible for controlling repertoire ontogeny, some of which are *Igh-1* linked and some of which are not.

3. Background Loci May Mediate V_H Gene Expression

Because both Igh-1^b homozygotes, C.B20, and (C.B20 × B10.D2)F_1, expressed developmental patterns similar to those of (BALB/c × B10.D2)F_1s, an Igh-1^b/Igh-1^a heterozygote, the possibility that background loci might exert their effects via mechanisms that mediate V_H gene expression could be inferred by allotypic analysis of the antibodies derived from (BALB/c × B10.D2)F_1s. The rationale for this experiment is twofold. First, it seemed that the "F_1-like" developmental pattern always occurred when BALB/c background loci were coupled with the Igh-1^b haplotype. Second, current evidence suggests that most V-C joining occurs cis rather than trans. Therefore, if the (BALB/c × B10.D2)F_1 preferentially draws its 12–14-day repertoire from the B10.D2 parents' structural gene contribution, as implied by the C.B20 and (C.B20 × B10.D2)F_1 repertoires, most of the antibodies should be of the Igh-1^b allotype.

Allotype analysis of all HA-specific antibodies derived from (BALB/c × B10.D2)F_1 neonates confirmed this possibility, because there was a clear skewing toward the Igh^b allotype, and all of the unique F_1 specificities which characterize the F_1-like pattern were of this allotype (Fig. 2).

D. SUMMARY AND PERSPECTIVE

These studies clearly indicate the action of multiple heritable elements in the control of antibody repertoire ontogeny. Certain aspects of these findings remain puzzling, however.

It is still uncertain whether the observed staging of clonotype appearance is mediated by intrinsic events which dictate the order of V-region gene expression, or instead reflects receptor-mediated clonal expansion and deletion. Several approaches may help resolve this issue. First, limiting dilution models of higher efficiency might prove valuable, because they would allow the characterization of low-frequency clonotypes. If reproducibility in clonal emergence is also seen among low-frequency clonotypes in such experiments, it would be difficult to accommodate the idea that differential clonal expansion is responsible for the apparently staged emergence of specificities. Alternatively, detailed characterization and comparison of the antibodies expressed at different ages might provide insight regarding potential mechanisms for sequential activation of V region genes.

With the same experimental approach, it should be possible to localize further the allotype-linked effects and map them to the right or left of IgCH genes by examining the 12–14-day repertoire of BAB.14 mice. The results discussed in Section V,B, which indicate that suppressor T-cell populations may shape repertoire phenotype, coupled with studies which have shown that certain T-cell markers also map in this region (Owen *et al.*, 1981; Owen, 1982), suggest that the allotype-linked component of clonotype emergence may reflect the action of genes which dictate the behavior of regulatory cells rather than V_H structural genes.

Regardless of the precise mechanism, it is reasonable to ask whether a knowledge of clonal emergence might be valuable in the human population. This question must be approached cautiously in light of our observations with F_1 individuals. Because F_1s differed from both parental strains, it is probable that in outbred populations, although similar mechanisms will be operative in terms of B-cell repertoire development, great variation may exist among individuals. It might be possible to "fix" the population's developmental expression of particular specificities temporally if ubiquitous, strong, selective pressures were active (e.g., clonotypes which recognize a prevalent pathogen), but these might be rarities. In addition, the multigenic nature of this process requires the correlation of several loci in order to perceive such staging within an outbred population. An obvious candidate at this time is the Ig allotype (from the above data), but additional loci are also clearly involved and await definition. Finally, although we have employed only $H-2^d$ homozygotes in our studies, should antigen-driven events be important (see Sections IV and V), MHC would, of course, be expected to be influential.

IV. Dynamics of the Emerging Primary B-Cell Pool

A. RAPID TURNOVER OF CLONOTYPES WITHIN A COMPARTMENT OF FIXED SIZE

The genetic studies discussed above demonstrate that the mechanisms controlling the emergence of specificities within the primary B-cell pool are heritable, leading to a predictable ontogenetic pattern given genetic identity. However, the effects of environmental stim-

TABLE II

Lymphocyte Composition of the Spleen During Ontogeny: FACS
Determinations

Age	Ig^{+a} (%)	Total number of nucleated cells per spleen ($\times 10^{-7}$)[b]	Calculated total number of B cells per spleen ($\times 10^{-7}$)[c]
Day 3	18.1 ± 2.0^{d}	0.95	0.17
Days 6–7	12.4 ± 2.4	5.6	0.69
Days 13–14	26.2 ± 1.9	8.2	2.1
Adult	53.7 ± 4.1	10.0	5.4

[a] Based on a minimum of four determinations. Splenic B cells were stained with anti-mouse Ig and analyzed for fluorescence and forward small-angle light scatter. Fluorescein-ated reagents used were Tago goat antimouse IgG (heavy and light chains), Meloy goat antimouse IgM, and Fab_2 goat antimouse Ig. All reagents gave comparable results. Fluorescence gain was between 2 and 4, and fluorescence above channel 10 or 15 was considered positive, depending on the individual experiment. Erythrocytes and dead cells were gated out on the basis of forward small-angle light scatter.

[b] Based on a minimum of three determinations. Variance caused by counting and sampling error is $\pm 20\%$.

[c] Calculated by multiplying the mean percentage of Ig^+ by the total number of nucleated cells.

[d] Figures are given ± 1 SD.

uli will differ greatly depending upon the kinetics and dynamics of emerging B-cell clones. Assessment of clonal dynamics within the responsive B-cell population is therefore essential prior to studying how an emerging repertoire of predictable composition is acted on by external perturbations. We have again used the HA-specific response to probe this question by characterizing the B-cell pool responsive to HA at several ages (Thompson and Cancro, 1982).

As a preliminary to these studies, the lymphocyte composition of spleens from BALB/c mice at 3, 6, and 14 days of age was assessed using a fluorescence-activated cell sorter (FACS). The results of this analysis are summarized in Table II and are in general agreement with earlier assessments of these parameters (Spear *et al.*, 1973; Sidman and Unanue, 1975). Following this, limiting dilution culture of HA-specific B cells was performed with mice at these ages, and the absolute number of HA-reactive B cells per spleen was calculated. These results are shown in Table III. The major conclusion which emerges from these studies is that, although the absolute number of B cells increases during this period, the number of HA-responsive B cells remains relatively constant. This is depicted graphically in Fig. 3.

TABLE III

Frequency of Viral and HA-Specific B Cells in Neonatal and Adult Mice

Age[a]	Virus-specific clones per 10^6 splenic B cells[b]	HA-specific clones per 10^6 splenic B cells[b]	Number of B cells per spleen ($\times 10^{-6}$)[c]	Calculated number of HA-specific B cells per spleen
Days 6–7	46.6	8.2	6.9	57
Days 13–14	14.8	3.3	21.2	70
Days 13–14: virus-exposed[d]	59.1	19.1	21.2	405
Adult	27.1	13.0	53.7	698

[a] Frequencies based on analysis of 2.74×10^9 cells from 127 1-week-old mice, 2.16×10^9 cells from 55 2-week-old mice, 6.41×10^8 cells from 2-week-old antigen-exposed mice, and 1.52×10^9 cells from adult spleens.

[b] Frequency estimates were obtained from splenic fragment cultures using PR8 as an antigen. Values given are after correction for homing efficiency (23). Monoclonal antibodies obtained were screened for virus and HA specificity by radioimmunoassay.

[c] From Table II.

[d] Mice were injected with UV-inactivated PR8 ip on days 3 and 6 after birth and sacrificed at 2 weeks of age.

RP analysis of antibodies derived from 6-day-old mice provides two additional pieces of information when compared to a similar analysis of antibodies from 12–14-day-old animals. First, the degree of diversity (i.e., the number of distinct RPs observed) at 6 days of age is comparable to that seen at 12–14 days of age. Thus, both the magnitude *and* the heterogeneity of the HA-reactive pool remain constant during this period. In contrast, the clonal composition changes markedly. This is evident from inspection of Fig. 4, where RP analyses of both 6- and 12–14-day-old BALB/c mice are compared. Several RPs characteristic of the 6-day repertoire are absent at 13 days of age; conversely, several RPs are observed at high frequency among 13-day-old animals that were not present at 6 days of age. These major compositional changes, given an HA-responsive compartment of similar size and diversity, necessarily imply a rapid turnover of specificities within the primary HA-responsive B-cell pool.

It is important to stress that the consistency of clonal composition between individuals again leads to the notion that the emerging repertoire's behavior is mediated by heritable control mechanisms. Otherwise, one would expect individuals to be out of phase with each other, precluding the visualization of turnover at the population level.

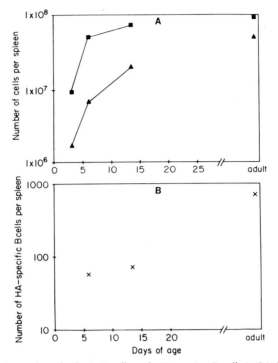

Fig. 3. Absolute number of splenic B cells and HA-reactive B cells in BALB/c mice during neonatal life. The absolute number of Ig⁺ lymphocytes in the spleens of BALB/c mice at several ages during early life (ontogeny) was determined by FACS analysis (A); ■——■, total nucleated cells per spleen; ▲——▲, B-cells per spleen. (B) shows the absolute number of HA-reactive B cells per spleen at the same ages, which was determined by limiting dilution culture analysis of precursor frequency (×). The graphs shown demonstrate that although the total number of B cells increases during this period, the number of HA-reactive primary B cells remains relatively constant.

In addition, the present results disagree with the notion that specificities observed late in development are actually only those present at low frequency. This is because the clones arising later are represented at similar frequencies and in the absence of those specificities present at earlier developmental points.

Finally, these findings again indicate a homeostasis in the degree of diversity present within the primary pool, as originally suggested by the data obtained when individuals heterozygous at *Igh-1* were examined (Section III,C). Further, this relative constancy of heterogeneity indicates that the primary pool may retain this property regardless of age.

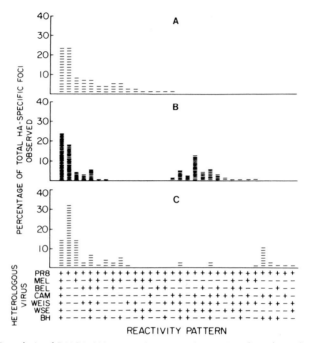

Fig. 4. RP analysis of BALB/c HA-responsive repertoires at 6 and 13 days of age. The HA-specific monoclonal antibodies derived from splenic fragment cultures were assayed for binding on six heterologous viruses by RIA. Each vertical bar shows the relative frequency of a given RP, and each horizontal line within a bar represents a single antibody. (A) shows the relative frequencies of all observed RP within the 6-day BALB/c repertoires (*n* = 73); the middle panel shows the 13-day BALB/c repertoire (*n* = 151); (C) shows the 13-day repertoire of BALB/c mice given 1000 HAU of PR8 virus ip at 3 and 6 days of age (*n* = 83). Only RP actually observed have been included on the horizontal axis, although 64 RP are possible with a panel of six heterologous viruses.

B. LIGAND EXPOSURE PERTURBS NORMAL TURNOVER
PATTERNS

The foregoing studies indicate that not only is the emerging repertoire's composition predictable at a given age among genetically identical individuals, but that the composition changes in a rapid and regular fashion. This observation suggests that the effects of external, receptor-specific stimuli (e.g., ligand) may be exquisitely time dependent. For example, antigenic exposure superimposed on the repertoire at 6 days of age may have profoundly different effects than similar exposure a week later.

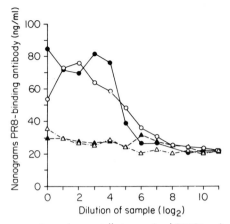

Fig. 5. PR8-specific serum titers of neonatally immunized BALB/c mice. Immediately before use as spleen cell donors, neonatally immunized mice, their unimmunized littermates, and their mother were bled. Doubling dilutions of serum were made and then assayed for PR8-specific antibody by RIA. O——O and ●——●, serum from 2-week-old mice given 1000 HAU of PR8 ip at 3 and 6 days of age; △---△, serum from an unimmunized littermate; ▲---▲, serum from the litter's mother.

In order to model these effects, we first asked whether normal patterns of clonal appearance and turnover are changed by deliberate antigenic exposure. BALB/c mice were immunized with PR8 at both 3 and 6 days of age, and subsequently used as spleen cell donors in limiting dilution culture when 13 days old. These immunizations resulted in demonstrable titers of PR8-specific antibody (Fig. 5). Serum titrations of the mothers showed that cross-immunization did not occur, minimizing the likelihood of induced maternal influences.

The frequency of HA-specific B cells among these neonatally immunized, 13-day-old mice was sixfold higher than observed among unimmunized mice. RP analysis of HA-specific antibodies derived from these mice is compared to analyses of normal 6- and 12–14-day-old mice in Fig. 4. It is evident from inspection that the majority of RPs characteristic of the normal 13-day repertoire are absent. Moreover, several of the RPs which are normally only transiently expressed at 6 days of age appear to have been preserved. It is important to note that these clonotypes not only persist but have been expanded, because they comprise a similar percentage of the repertoire of the antigen-exposed mice, in which the absolute number of HA-reactive cells has increased sevenfold over that of 6-day-old mice.

V. Longevity and the Basis of Ligand-Induced Effects

A. LIGAND-INDUCED OLIGOCLONAL PHENOTYPE PERSISTS TO ADULTHOOD

Although the studies with immunized neonates provide evidence for at least short-term effects upon repertoire phenotype, they address neither the potential of these effects upon adult repertoire phenotype nor the predictability of these effects vis-à-vis the developmental stage at which initial exposure occurs. To determine the longevity and predictability of antigen-driven effects, neonatal mice were immunized with PR8 initially at either 3 and 6 days or 12 and 15 days of age. In addition, each of these groups was divided into a "chronically" treated group, which received additional immunizations at weekly intervals, and an "acute" group, which received only the two initial doses of antigen. These animals were allowed to reach exactly 7 weeks of age and were then used as donors in limiting dilution culture.

TABLE IV

Frequency of HA-Specific B Cells Among Normal and Immunized BALB/c Mice[a]

Age	Age at initial PR8 immunizations[b]	Immunization[c] regimen	HA-specific[d] cells per 10^6 splenic B cells
6 days	—	—	8
12–14 days	—	—	3
13–14 days	Days 3–6	Acute	19
Adult	—	—	13
Adult	Day 3–6	Chronic	321
Adult	Day 3–6	Acute	76
Adult	Day 12–15	Chronic	312

[a] The frequency of HA-responsive splenic B cells was determined by limiting dilution splenic fragment culture.

[b] Mice were either unimmunized or initially immunized with 1000 HAU of UV-inactivated PR8 at the age shown.

[c] Among immunized mice, either chronic or acute dose regimens were employed. Acutely immunized mice were given the initial dose of PR8 only. Chronically immunized mice received 1000 HAU of UV-inactivated PR8 weekly following initial immunization. They received their final dose of virus 6 days prior to use as spleen cell donors in limiting dilution culture.

[d] The values given are after correction for the proportion of B cells in the inoculum (17), as well as homing and cloning efficiency (30).

The frequencies of HA-responsive B cells in each of these groups (Table IV) indicate 25- and 6-fold expansion of the HA-responsive population in chronically and acutely immunized mice, respectively. RP analyses of each group's HA-specific repertoires are compared to those of normal neonates in Fig. 6. Several conclusions emerge from examination of these results. First, neonatal antigen exposure generally leads to an adult which displays dominance of a restricted number of HA-reactive clonotypes when compared to an unimmunized adult population. Second, given a knowledge of the composition of the available primary pool at the time of initial exposure, the clones which become dominant are predictable. Third, there is a paucity of clonotypes which would otherwise have emerged subsequent to antigenic exposure. Finally, both the chronic and acute regimens appear capable of inducing such effects, but the chronic treatment appears to expand the dominant clonotypes to a greater extent, as might be expected.

Thus, neonatal antigen-driven events exert profound effects upon individual phenotype which persist into adulthood. Further, the precise effects are not only time dependent but predictable, given a knowledge of the emerging repertoire's dynamics and composition at the time of antigen exposure.

B. MECHANISMS OF THE NEONATALLY INDUCED OLIGOCLONAL PHENOTYPE

Preliminary studies of the mechanisms responsible for these effects have focused on two areas: First, are the stimulated B cells that assume dominance functionally altered in any fashion? Second, are suppressive circuits, mediated by T lymphocytes, responsible for the apparent lack of those HA-reactive clonotype which would have arisen had no antigen been given?

1. Changes in B-Cell Subset Occur Following Immunization

In these experiments the hybridoma antibody, J11d, was used to assess surface phenotype of B cells. The marker defined by this antibody was shown to be nonpolymorphic and present on primary but not secondary splenic B cells specific for sheep red blood cells or TNP (Bruce et al., 1981).

In our experiments, splenic B cells from either normal or neonatally immunized BALB/c mice were treated with J11d and complement,

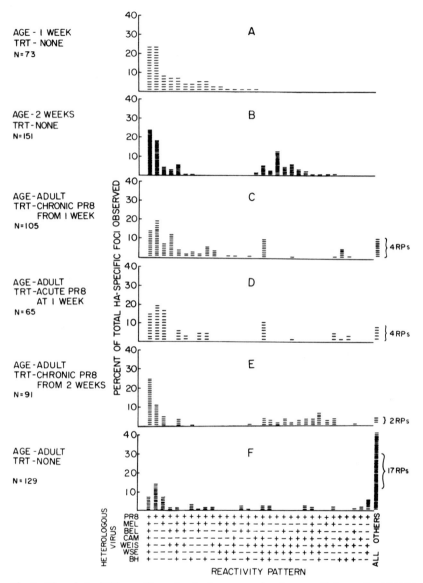

Fig. 6. RP analysis of HA-specific antibodies from normal and neonatally immunized BALB/c mice. The HA-specific monoclonal antibodies derived from splenic fragment cultures were assayed for binding on six heterologous viruses by RIA. (A) and (B) show the HA-responsive repertoires of unimmunized BALB/c mice at 3–6 and 12–14 days of age, respectively; (C) and (D) show the repertoires of adult mice that had been either chronically or acutely immunized beginning at 3–6 days of age; (E) shows the repertoire of adult mice which had been chronically immunized beginning at 12–14 days of age; and the repertoire observed among a sample of unimmunized adults is shown in (F).

TABLE V

Frequency of HA-Responsive, J11d⁻ B Cells in
Normal and PR8-Immune BALB/c Mice[a]

Experiment	HA-specific foci per 10^7 injected J11d⁻ splenic cells from	
	Normal BALB/c	PR8 immune BALB/c
1	2.2	53.3
2	0.5	80.0

[a] Splenic J11d⁻ cells were prepared from either normal BALB/c adults or age-matched animals which had been immunized with 1000 HAU of PR8 at 3 and 6 days of age and weekly thereafter. Splenic J11d⁻ cells were pooled from several individuals, and either 2×10^7 cells from normal mice or 5×10^5 cells from immunized mice were adoptively transferred to recipients for limiting dilution splenic fragment culture.

leaving the J11d⁻ cell population. These cells were then used in limiting dilution cultures, and their HA-specific responses were assessed. The frequencies of HA-responsive B cells among splenic J11d⁻ cells from these mice are shown in Table V.

There is a 20- to 120-fold increase of HA-specific B cells in the J11d⁻ compartment after chronic immunization.

2. Induction of Differential Suppression

The ability of T cells from either normal or neonatally immunized mice to suppress PR8-specific responses *in vivo* was tested. In these experiments, suppression of both primary and secondary responses was examined (Table VI). At the dosages used, lymph node T cells from normal adult mice exert little effect upon the ability of adoptive recipients to respond to PR8. In contract, T cells derived from chronically immunized mice are able to suppress primary but not secondary HA-specific responses. Finally, the suppressive ability of the transferred cells is completely abolished by either irradiation (1500 rads) or treatment with anti Lyt-2 and complement.

The specificity of the T suppressor cells generated was initially tested by transferring T cells from mice chronically immunized with PR8 to recipients which were subsequently immunized with CAM. CAM (H1N1) has an HA of a different type than PR8 and is recognized by very few of the PR8-HA-specific clonotypes known to be present in neonatal and chronically exposed mice. The results are shown in Ta-

TABLE VI

Neonatal Antigen Challenge Induces Suppressors Capable of Ablating Primary
But Not Secondary HA-Specific Humoral Responses *in Vivo*

Donor L.N.[a] cells	Donor[b] treatment	Recipient[c]	HA-specific antibody (μg/ml)[d]
—	—	Normal	65, 130, 190
—	—	PR8	350, 250, 360, 175
1×10^7 T	Chronic PR8	Normal	<10, <10, <10, 30
1×10^6 T	Chronic PR8	Normal	<10, 50, <10, 30
5×10^5 T	Chronic PR8	Normal	75, 175
1×10^7 T	Chronic PR8	PR8	350, 375
1×10^6 T	Chronic PR8	PR8	350, 750, 750, 750
1×10^7 T	None	Normal	90, 180, 165, 90, 260
1×10^7 T	None	PR8	350, 700, 750, 750
1×10^7 T after anti Lyt-2 and C'	Chronic PR8	Normal	150, 175
1×10^7 T after irradiation	Chronic PR8	Normal	180, 260

[a] All lymph node cells were treated with anti-I-A and J11d plus complement to yield a 97% Thy-1$^+$ cell population. In the last treatment groups, these cells were also treated with a monoclonal anti-Lyt-2 reagent and C', which kills 22% of LNT cells, or were irradiated (1500 rads).

[b] BALB/c donor mice were either untreated or had received UV-inactivated PR8 chronically (1000 HAU/week) beginning 3–6 days after birth.

[c] Recipients were either normal BALB/c mice or age-matched, PR8-immunized BALB/c mice. All recipients received 1000 HAU of PR8 i/p 2 days after T-cell transfer and were bled at days 6, 8, and 10 after immunization.

[d] HA-specific antibody was determined by hemagglutination inhibition. This allows the detection of HA-specific antibody but not antibodies directed to other viral antigens. Each number represents the mean of three determinations on an individual animal.

ble VII. The transferred cells suppress primary responses to the HAs of both CAM and PR8 equally well.

Taken together, the results of these experiments suggest that neonatal immunization results in the stimulation, expansion, and differentiation of extant primary B-cell clones to a serologically distinguishable suppression-resistant state and simultaneously induces T suppressor cells which effectively suppress primary but not secondary B-cell populations.

Because this conclusion logically implies that J11d$^-$ cells from immunized mice are a suppression-resistant subset, it seemed reasonable to test this directly (Table VIII). Splenic B cells and lymph node T cells were obtained from the same mice and cotransferred to irradi-

TABLE VII

Suppressors Generated by PR8 Immunization Ablate Primary B-Cell
Responses to Heterologous Influenza Viruses

Donor L.N. cells[a]	Donor treatment[b]	Immunizing antigen[c]	HA-specific antibody (μg/ml) reactive with [d]	
			PR8	CAM
—	—	PR8	130, 200	<10, 30
—	—	CAM	40, 20	200, 110
1×10^7	Chronic PR8	PR8	20, <10	<10, <10
1×10^6	Chronic PR8	PR8	20, 20	<10, <10
1×10^7	Chronic PR8	CAM	<10, <10	<10, <10
1×10^6	Chronic PR8	CAM	<10, <10	<10, <10
1×10^7	None	PR8	100, 80	40, <10
1×10^7	None	CAM	40, 20	200, 110

[a] Lymph node cells were prepared as in Table VI.
[b] Donor mice were treated like those in Table VI.
[c] Recipients were normal (unimmunized) BALB/c mice at 6–8 weeks of age. Each recipient received 1000 HAU of either PR8 or CAM 2 days after T-cell transfer. Sera were taken at days 6, 8, and 10 after immunization.
[d] HA-specific antibody was determined by hemagglutination inhibition. For each recipient, titration was performed for both PR8- and CAM-reactive antibody by using the appropriate virus in the hemagglutination inhibition assay.

ated recipients. Various mixtures of these cells were tested for their ability to reconstitute the recipient's response to PR8. Neither whole nor J11d⁻ splenic B cells from unimmunized animals respond without cotransferred T cells. Further, J11d⁻ B cells from unimmunized mice also fail to reconstitute serum responses even when normal T cells are cotransferred, whereas whole splenic B-cell populations yield good responses under these conditions. This finding strengthens the notion that most HA-responsive B cells in unimmunized mice reside within the J11d⁺ pool. The key treatment groups of this experiment are those that show that J11d⁻ B cells from immunized mice respond even in the presence of T cells which abolish the responses of splenic B cells from normal individuals. This indicates that the J11d⁻ B-cell pool of immunized mice both contains HA-reactive cells and is resistant to suppressor T cells generated by immunization.

Interpretive caution must be exercised with respect to the J11d marker. First, although the precursor frequency studies clearly demonstrate changes in the *distribution* of B cells within J11d⁺ versus J11d⁻ subsets following immunization, it is not clear whether this is a

TABLE VIII

HA-Reactive, J11d⁻ B Cells from Immunized Mice Are Resistant to
Antigen-Induced Suppression[a]

Spleen cell donor	Spleen cell treatment	Lymph node T-cell donor	Recipient serum HA-specific antibody after challenge (μg/ml)[b]
—	—	Normal	<10
—	—	Chronic PR8	<10
Normal	Thy-1	—	<10
Chronic PR8	Thy-1	—	130, 65
Normal	Thy-1	Normal	130, 130
Normal	Thy-1	Chronic PR8	<10, <10, <10
Chronic PR8	Thy-1	Normal	735
Chronic PR8	Thy-1	Chronic PR8	520
Chronic PR8	Thy-1/J11d	Normal	520, 1040
Chronic PR8	Thy-1/J11d	Chronic PR8	370, 735, 1040
Normal	Thy-1/J11d	Normal	30, <10
Normal	Thy-1/J11d	Chronic PR8	<10, <10

[a] Spleen and lymph node cells were prepared from either normal BALB/c mice or BALB/c mice that had been immunized chronically with PR8 beginning at 3–6 days of age. All donors were 7–8 weeks of age. Spleens and nodes were taken from the same animals. Lymph node T cells were prepared by treatment with monoclonal anti-I-A and J11d, as described. Spleen cells were treated with either anti-Thy-1 only or with both anti-Thy-1 and J11d. These cells were transferred intravenously to irradiated (950 rads) BALB/c mice. In all cases, doses of 2.5×10^7 B cells and 1×10^7 T cells were used.

[b] Two days after transfer, recipients were immunized with 1000 HAU of UV-inactivated PR8 intraperitoneally. Serum was collected on days 6, 8, and 10 after immunization and assayed for PR8-specific antibody by both radioimmunoassay and hemagglutination inhibition. The figures given are based on the day 6 sera.

loss of the J11d marker through differentiation of previously J11d⁺ cells or a differential expansion of HA-reactive cells already in the J11d⁻ pool. Although we favor the former idea based upon the reconstitution studies, this remains debatable. Second, the J11d marker's association with susceptibility to T-mediated suppression may be coincidental rather than absolute. For example, transition from J11d⁺ to J11d⁻ may reflect stimulation by certain types of priming (e.g., thymus-dependent versus thymus-independent antigens), whereas functional changes may occur under all immunization conditions. Additional experiments are necessary to probe these possibilities.

C. SUMMARY AND PERSPECTIVE

These studies demonstrate several aspects of the behavior and maintenance of the primary repertoire not previously appreciated. First, the primary repertoire, in the apparent absence of ligand-driven events, changes rapidly and regularly. Again, the *regularity* of these compositional changes implies a heritable basis for initial primary repertoire expression. Second, these observations lead to the idea that ligand-driven events may exert vastly different effects upon repertoire phenotype depending on the developmental   point at which initial challenge occurs. Third, the nature of ligand-driven events seems to be the "fixation" of those primary clonotypes currently available and the suppression of subsequently arising clonotypes responsive to the same or similar antigens. Fourth, this fixation of phenotype is long lived, persisting to adult life. Finally, the mechanisms of phenotype fixation entail at least two elements: (1) the movement of activated B cells to functionally distinct differentiation subsets, and (2) the concomitant generation of T-cell-mediated suppression which acts differentially on primary versus secondary B cells.

Several aspects of this phenomenon are presently unclear, but are approachable experimentally.

First, the exact nature of the normal turnover observed among emerging primary specificities is not revealed by these studies. Primary B cells may have intrinsically short half-lives, so that cell death may provide a basis for the turnover. Rapid turnover in the B-cell compartment is implied by the work of Osmond *et al.* (1974), as well as by more recent studies (deFreitas and Coutinho, 1981). Alternatively, this turnover may reflect the further differentiation of B cells to states which are unresponsive in the limiting dilution system employed. Finally, the constitutive generation of idiotype-specific suppression could be responsible for this apparent loss of specificities. Although suppressive cells have been reported in neonatal mice in the absence of any deliberate antigenic exposure (Mosier and Johnson, 1975), these cells were apparently antigen specific and would thus fail to explain the present observations.

Second, the specificity of the suppression generated during antigenic exposure is presently under investigation. Evidence suggests that this suppression is antigen specific rather than idiotype specific. Transfer of T suppressor cells virtually ablates the primary serum response to PR8-HA, suggesting that the suppression affects most HA-specific primary B cells. Because these include specificities not activated (perhaps not even present) in the chronically immunized mice which donated the suppressors, it is difficult to imagine how the suppressors could be recognizing B-cell idiotype per se. The experiment demonstrating suppression of the primary response to CAM by T cells from mice chronically exposed to PR8 also addresses the question of specificity. Although few clonotypes responsive to CAM are present in the donors of the T cells, the CAM response as well as a primary PR8 response is suppressed, again suggesting a T suppressor population which has broad antigen specificity. Alternatively, it is possible that many HA-reactive clonotypes share those idiotopes important to T-cell-mediated suppression. Although the extensive potential diversity of the HA-specific repertoire (Cancro *et al.*, 1978b; Staudt and Gerhard, 1982) makes this seem unlikely, it is clear that large arrays of antibodies sometimes share V-region determinants (Marshak-Rothstein *et al.*, 1980).

A third question raised by these data is the mechanism, at a cellular and molecular level, whereby suppressor cells may show preferential activity upon primary versus secondary B-cell responses. Similar general phenomena have previously been reported in several experimental systems (Owen and Nisonoff, 1978; Owen *et al.*, 1977; Pierce and Klinman, 1977), but these studies also fail to provide a mechanistic explanation. Resolution of this problem will require precise assessment of what stage in the B-cell activation or maturation process is interfered with by these regulatory cells, as well as the recognitive elements of the suppressors themselves.

VI. The "Moving Window" Model of Primary Repertoire Phenotype Expression

Although certain mechanistic details remain unclear, the work reviewed above leads us to propose the following model for early primary repertoire expression. This general model may be outlined as follows:

1. Antigen responsive primary B-cell specificities appear in a staged fashion resulting from the interaction of multiple heritable factors.
2. For a given determinant or antigen, the *available responsive* primary repertoire at any time is only a subset of the potential repertoire (afforded by the genotype).

3. The specificities within this subset undergo turnover, such that the primary B-cell pool's composition fluctuates rapidly and regularly. Among individuals who are identical at the loci responsible for this process, similar changes occur regularly at the same age.
4. Antigen challenge at a given developmental point perturbs this process by precipitating several events:
   a. Activation of the presently available responsive primary B-cell clonotypes, and their concomitant expansion and differentiation to a functionally distinct B-cell subset(s?).
   b. Induction (and expansion?) of suppressor T cells that can effectively prevent primary B cells, but not *previously activated B cells*, from participating in subsequent responses to the inducing antigen or closely related antigens.
5. These ligand-driven events have the net effect of preserving those clonotypes present in the responsive primary pool at the time of initial challenge and maintaining them as the individual's usable B-cell repertoire to this and closely related antigens, thus "fixing" the phenotype.

Several implications are inherent in this general scheme which warrant discussion in light of their relationship to existing concepts and information, as well as in regard to their critical experimental analysis.

First, initial antigenic experiences should, to a great extent, determine an individual's available repertoire to closely related antigens. An intriguing phenomenon exists in human responses to influenza virus which might be interpreted as exemplary of this occurrence. In a classic study, Fazekas de St. Groth and Webster (1966) showed that children previously immunized to one strain of influenza tended, upon secondary challenge with a heterologous strain, to produce antibodies of greater avidity for the virus used in the primary rather than the secondary challenge. Our work (Section V,B,2) regarding the suppression of primary responses to heterologous viruses closely parallels this observation and may provide a mechanistic explanation for this phenomena, termed "original antigenic sin." Although the classical explanation for this phenomenon, stimulation of cross-reactive, previously expanded B-cell clones to the exclusion of specific primary clones, may in part be true, our results indicate that active suppression may be a major contributing factor. Should additional studies uphold this idea, it might be advantageous to explore vaccination regimens which avoid the induction of suppressor circuits. Recent studies with synthetic B-cell immunogens might provide the basis for approaches to this problem (Lerner, 1982).

Aside from suggesting a mechanistic model for this perplexing problem of influenza immunization, the results detailed in the previous section raise the more general issue of precisely how induced suppressive circuits control the adult's responsive repertoire. Although much work now indicates the importance of such circuits, the present observations and concepts raise a cautionary note regarding assessments of suppressor specificity. Ligand challenge not only induces suppressor circuits but simultaneously causes the movement of B cells to novel differentiation subsets in a *clonotype-specific* fashion. Thus, only B-cell specificities extant at the time of challenge move to suppression-resistant subsets. This compartmentalizes B-cell clonotypes in a way which, under certain circumstances, could lead to apparent clonotype-specific suppression, although the specificity would actually reflect the distribution of antigen-responsive clonotypes among suppression-sensitive versus suppression-resistant subsets.

An interesting implication of this model is that among genetically identical individuals, whose temporal patterns of clonal emergence are necessarily similar, the ubiquitous introduction of a given antigen at the same time will fix each individual's repertoire similarly. Interestingly, several situations of "natural" clonal dominance in mice involve ubiquitous environmental antigens, although additional experiments are required to establish the relationship of these observations to the studies described here. Conversely, the same antigen encountered either at different times or by genetically disparate individuals will result in varying dominant clonal profiles. This concept bears strongly on the potential effects of either vaccination or natural immunization with respect to both efficacy and potentially harmful effects.

A third set of predictions from the model concerns how the establishment of dominance may be reversed or prevented. It seems probable that effective reversal would necessarily entail destruction of existing T-cell suppressor circuits, as well as the expanded secondary B cells resistant to suppression.

Alternatively, existing circuits for a given determinant might be circumvented by stimulation with the same determinant on a *different* carrier structure. This is suggested by the experiments which indicate that responses to heterologous viruses are effectively ablated by PR8-induced suppressors, implying that suppression may be specific for structures associated with but not identical to B-cell epitopes.

In terms of preventive manipulations, it seems likely that any operation which interferes with the interaction between ligand and extant primary B-cell clones should prevent the fixation of those clonotypes in the repertoire during that exposure. At least three major sources of such interference are evident: (a) the introduction of competitive, nonimmunogenic ligand; (b) the introduction of idiotype-specific antibody, which should have similar effects, but with greater precision regarding the particular B-cell clones acted up; and (c) the presence of passively acquired antibody that effectively competes with B-cell receptors for antigen, which under natural circumstances might be maternally derived.

The conclusion that early antigen-driven events dictate the composition of the adult repertoire has interesting clinical implications. Unfortunately, the result of neonatal antigen exposure at a particular age cannot be predicted in the outbred human population as easily as among the inbred mouse strains. From a theoretical standpoint, however, one can imagine both beneficial and detrimental results from predictable neonatal antigen exposure. If a clonotype with high affinity for a virulent pathogen naturally arises at the time most children are first exposed to the pathogen, then the high-affinity clonotype will expand in response to exposure and confer protection. Such a fortuitous interaction may be selected for evolutionarily. Alternatively, if an antigen is encountered at a time in development when a primary clonotype exists which reacts both with the antigen and with a self-component, then a potentially autoimmune phenotype might be fixed or fostered. This may explain the loose association of many autoimmune diseases with various viral or bacterial antecedents.

Further resolution of genetic loci which control the B-cell repertoire's initial expression and dynamics, coupled with an appreciation of how these elements interact with ligand-driven events to determine phenotype, should render these speculative possibilities amenable to experimental analysis.

Acknowledgments

The expert technical assistance of Mrs. Geraldine Ball and Mrs. Ada Gomelsky in all of the studies discussed herein is gratefully acknowledged, as are the expert manuscript preparation skills of Ms. Ellen Schwartz.

The work described in the chapter was in part supported by USPHS grants CA-15822 and 5-T32-GMO7170 and ACS grant IM-288.

References

Bona, C., Mond, J. J., Stein, K. E., House, S., Lieberman, R., and Paul, W. E. (1979). Immune responses to levan. III. The capacity to produce anti-insulin antibodies and cross-reactive idiotype appears late in ontogeny. *J. Immunol.* **123**, 1484.

Bracialle, T. J., Gerhard, W., and Klinman, N. R. (1976). Analysis of the humoral immune response to influenza virus *in vitro. J. Immunol.* **116**, 827.

Bruce, J., Symington, F. W., McKearn, T. J., and Sprent, J. (1981). A monoclonal antibody discriminating between subsets of T and B cells. *J. Immunol.* **127**, 2496.

Cancro, M. P. (1981). Developmental genetics of the B-cell repertoire: The role of allotype-linked loci. *In* "B Lymphocytes in the Immune Response: Functional, Developmental, and Interactive Properties" (N. Klinman, D. Mosier, E. Scher, and E. Vitetta, eds.), p. 55. Elsevier/North-Holland, New York.

Cancro, M. P. (1982). Multiple loci mediate B-cell repertoire ontogeny: Analysis of the hemagglutinin-specific repertoires in neonatal C.B20 and (C.B20 × B10.D2)F_1 mice. *J. Immunol.* **128**, 1307.

Cancro, M. P., and Klinman, N. R. (1980). B-cell repertoire ontogeny: Heritable but dissimilar development of parental and F_1 repertoires. *J. Immunol.* **126**, 1160.

Cancro, M. P., Sigal, N. H., and Klinman, N. R. (1978a). Differential expression of an equivalent clonotype among BALB/c and C57BL/6 mice. *J. Exp. Med.* **147**, 1.

Cancro, M. P., Gerhard, W., and Klinman, N. R. (1978b). The diversity of the influenza-specific primary B-cell repertoire in BALB/c mice. *J. Exp. Med.* **147**, 776.

Cancro, M. P., Wylie, D. E., Gerhard, W., and Klinman, N. R. (1979). Patterned acquisition of the antibody repertoire: Diversity of the hemagglutinin specific B-cell repertoire in neonatal BALB/c mice. *Proc. Natl. Acad. Sci. U.S.A.* **76**, 6577.

deFreitas, A. A., and Coutinho, A. (1981). Very rapid decay of mature B lymphocytes in the spleen. *J. Exp. Med.* **154**, 994.

Du Pasquier, L., and Wabl, M. R. (1978). Antibody diversity in amphibians: Inheritance of isoelectric focusing antibody pattern in isogenic frogs. *Eur. J. Immunol.* **8**, 482.

Du Pasquier, L., Blomberg, B., and Bernard, C. C. A. (1979). Ontogeny of immunity in amphibians: Changes in antibody repertoire and appearance of adult major histocompatibility antigens in *Xenopus. Eur. J. Immunol.* **9**, 900.

Early, P., Huang, H., David, M., Calame, K., and Hood, L. (1980). An immunoglobulin heavy chain variable region gene is generated from three segments of DNA: V_H, D, and J_H. *Cell* **19**, 981.

Fazekas de St. Groth, S., and Webster, R. G. (1966). Disquisitions on original antigenic sin. I. Evidence in man. *J. Exp. Med.* **124**, 331.

Fernandez, C., and Möller, G. (1978). Immunological unresponsiveness to native dextran B512 in young animals of dextran high responder strains is due to lack of Ig receptor expression: Evidence for a non-random expression of V-genes. *J. Exp. Med.* **147**, 645.

Gearhart, P. J., Johnson, N. D., Douglas, R., and Hood, L. (1981). IgG antibodies to phosphorylcholine exhibit more diversity than their IgM counterparts. *Nature (London)* **291**, 29.

Gerhard, W. (1976). The analysis of the monoclonal immune response to influenza virus. II. The antigenicity of the viral hemagglutinin. *J. Exp. Med.* **144**, 985.

Hiernaux, J., Bona, C., and Baker, P. J. (1981). Neonatal treatment with low doses of anti-idiotypic antibody leads to the expression of a silent clone. *J. Exp. Med.* **153**(4), 1004–1008.

Huang, H. V., and Dreyer, W. J. (1978). Bursectomy *in ovo* blocks the generation of immunoglobulin diversity. *J. Immunol.* **121**, 1738.

Klinman, N. R., and Press, J. L. (1975a). The characterization of the B-cell repertoire specific for 2,4-dinitrophenyl and 2,4,6-trinitrophenyl determinants in neonatal BALB/c mice. *J. Exp. Med.* **141**, 1133.

Klinman, N. R., and Press, J. L. (1975b). The B-cell specificity repertoire: Its relationship to definable subpopulations. *Transplant. Rev.* **24**, 41.

Klinman, N. R., Press, J. L., Sigal, N. H., and Gearhart, P. J. (1976). The acquisition of the B-cell specificity repertoire: The germ-line theory of predetermined permutation of genetic information. *In* "The Generation of Antibody Diversity: A New Look" (A. J. Cunningham, ed.), pp. 127–147. Academic Press, New York.

Klinman, N. R., Wylie, D. W., and Cancro, M. P. (1980). Mechanisms that govern repertoire expression. *Prog. Immunol.* **4**, 124.

Köhler, G. (1976). Frequency of precursor cells against the enzyme galactosidase. An estimate of the BALB/c strain antibody repertoire. *Eur. J. Immunol.* **6**, 340.

Kreth, H. W., and Williamson, A. R. (1973). The extent of diversity of anti-hapten antibodies in inbred mice: Anti-NIP (4-hydroxy-5 iodo-3-nitrophenacetyl) antibodies in CBA/H mice. *Eur. J. Immunol.* **3**, 141.

Kurosawa, Y., and Tonegawa, S. (1982). Organization, structure and assembly of immunoglobulin heavy chain diversity DNA segments. *J. Exp. Med.* **155**, 201.

Lerner, R. A. (1982). Tapping the immunological repertoire to produce antibodies of predetermined specificity. *Nature (London)* **299**, 592.

Mac, E. E., Seidman, J. G., and Leder, P. (1979). Sequences of five potential recombination sites encoded close to an immunoglobulin K constant region gene. *Proc. Natl. Acad. Sci. U.S.A.* **76**, 3450.

Marshak-Rothstein, A., Seikevitz, M., Margolies, M. N., Mudgett-Hunter, M., and Geffner, M. L. (1980). Hybridoma proteins expressing the predominant idiotype of the antiazophenyarsonate response of A/J mice. *Proc. Natl. Acad. Sci. U.S.A.* **77**(2), 1120–1124.

Mosier, D. E., and Johnson, D. M. (1975). Ontogeny of mouse lymphocyte function. II. Development of the ability to produce antibody is modulated by T lymphocytes. *J. Exp. Med.* **141**, 216.

Osmond, D. G., and Nossal, G. J. V. (1974). Differentiation of lymphocytes in mouse bone marrow. II. Kinetics of maturation and renewal of anti-globulin binding cells studied by double labeling. *Cell. Immunol.* **13**, 132.

Owen, F. L. (1982). Products of the Ig T-C region of chromosome 12 are maturational markers for T-cells. *J. Exp. Med.* **156**(3), 703–718.

Owen, F. L., and Nisonoff, A. (1978). Effect of idiotype-specific suppressor T cells on primary and secondary responses. *J. Exp. Med.* **148**:182.

Owen, F. L., Ju, S.-T., and Nisonoff, A. (1977). Presence on idiotype-specific suppressor T cells of receptors that interact with molecules bearing the idiotype. *J. Exp. Med.* **145**, 1559.

Owen, F. L., Riblet, R., and Taylor, B. A. (1981). The T suppressor cell alloantigen Tsu[d] maps near immunoglobulin allotype genes and may be a heavy chain constant-region markers on a T-cell receptor. *J. Exp. Med.* **153**, 801–810.

Pierce, S. K., and Klinman, N. R. (1977). Antibody-specific immunoregulation. *J. Exp. Med.* **146**, 509.

Rowlands, D. T., Blakslee, D., and Angala, E. (1974). Acquired immunity in opossum (Didelphis Virginiana) embryos. *J. Immunol.* **112**, 2148.

Sherwin, W. K., and Rowlands, D. T. (1975). Determinants of the hierarchy of humoral immune responsiveness during ontogeny. *J. Immunol.* **115**, 1549.

Shimizu, A., Takahashi, N., Yaoita, Y., and Honjo, T. (1982). Organization of the constant-region gene family of the mouse immunoglobulin heavy chain. *Cell* **28**, 499.

Sidman, C. L., and Unanue, E. R. (1975). Development of B lymphocytes I. Cell populations and a critical event during ontogeny. *J. Immunol.* **114**, 1730.

Sigal, N. H. (1977). The frequency of p-azophenylarsonate and dimethylamino-naphthalene-sulfonyl-specific B cells in neonatal and adult BALB/c mice. *J. Immunol.* **119**, 1129.

Sigal, N. H. (1982). Regulation of azophenylarsonate-specific repertoire expression. I. Frequency of cross-reactive idiotype-positive B cells in A/J and BALB/c mice. *J. Exp. Med.* **156**, 1352.

Sigal, N. H., and Klinman, N. R. (1978). The B-cell clonotype repertoire. *Adv. Immunol.* **26**, 255.

Sigal, N. H., Press, P. J., and Klinman, N. R. (1976). Late acquisition of a germline specificity. *Nature (London)* **259**, 51.

Sigal, N. H., Pickard, A. R., Metcalf, E. S., Gearhart, P. J., and Klinman, N. R. (1977). Expression of phosphorylcholine-specific B cells during murine development. *J. Exp. Med.* **146**, 933.

Silverstein, A. M., Uhr, J. W., Kraner, K. L., and Lukes, R. J. (1963). Fetal response to antigenic stimulus. II. Antibody production by the fetal lamb. *J. Exp. Med.* **117**, 799.

Soper, K. (1980). "Use of Simpson's Index of Diversity to Compare Multinominal Populations with Small Samples," Res. Memo. DV2. Dept. of Research Medicine, University of Pennsylvania, Philadelphia.

Spear, P. G., Wang, A., Rutishauser, U., and Edelman, G. M. (1973). Characterization of splenic lymphoid cells in fetal and newborn mice. *J. Exp. Med.* **138**, 557.

Staudt, L., and Gerhard, W. (1982). The generation of antibody diversity in the immune response to influenza virus hemagglutinin. *J. Exp. Med.* **157**, 687.

Thompson, M. A., and Cancro, M. P. (1982). Dynamics of B-cell repertoire formation: Normal patterns of clonal turnover are altered by ligand interaction. *J. Immunol.* **129**, 2372.

Weigert, M., Perry, R., Kelly, D., Hunkapillar, T., Schilling, J., and Hood, L. (1980). The joining of V and J gene segments creates antibody diversity. *Nature (London)* **282**, 497.

Wybrow, G. M., and Berryman, I. L. (1973). Estimation of the pool size of different anti-NIP antibodies for the CBA/H strain. *Eur. J. Immunol.* **3**, 146.

Chapter 10

Ontogeny of Antilevan and Inulin Antibody Responses[1]

Constantin A. Bona and Carol Victor

Department of Microbiology
Mount Sinai School of Medicine
New York, New York

I. Introduction

The generation of the antibody repertoire occurs concomitantly with the development of the B-lymphocytic lineage. Pluripotential stem cells located within the hemopoietic sites in fetal liver generate the stem cell precursors of B cells, which first differentiate into pre-B cells and ultimately into virgin lymphocytes carrying Ig receptors. The differentiation of the B lineage from pluripotential stem cells to virgin lymphocytes is a genetically programmed as well as an antigen-independent process.

Recent observations have suggested that the rearrangement of the V, D, and J genomic segments which comprise the V_H gene from IgM probably occurs during the first stages of differentiation because pre-B

[1] This work was supported by grants PCM81105788 of National Science Foundation. Carol Victor is a Fuller Foundation Fellow.

cells are already clonally restricted and capable of synthesizing an intact μ-chain (Siden *et al.*, 1981). However, numerous studies on the ontogeny of the immune responses against various antigens have demonstrated a sequential activation mechanism for the expression of V genes. Silverstein (1977) observed in lambs that the immune responses to certain antigens such as ferritin, ovalbumin, and hemocyanin could be obtained during fetal life, whereas responses to diphtheria toxoid and BCG occurred only after 40 days of postnatal life. Numerous examinations of the idiotypy of various antibody responses in mice have revealed that only a fraction of the repertoire is expressed at birth. Thus, X24Id$^+$ antigalactan and 384Id$^+$ anti-LPS responses can be elicited in 1-day-old BALB/c mice subsequent to immunization with gum ghatti or *Salmonella tranaroa* LPS, respectively (Bona, 1980). In contrast, T15Id$^+$ antiphosphocholine and CRI$^+$ antiarsonate responses occur relatively late in the neonatal period and can be induced only 4–7 days after birth (Siegal *et al.*, 1976; Nutt *et al.*, 1979). Furthermore, the anti-α1-6 dextran response can be obtained only in adult mice (Fernandez and Moller, 1978). Taken together, these observations suggest that there is a sequential activation of V-region genes in various mammalian species. This phenomenon can be attributed to a preferred order of expression of V-gene families which may be a consequence of the order of these genes in embryonic DNA or, alternatively, of regulatory mechanisms. The study of the ontogeny of the antibacterial levan antibody response provides a useful model with which to investigate the cellular and genetic mechanisms responsible for the expression of V genes.

II. Characteristics of the Antibacterial Levan Immune Response

Levan and Inulin are polyfructosans that are especially suitable for studying an immune response, because they evoke a vigorous production of antibodies in various strains of mice. Bacterial levan (BL) is a β2-6 polyfructosan with β2-1 branch points, whereas Inulin (Inu) is a β2-1 linked polyfructosan. BL induces a T-independent immune response, as was concluded on the basis of a study of this response in nude mice (Bona *et al.*, 1978). Although Inulin itself is not immunogenic, it can elicit an antibody response when coupled to various carriers such as *Brucella abortus* (Bona *et al.*, 1978). BALB/c mice immunized with BL produce two types of antibodies. One family of antibodies displays specificity for both the β2-1 and β2-6 epitopes

(Bona *et al.*, 1978) and shares cross-reactive idiotypes (IdX) with several Inu-binding myeloma proteins.

Of 13 known polyfructosan-binding myeloma proteins, 11 bind both β2-1 and β2-6 epitopes. The IdX system of the Inu-binding myeloma proteins is polymorphic and composed of several IdXs, that is, IdXA, B, and G (Lieberman *et al.*, 1975). Both heavy and light chains appear to be required to express these IdXs (Lieberman *et al.*, 1977). The expression of these IdXs is under the control of *IghC* genes; however, the diversity of the repertoire is controlled by an autosomal gene, *Sr-1*. This gene is not linked to either the *MHC* or *IghC* gene complexes (Stein *et al.*, 1980).

The second family of antibodies binds only β2-6 fructosans. These antibodies do not share the IdXs of Inu-binding myeloma proteins (Bona *et al.*, 1978) or those of ABPC48 and UPC10, which bind only to β2-6 fructosan epitopes (Lieberman *et al.*, 1976). However, we have shown that A48 Id$^+$-bearing anti-β2-6 antibodies can be obtained in nude mice that have been IdX suppressed by administration of homologous anti-IdX antibodies (anti-E109Id) before immunization with BL. This observation strongly suggests that a fraction of the anti-β2-6 antibodies, particularly those that bear the A48Id, is silent in normal BALB/c mice.

Furthermore, our studies have shown that the anti-β2-6 fructosan antibody response can be obtained in 1-day-old BL immune mice, whereas the anti-β2-1 fructosan response can only be obtained 1 month later. A clear ontogenic dissociation exists between clones reactive for the two different eiptopes. Therefore, by studying the ontogeny of the anti-BL response, we are fortuitously provided with an excellent model with which to investigate the ontogeny of clones which recognize two different epitopes carried on the same molecule, that is, β2-6 and β2-1 fructosan epitopes.

III. Ontogeny of the β2-6 Fructosan Response

Immunization of 1- and 9-day-old mice with BL elicits the production of anti-BL antibodies, as demonstrated by an increased HA titer as well as the appearance of a number of anti-BL PFC. These antibodies lack the ability to bind to β2-1 fructosan epitopes and do not express the E109-IdX, indicating that they are directed solely against the β2-6 fructosan epitope (Bona *et al.*, 1979). In addition, these anti-β2-6 fructosan antibodies do not express A48Id or UPC10Id, which are also not present in adult mice. Because of the early appearance of the anti-B2-6 fructosan response, we assumed that the precursors of A48Id silent clones occur simultaneously with the precursors of A48Id⁻ anti-β2-6 fructosan clones. Therefore, we studied the activation of A48Id silent clones by injection at birth of A48Id-bearing monoclonal proteins, as well as by administration of anti-A48Id antibodies.

A. ACTIVATION OF A48Id CLONES BY PARENTERAL ADMINISTRATION AT BIRTH OF A48Id-BEARING MONOCLONAL PROTEINS

Administration at birth of A48Id-bearing monoclonal antibodies (10 μg) has a profound effect on the expansion of the precursors of the A48Id⁺ anti-β2-6 fructosan antibody-forming cells in BALB/c mice (Rubinstein *et al.*, 1982). Treatment with the monoclonal protein neonatally or even during the first weeks after birth led to the dominance of the A48Id in the anti-β2-6 fructosan antibody response. The A48 idiotype, which is expressed on the myeloma protein ABPC48, is probably composed of several idiotypes, some of which are shared by UPC10, another β2-6 fructosan-binding protein, as well as by monoclonal antibodies which we have recently prepared from animals producing anti-(anti-A48) idiotype antibodies (i.e., 76-Ab3-42). Treatment at birth with UPC10 or 76-Ab3-42 also led to a predominance of A48Id anti-β2-6 fructosan-binding antibodies. Rubinstein *et al.* (1982) showed that the activation of A48Id-producing clones subsequent to the administration at birth of A48Id-bearing monoclonal protein requires antigenic stimulation, because only those animals immunized with BL exhibited antibodies bearing A48 idiotypes. This phenomenon is idiotype specific as well. Indeed, in the sera of animals treated at birth with A48 monoclonal protein followed by immunization with BL and TNP-Ficoll, A48Id⁺ molecules but not 460Id⁺ were detected. Conversely, in mice treated at birth with MOPC460 and subsequently immunized with BL and TNP-Ficoll, only the level of the 460Id was increased as compared to a normal animal (Table I). Therefore, our results showed that the activation of A48Id silent clones achieved by administration at birth of A48Id monoclonal antibodies is idiotype specific and requires antigenic stimulation.

Two monoclonal antibodies have been obtained from BALB/c mice treated with A48 monoclonal protein, which bear only those A48 idiotypes not shared with the UPC10 monoclonal protein. Surprisingly, these two monoclonal antibodies bind to both β2-6 and β2-1 fructosan epitopes. Therefore, the binding specificity of these two monoclonal antibodies is very different from that of both A48 and

TABLE I

Specificity of Activation of A48Id Clones by Administration at Birth of
A48Id Monoclonal Protein[a]

Pretreatment at birth	Immunization with BL	Anti-BL response		Anti-TNP response	
		BL	A48Id	TNP	M460Id
—	—	—	—	nd	nd
—	BL	+++	—	nd	nd
A48	—	—	—	nd	nd
A48	BL	+++	+++	nd	nd
M460	BL	+++	—	—	—
M460	TNP Ficoll	—	—	+++	++

[a] The degree of response designated in a scale of − to +++ was determined by PFC response and RIA (Rubinstein et al., 1982). nd = not done.

UPC10, which bind only the β2-6 fructosan epitope. This strongly suggests that the A48Id can be shared by clones with different binding specificities.

B. GENETICS OF ACTIVATION OF A48Id SILENT CLONES

The genetic control of the activation of A48Id silent clones was studied in various BALB/c congenic strains of mice. Rubinstein and Bona (1983) showed that the activation of A48Id clones subsequent to the treatment of mice with 10 μg A48 monoclonal protein at birth is independent of *MHC* and *IghC* gene complexes (Table II). Interestingly, A48Id-bearing molecules occurred in strains bearing V_H^a genes (i.e., BALB/c, BAB.14, BALB.B, and BALB.K), as well as in strains bearing V_H^b genes (i.e., C.B20 and CBB R4) or V_H^d genes (i.e., CAL.20).

The A48Id seems to be encoded by a germline gene which is present in various strains of mice.

C. ACTIVATION OF A48Id SILENT CLONES IS RELATED TO THE EXPRESSION OF A48Id-SPECIFIC HELPER T CELLS

In response to immunization with BL, the production of A48Id-bearing antibodies is not seen in irradiated mice that have been in-

TABLE II

Genetics of Activation of A48Id Silent Clones[a]

Strain of mice	H-2	V_H	C_H	Treatment at birth	Anti-BL response			
					HA titer (log 2 units)	PFC response (per spleen)	A48Id (%)	RIA (A48Id µg/ml)
BALB/c	d	a	a	Nil	5.5 ± 0.3	7,833 ± 2,748	8 ± 4	<0.3
				A48	5.7 ± 0.6	21,133 ± 2,245	95 ± 1	82.4 ± 47.6
BALB.B	b	a	a	Nil	4.8 ± 1.1	24,067 ± 2,875	13 ± 7	0.7 ± 0.2
				A48	4.1 ± 0.7	869 ± 238	55 ± 14	32 ± 14.6
BALB.K	k	a	a	Nil	7.0 ± 3.0	16,100 ± 9,300	ND	ND
				A48	3.0 ± 1.1	ND	ND	18.3 ± 9.0
BAB.14	d	a	b	Nil	6.1 ± 0.4	18,975 ± 7,157	5 ± 5	ND
				A48	3.7 ± 1.2	4,511 ± 1,223	47 ± 12	15.2 ± 4.2
CCB.R4	d	b	a	Nil	28.0	8,050	0	ND
				A48	4.6 ± 0.5	1,811 ± 629	26 ± 8	27.1 ± 10.4
CAL.20	d	d	d	Nil	3.4 ± 0.2	7,028 ± 3,225	ND	<0.3
				A48	4.5 ± 0.5	1,375 ± 125	ND	63.0 ± 22

[a] Mice were injected at birth with 10 µg ABPC48 monoclonal protein and immunized 4–6 weeks later with 20 µg BL. The BL response was tested 5 days after immunization.

fused with B cells from mice treated at birth with A48. In contrast, the infusion of irradiated recipients with a mixture of T and B cells from A48-treated mice restored the ability to produce A48Id antibodies. The cells responsible for this effect bear Lyt1.2 alloantigens.

The subset of Lyt1.2$^+$ cells responsible for the predominance of the A48Id$^+$ response probably are themselves specific for the A48Id. Indeed, the activity of these cells can be ablated by incubation with A48+C'. Furthermore, on transfer into nude mice, they can help these animals mount an anti-TNP B-cell response subsequent to immunization with an A48-TNP$_{18}$ conjugate (Rubinstein *et al.*, 1982).

Therefore, these results suggest that treatment with A48 monoclonal protein at birth activates A48Id-specific helper T cells that select for the expansion following antigenic stimulation of those clones which express the A48Id on their Ig receptor.

IV. Ontogeny of the β2-1 Fructosan Response

The study of the ontogeny of the β2-1 fructosan response and of the IdXs of Inu-binding myeloma proteins shared by these antibodies has revealed that a substantial delay occurs in the activation of the V-gene family encoding them.

In 1–2-week-old BALB/c mice, we have detected Ig molecules bearing IdXA and IdXB. The titer of these antibodies was not affected by immunization with BL or In-BA. Furthermore, the IdXA$^+$- or IdXB$^+$-bearing molecules could not be removed with either Inu or levan-SRBC (Bona *et al.*, 1979), indicating either that they were devoid of β2-1- and β2-6-binding activity or that they were not associated with high-affinity antibodies. The precursors of such IdXA$^+$-secreting cells found in 1-week-old mice are interesting candidates for the antecedents of IdXG$^+$-, A$^+$-, and B$^+$-bearing anti-Inu antibodies, which are indeed produced by older BALB/c mice subsequent to immunization with BL. However, the possibility cannot be excluded that the cells producing these antibodies represent an independent lineage which synthesizes a parallel set with a different antigen-binding activity.

Study of the ontogeny of the IdXA, B, and G anti-β2-1 antibody response in BALB/c mice by hemagglutination (HA), plaque-forming cells (PFC), and isoelectric-focusing (IEF) assays indicated that they occur long after birth. A weak anti-β2-1 fructosan PFC response was first observed in 21-day-old mice, with a substantial increase at 28 days. The majority of anti-β2-1 fructosan antibodies bear IdXA, B, and G in adult mice.

Several experimental findings support the concept that the late oc-currence of anti-β2-1 fructosan antibodies is related to a true onto-genic delay in the activation of the precursor of antibody-forming cells. Thus, *in vitro* stimulation with B-cell mitogens of spleen cells from young BALB/c mice failed to elicit an anti-β2-1 fructosan re-sponse. It is known that B-cell polyclonal activators could activate precursors in their very early stages (Anderson *et al.*, 1977) and even induce their proliferation in mice tolerized to polysaccharide antigens (i.e., α1-6 dextran) (Fernandez *et al.*, 1979) or to various allotypes (Bona and Cazenave, 1977). We studied the occurrence of anti-Inu PFC after stimulating cells from 1–4-week-old BALB/c mice *in vitro* with NWSM. Although a significant [^{3}H]thymidine incorporation by the spleen cells of 1-week-old mice was observed, an anti-β2-1 fructo-san response was not detected until the donors were 4 weeks of age.

In order to investigate whether the failure of young BALB/c mice to produce anti-β2-1 fructosan antibodies could be attributed to a prob-lem with the presentation of the antigen, we studied whether Inu or BL conjugated to carriers known to stimulate B cells might induce their appearance. Inu or BL conjugated to *Brucella abortus*, NWSM, or SRBC were ineffective in eliciting a β2-1 fructosan response in young BALB/c mice. These results suggested that the anti-β2-1 fructo-san antibody response is not related to the presentation of antigen to the specific antibody-forming cells.

Furthermore, we showed in transfer experiments that this onto-genic delay is not caused by the absence of environmental antigens. We found that the IdX$^+$ anti-β2-1 fructosan response of 1-week-old BALB/c spleen cells infused into a 300-rad-irradiated adult C.B20 mouse was delayed until 7–14 days after cell transfer. The C.B20 strain is an H-2^d congenic BALB/c mouse that bears the IghV^b and IghC^b and is therefore unable to develop an IdX$^+$ anti-β2-1 fructosan response. The infusion of 1-week-old BALB/c lymphocytes into adult C.B20 mice caused the recipients to develop an anti-β2-1 fructosan response and corresponded to the time required for the maturation of the response in BALB/c mice. Therefore, these results indicated that the lack of an anti-β2-1 fructosan antibody response was not related to the expansion of precursors induced by environmental antigens or to the lack of maturity of accessory cells.

Finally, this substantial ontogenic delay was not related to an active cell-mediated suppressive mechanism functioning in young mice. The transfer of 1-day-old spleen cells into adult BALB/c mice did not alter the anti-β2-1 fructosan response of the recipients. Conversely, the transfer of adult cells into neonates did not prevent the development of an IdX^+ anti-β2-1 fructosan response (Bona *et al.*, 1979). However, a study on the influences of anti-Id antibodies, via *in utero* exposure or neonatal injection, demonstrated that they exert a profound effect on the activation of clones capable of producing IdX^+ anti-β2-1 fructosan antibodies.

The influence of maternal idiotype suppression was studied in the progeny of C.B20 females immunized with the E109 monoclonal protein ($IdXG^+$, A^+, B^-) prior to their mating with BALB/c males. The anti-β2-1 response of these mice was studied at 1 month of age, subsequent to their immunization with BL, and was compared to the response obtained either from normal (C.B20 × BALB/c)F_1 mice or from mice originating from a cross of a C.B20 female immunized with XRPC24 (a galactan-binding myeloma protein of unrelated idiotype) prior to being mated to a BALB/c male. The anti-β2-1 response was completely suppressed in these mice, as assessed by HA, IEF, and PFC assays (Bona *et al.*, 1979). Although no $IdXA^+$, B^+, and G^+ β2-1 fructosan-binding molecules have been detected, we have found in these mice IdXA-bearing Ig molecules devoid of Inu-binding activity. The presence of IdXA-bearing Ig molecules in maternally idiotype-suppressed mice suggested that *in utero* exposure to anti-Id antibodies did not entirely affect the β2-1 fructosan idiotype repertoire. This observation is consistent with our previous finding of $IdXA^+$ molecules devoid of anti-Inu activity in 1–2-week-old BALB/c mice. The clones secreting such molecules can represent a parallel set under the control of completely different regulatory mechanisms.

An equally long-lasting suppression was also obtained by injection of anti-E109 or anti-W3082 (an $IdXG^+$, A^+, B^+ monoclonal protein) idiotypic antibodies into 1-day-old BALB/c mice. Animals treated as neonates with A/J anti-E109Id antibodies did not produce $IdXA^+$ and $IdXG^+$ anti-β2-1 fructosan antibodies until 80 days of age, and those injected with anti-W3082 idiotypic antibodies were suppressed even longer (Bona *et al.*, 1979).

Suppression of the IdX^+ anti-β2-1 fructosan response by *in utero* exposure or parenteral neonatal administration of anti-IdX antibodies is at first somewhat surprising in view of the ontogenic delay of the anti-β2-1 fructosan response.

In the BL-Inu system, we do not yet have information regarding the cellular mechanisms responsible for maternal or neonatal suppression. By contrast, we have recently observed alterations in the cellular expression of the J558 Id of α1-3 dextran-specific antibodies in (A/J × BALB/c)F_1 mice originating from A/J females immunized with the J558 monoclonal protein prior to their mating with BALB/c males. A long-lasting suppression of the total anti-α1-3 dextran response was observed in J558 Id maternally suppressed mice (Victor *et al.*, 1983b). However, in spite of the profound suppression of the J558 Id$^+$, anti-α1-3 dextran response, we observed a high percentage of lymphocytes fluorescently staining with the monoclonal anti-J558 IdI-specific antibody, EB 3-7-2.

A high frequency of Id-bearing cells was also reported in maternally 460Id-suppressed mice. The increased percentage of 460Id-bearing cells was attributed to the polyclonal effect of anti-460Id antibodies, which presumably induced the proliferation of lymphocytes bearing 460Id-like structures on the mitogen receptors (Bernabe *et al.*, 1981).

Surprisingly, in the J558 system, we found that lymphocytes bearing the J558Id belong to both the T and B subpopulations. Indeed, we found that 3% of lymphocytes were costained with anti-Thy-1.2 monoclonal antibody and that the remaining 2.5% of lymphocytes bearing the J558IdI receptor were cocapped with monoclonal anti-IgM and anti-IgD antibodies. Furthermore, the J558IdI$^+$ T cells exhibited Lyt2.2 alloantigens and were able to suppress 60% of the total anti-α1-3 dextran response when transferred in normal (A/J $\times$ BALB/c)F$_1$ mice. These results indicate that *in utero* exposure to anti-Id antibodies has a profound effect on clones bearing the corresponding Id$^+$ receptor. These antibodies induce a strong expansion of IdI-bearing precursors of both T and B lymphocytes despite the long-lasting suppression of the J558IdX and IdI anti-α1-3 dextran responses. The expansion of J558IdI-bearing suppressor T cells probably is responsible for the observed suppression of the anti-α1-3 dextran response because these cells were identified only in idiotype-suppressed mice. Indeed, the expanded population of IdI$^+$ B cells are probably being stimulated by dextran but are being prohibited to respond by their IdI$^+$ T-cell counterparts. Id$^+$ T cells exhibiting suppressor activity were identified in other antigenic systems such as T15, antilysozyme, (T,G)A-L,A5AId$^+$ anti-A-CHO antibody responses (Kim, 1979; Adorni *et al.*, 1979; Mozes and Haimovich, 1979; Eichmann *et al.*, 1978).

The failure of the EB3-7-2 anti-J558IdI monoclonal antibody to induce the proliferation of adult spleen cells or of various LPS-sensitive Abelson lines (Victor *et al.*, 1983) strongly indicates that the expansion of IdI-bearing cells subsquent to *in utero* exposure to anti-Id antibodies is not mediated through an interaction of the anti-Id antibodies with an Id$^+$ Ig$^-$ receptor.

V. Conclusions

The ontogeny of the BL response was studied in an attempt to investigate the role that cellular factors as well as genetic influences play in the activation and expression of V-region genes. BL, a β2-6-linked polyfructosan with β2-1 linked branch points, evokes in BALB/c mice an immune response which is characterized by two distinct families of antibodies, each demonstrating a unique ontogenic schedule. The first family is composed of antibodies that are specific for the β2-1 and β2-6 epitopes of BL and display the IdXs shared by 11 Inu-binding myeloma proteins (i.e., IdX A, B, and G) and are first detected in the sera of BL-immune animals that are at least 1 month old. The second group is typified by antibodies that are specific only for the β2-6 epitope, do not express any of the IdXs that are associated with β2-6 polyfructosan-binding myelomas such as ABPC48 and UPC10, and are evocable in 1-day-old mice immunized with BL. Our studies on the ontogeny of this latter family of antibodies indicated that although those antibodies under normal circumstances never express the A48Id, BL-reactive clones displaying this idiotype do exist but are simply not expressed. These clones can be activated by treating the mice with a mere 10 μg of the A48Id-bearing monoclonal proteins. This activation is independent of either *MHC* or *IghC* gene complexes and appears to be mediated via an A48Id-specific Ly1.2$^+$ T helper cell. In contrast to this group, studies on the ontogeny of the first group of antibodies have been directed at elucidating the reason this response appears so late in the ontogeny. Although IdXA$^+$ and B$^+$ molecules have been detected in the sera of 1–2-week-old mice, they are devoid of any β2-1 or β2-6 binding activity, and their titers remain refractory to the effects of immunization with BL. These clones can represent either forebears of the BL-reactive ones or simply members of a parallel set under separate control. Our observations definitely established that the ontogenic delay of β2-1 fructosan clones is not attributable to the lack of stimulation by environmental antigens, an immaturity of accessory cells, or an active suppressive mechanism prevalent in young mice. Curiously enough, in spite of the substantial ontogenic delay in the expression of β2-1 fructosan-binding antibodies bearing the relevant idiotypes, these clones can be expressed by exposure *in utero* or neonatally to anti-Id generated against E109 or W3082 monoclonal proteins.

Among the many hypotheses that can be suggested to explain how this suppression occurs is the possibility that anti-E109Id antibodies persist until the precursors appear, or alternatively, that the precursors are present in the young animal and are only sensitive to tolerogenic stimuli.

The third hypothesis is that of an anti-Id generation of suppressor T cells, which has in fact been rigorously demonstrated in the α1-3 dextran system. Indeed, CAF_1 mice born of A/J females with anti-J558Id immunity exhibited a long-lasting suppression of the α1-3 dextran response as well as a marked increase in the percentage of lymphocytes bearing J558Id on their membranes. The J558Id$^+$ cells included cells from the B lineage as well as Lyt2.2$^+$ T cells that were capable of transferring the suppression to naive hosts. In contrast to the B cells that bore the J558IdX and IdI, the T cells displayed only the IdI, a determinant known to lie in the third hypervariable region at amino acids 100 and 101 and to be encoded by the D segment. By not expressing the IdX, known to be encoded by the V gene at amino acids 54 and 55 in the second hypervariable region, these cells may indeed display no VDJ gene rearrangement, but only a DJ rearrangement leading to the expression of IdI which has been presumed to be nonfunctional.

Our data suggest that this D-J rearrangement may contribute significantly to the construction of the T-cell receptor.

References

Adorni, L., Harvey, M., and Sercarz, E. E. (1979). *Eur. J. Immunol.* **9**, 900.

Anderson, J., Coutinho, A., and Melchers, F. (1977). *J. Exp. Med.* **145**, 1577.

Bernabe, R. H., Coutinho, A., Cazenave, P.-A., and Forni, L. (1981). *Proc. Natl. Acad. Sci. U.S.A.* **78**, 6416.

Bona, C. (1980). *Am. J. Reprod. Immunol.* **1**, 35.

Bona, C., and Cazenave, P.-A. (1977). *J. Exp. Med.* **146**, 881.

Bona, C., Lieberman, R., Chien, C. C., Mond, J., House, S., Green, I., and Paul, W. E. (1978). *J. Immunol.* **120**, 1436.

Bona, C., Mond, J. J., Stein, K. E., House, S., Lieberman, R., and Paul, W. E. (1979). *J. Immunol.* **123**, 1484.

Bona, C., Stein, K. E., Lieberman, R., and Paul, W. E. (1979). *Mol. Immunol.* **16**, 1093.

Eichmann, K., Falk, I., and Rajewsky, K. (1978). *Eur. J. Immunol.* **8**, 853.

Fernandez, C., and Möller, G. (1978). *J. Exp. Med.* **147**, 645.

Fernandez, C., Hammarström, L., Möller, G., Primi, D., and Smith, E. (1979). *Immunol. Rev.* **43**, 3.

Kim, B. S. (1979). *J. Exp. Med.* **149**, 1371.

Lieberman, R., Potter, M., Humphrey, W., Jr., Mushinski, E. B., and Vrana, M. (1975). *J. Exp. Med.* **142**, 106.

Lieberman, R., Potter, M., Humphrey, W., Jr., and Chien, C. C. (1976). *J. Immunol.* **117**, 2105.

Lieberman, R., Vrana, M., Humphrey, W., Jr., Chien, C. C., and Potter, M. (1977). *J. Exp. Med.* **146**, 1234.

Mozes, E., and Haimovich, J. (1979). *Nature (London)* **278**, 56.

Nutt, N. B., Weisel, A. N., and Nisonoff, A. (1979). *Eur. J. Immunol.* **9**, 864.

Rubinstein, L. J., and Bona, C. A. (1983). *Ann. N.Y. Acad. Sci.* **418**, 97.

Rubinstein, L. J., Yeh, M., and Bona, C. A. (1982). *J. Exp. Med.* **156**, 506.

Siden, E., Alt, F. W., Shinefeld, L., Sato, V., and Baltimore, D. (1981). *Proc. Natl. Acad. Sci. U.S.A.* **78**, 1823.

Siegal, N. H., Gerhart, P. J., Press, J. L., and Klinman, N. R. (1976). *Nature (London)* **259**, 51.

Silverstein, A. M. (1977). *In* "Development of Host Defense" (M. Cooper and D. Dayton, eds.), pp. 1–19. Raven Press, New York.

Stein, K. E., Bona, C. A., Lieberman, R., Chien, C. C., and Paul, W. E. (1980). *J. Exp. Med.* **151**, 1088.

Victor, C., Bona, C. A., and Pernis, B. (1983a). *J. Immunol.* **130**, 1819.

Victor, C., Bona, C. A., and Pernis, B. (1983b). *Ann. N.Y. Acad. Sci.* **418**, 220.

Chapter 11

Selective Alteration of the Humoral Response to α1-3 Dextran and Phosphorylcholine by Early Administration of Monoclonal Antiidiotype Antibody

Brian A. Pollok, Robert Stohrer, and John F. Kearney

Cellular Immunobiology Unit of the Tumor Institute
The Comprehensive Cancer Center and Department of Microbiology
University of Alabama in Birmingham
Birmingham, Alabama

I. Introduction

The capacity of antiidiotype (anti-Id) immunoglobulin to ablate chronically the corresponding B-cell response in mice exposed during the early stages of life has been documented by a host of investigators in several antigen–idiotype systems. In most of these studies, the anti-Id reagents used to manipulate a particular immune response were heterologous preparations (of xenogeneic or allogeneic origin) which probably contain antibodies recognizing a variety of idiotypic determinants such as (a) V_L- and V_H-associated idiotopes (possibly reactive with T cells; Eichmann, 1978), (b) framework-localized idiotypic determinants, and (c) binding site-associated idiotypes (requiring paired V_H–V_L chains). The immunoglobulin subclasses of the anti-Id antibodies in most heterologous anti-Id preparations are often not characterized; because certain isotypes appear to exhibit distinct immunoregulatory activities (Eichmann, 1974; Kelsoe et al., 1981), it is obviously important that the different functional properties of immunoglobulin isotypes be considered.

The above issues can be circumvented by the use of monoclonal antiidiotype antibodies (MAIDs) to induce idiotype-specific unresponsiveness in vivo. We have used panels of hybridomas secreting well-defined MAIDs reactive with the dominant T15 idiotype present in the antiphosphorylcholine (PC) response and with major idiotypes found in the anti-α1-3 dextran (DEX) response to establish an idiotype-specific suppressed state in neonatal mice (directly and maternally). The pattern and mechanism of B-cell unresponsiveness resulting from both direct and maternal administration of these MAIDs are discussed.

II. Description of Methodology

A. GENERATION AND SPECIFICITIES OF MAIDs

Monoclonal allogeneic (A/J, SJL) and syngeneic (BALB/c) antiidiotype antibodies were constructed by fusing the nonsecreting BALB/c plasmacytoma line P3x63Ag8.653 (Kearney et al., 1979) with lymph node cells from mice immunized with the myeloma proteins HOPC 8 (for anti-T15 Id), J558 (for anti-J558 Id), or MOPC 104E (for anti-M104 Id). The specificity and isotype of each MAID used in these studies are given in Table I. The BALB/c anti-anti-T15 Id antibody MM-60, which is specific for the anti-T15 MAID GB4-10, was derived from a fusion of Streptococcus pneumoniae strain R36A-immunized spleen cells and Ag8.653 (Pollok et al., 1982).

B. EXPERIMENTAL PROCEDURES

1. Treatment with MAID in Vivo

To induce T15 idiotype-specific unresponsiveness directly in neonatal BALB/c mice, 2 μg of MAID was given ip 24–48 h after birth. In

TABLE I

Specificity of Monoclonal Antiidiotype Antibodies

PC system

Anti-PC antibodies

| MAID | Isotype | T15+ | | | | | T15− | | | Id-positive anti-PC IgM (%) | |
		TEPC15	HOPC8	HPCG11	C3	PC123	M511	M603	HPCM3	Hybridomas	Serum antibody
ABI-2	$\gamma_1\kappa$	■	■	■	■	■				85	86–100
GB4-10	$\gamma_1\kappa$	■	■	■	■					80	83–100

α1-3 DEX

Anti-DEX antibodies

| MAID | Isotype | J558+ | | | | | J558− | | Id-positive anti-DEX Ig (%) | |
		J558+	HDEX-9	3-19	1-8	1-21	HDEX-36	M104	Hybridomas	Serum antibody
CD3-2	$\gamma_1\lambda$	■	■	■	■	■	■		81	Variable[a]
EB3-7	$\gamma_1\kappa$	■	■	■	■	■			57	5–95
EB3-16	$\gamma_1\kappa$	■	■	■	■				5	0–90
SJL18-1	$\mu\kappa$							■	35	1–85

[a] CD3-2 levels cannot be accurately quantitated.

the DEX system, Id-specific unresponsiveness was achieved by injecting 50 μg of MAID on alternate days from day 1 to day 15. Exposure of neonates to MAID via the mother was accomplished either (a) *in utero*, with 100 μg of MAID delivered ip 2 days prior to the birth of the litter, or (b) postpartum, in which case the mother was given 100 μg of MAID ip 24 h after giving birth. In all three cases, the MAID-treated mice were reared for at least 6 weeks prior to challenge with antigen. Control and experimental mice (a minimum of five per group) were always age matched.

2. Assay for Immunologic Unresponsiveness

MAID-exposed mice were challenged ip at 6–8 weeks with the appropriate T-independent type 2 antigen. In the PC–T15 system, 2×10^8 heat-killed *S. pneumoniae* R36A cells were given, and in the DEX system, 100 μg of dextran B1355S was injected. Mice were bled from the retroorbital plexus on days 5 and 7 after challenge, respectively. Antigen-binding and idiotype-bearing immunoglobulin levels present in the serum samples from suppressed and control mice were quantitated using a solid-phase enzyme-linked immunosorbent assay (ELISA) (Kearney *et al.*, 1981).

3. Adoptive Transfer

Cell-transfer experiments were carried out using the procedures described by Owen *et al.* (1977). All irradiated (200 rads) recipients received a total of 2×10^7 donor cells and were then challenged 3 days after transfer with a single dose of R36A vaccine; their serum antibody was assayed 5 days afterward, as described. T lymphocytes were depleted using complement in conjunction with monoclonal AKR anti-Thy-1.2 (a gift from Dr. G. Hammerling). B lymphocytes were depleted by two successive panning cycles on plastic Petri dishes coated with purified goat antimouse Ig, resulting in <3% B cells remaining (Mage *et al.*, 1977).

4. Splenic Focus Assay

Spleen cells from normal or EB3-7-suppressed BALB/c mice were transferred at limiting dilutions (about 3×10^7 cells) to normal irradiated (1400 rads) recipient BALB/c mice (65 and 6 recipients, respectively). From 18 to 24 h later, recipient spleens were diced into 1-mm cubes and cultured in complete Dulbecco's modified Eagle's medium (DMEM) with 10% fetal calf serum and 2 ng/ml dextran B1355S in sterile 96-well microtiter plates (Ward and Kohler, 1981). Culture supernatants were collected every 4 days and assayed for DEX-binding antibody, isotype expression, and idiotype expression by ELISA.

III. Id-Specific B-Cell Unresponsiveness after MAID Exposure

A. DIRECT TREATMENT OF NEONATES

The panel of MAIDs used in this study of BALB/c anti-DEX responses is specific for individual idiotopes on either J558 or M104E myeloma proteins (IdI) or for idiotopes present on both proteins (IdX), as shown by Clevinger *et al.* (1980). Table II shows the effects on the

TABLE IIA

DEX-Specific Antibody Levels after Direct Neonatal
Exposure to MAIDs

MAID	λ^+ Serum Ig (μg/ml $\pm$ SE)[a]			
	Anti-DEX	EB3-7$^+$	EB3-16$^+$	SJL18-1$^+$
CD3-2	75.6 (1.5)	0.8 (1.3)	3.6 (2.6)	<0.5
EB3-7	166.4 (1.5)	<0.5	<0.5	138.1 (1.6)
EB3-16	218.9 (1.4)	31.8 (1.4)	<0.5	9.8 (1.9)
SJL18-1	344.8 (1.2)	54.0 (1.6)	26.5 (2.6)	<0.5
Saline	663.1 (1.2)	379.6 (1.1)	5.8 (1.7)	50.8 (1.4)

[a] Geometric mean (all tables).

TABLE IIB

PC-Specific Antibody Levels after Direct Neonatal
Exposure to MAIDs

MAID	Serum IgM (μg/ml $\pm$ SE)[a]		
	Anti-PC	AB1-2$^+$	GB4-10$^+$
AB1-2	28.3 (3.7)	<0.1	<0.1
GB4-10	31.4 (3.7)	2.4 (1.0)	<0.1
MM-60	18.5 (3.8)	5.1 (1.4)	4.8 (1.4)
Saline	22.5 (2.7)	22.0 (3.1)	21.3 (2.6)

[a] Arithmetic mean (all tables).

adult anti-DEX response after administration of these MAIDs during the first 14 days of life. Treatment of neonatal mice with EB3-7 resulted in complete and chronic suppression of the J558 IdI portion of the anti-DEX response. The M104E IdI and IdX portions of the response were unaffected by EB3-7 treatment, as were the total λ-bearing anti-DEX levels. There was no detectable EB3-7-positive antibody observed after DEX challenge for periods of up to 1 year after treatment. Analysis of DEX-binding hybridomas shows that EB3-7 defines a large subset of J558 IdI-positive hybridoma antibodies (Clevinger *et al.*, 1981), whereas the idiotopes defined by EB3-16, BD5-3, and AB3-7 are expressed on smaller subsets of J558 Id$^+$ anti-DEX antibodies and are always associated with the EB3-7 idiotope (R. Stohrer and J. F. Kearney, unpublished). Neonatal exposure to EB3-7 completely abolishes expression of these idiotopes in the anti-DEX response (20–50% of control mice express high levels of the EB3-16, BD5-3, and AB3-7 idiotopes). When EB3-16 is injected into neonates, expression of the EB3-16$^+$ portion of the anti-DEX response is ablated, along with the expression of the idiotopes defined by BD5-3 and AB3-7. The EB3-7 and SJL18-1 idiotope levels also appear to be lowered, although they are still within control ranges. The total amount of λ-bearing anti-DEX antibody was similar to control levels.

An opposing pattern of unresponsiveness is obtained when neonatal mice are suppressed with SJL18-1, which recognizes a M104E IdI determinant. When SJL18-1-treated mice are challenged at 6–8 weeks of age, the M104E IdI levels (defined by SJL18-1) are undetectable. The J558 IdI, IdX, and total λ-bearing anti-DEX antibody are all unaffected, and their levels are comparable to those found in control mice.

The results obtained by neonatal suppression with IdI-specific MAIDs contrast to the effects produced by CD3-2, which recognizes a cross-reactive idiotope expressed on J558, MOPC 104E, and most λ-bearing anti-DEX antibodies. Neonatal treatment with CD3-2 results in a slight depression of the λ-bearing anti-DEX antibody level, accompanied by a complete failure in most mice to produce anti-DEX antibodies expressing the EB3-7, BD5-3, AB3-7, and SJL18-1 idiotopes. The EB3-16 idiotope is expressed at high levels in approximately 29% of suppressed individuals, and in these cases accounts for nearly all of the anti-DEX antibody. It is apparent that the EB3-16 idiotope can be expressed on CD3-2-negative antibody and that clones expressing this idiotopic profile are expanded in CD3-2-suppressed mice.

When certain idiotopes on anti-DEX antibodies are associated, they are concomitantly suppressed by a MAID directed against the inclusive idiotope, whereas the expression of nonassociated idiotopes is unaffected. EB3-7 and SJL18-1 exhibit distinct specificities for anti-DEX myeloma and hybridoma proteins of the J558 and M104E idiotype families, respectively. Because these MAIDs affect only those portions of the anti-DEX response for which they are specific, it may be inferred that the cellular mechanisms involved in maintaining unresponsiveness into adult life exhibit the exquisite specificities characteristic of this panel of MAIDs.

In the PC system, treatment of BALB/c neonates with the monoclonal antiidiotype AB1-2 consistently produced complete and chronic suppression of the T15 component of the anti-PC response, although the total response was only slightly diminished (Table II). The difference in anti-PC antibody levels between the two groups after primary challenge is lost as the mice age or after they receive a secondary challenge of antigen. Preimmune and immune sera from these mice also do not contain significant amounts of classically defined T15-positive antibody ($<1\%$ of the total amount of anti-PC serum antibody), which was determined by using a goat anti-T15 Id antibody preparation in the solid-phase ELISA (data not shown). Because the idiotope specificity of AB1-2 appears to encompass all immunoglobulins belonging to the T15 group of anti-PC antibodies (Kearney *et al.*, 1981), the pattern of unresponsiveness following neonatal treatment with AB1-2 was expected to parallel that found using heterologous anti-"pan" T15 reagents (Augustin and Cosenza, 1976).

Neonatal treatment with GB4-10, a distinct anti-T15 MAID, provides more insight into the nature of T15 idiotype-specific unresponsiveness that can be induced in this system. Mice treated neonatally with this antibody usually produce a significant proportion of T15$^+$ antibody within the total serum anti-PC IgM pool, but produce undetectable levels of anti-PC immunoglobulin expressing the GB4-10 idiotope. Evidently, the small set of T15$^+$ B cells which lack the GB4-10 idiotope are not inactivated by neonatal treatment with GB4-10 and expand in response to PC antigen to produce anti-PC antibodies of the AB1-2$^+$, GB4-10$^-$ phenotype [this situation can also be generated by treating adult mice with GB4-10, followed by repeated immunization with PC antigen (Kearney *et al.*, 1981)].

The induction of idiotype suppression, discussed above, resulted from administration of MAIDs. However, T15 Id-specific unresponsiveness can also be accomplished by treating neonates with MM-60 ($\mu\lambda$), a monoclonal BALB/c anti-anti-T15 antibody that recognizes an idiotope on the GB4-10 molecule (Pollok *et al.*, 1982). An important difference between the suppression protocols required when using

MM-60 as compared with AB1-2 is that MM-60 must be administered to the neonate after day 4 of life in order to detect subsequent MM-60-dependent immunoregulatory effects on the anti-PC responses of adult mice. This requirement probably results from the need for MM-60 to be introduced *in vivo* at a point during the ontogeny of the "GB4-10" anti-T15 B-cell clone when it is functional, because clearance of MM-60, an IgM molecule, will be much more rapid than that of IgG (Waldmann and Strober, 1969). The suppression of T15$^+$ immunoglobulin production in adult mice given MM-60 as neonates is neither as complete nor as permanent as that resulting from the neonatal treatment with anti-T15 MAIDs. Partial recovery of responsiveness among T15$^+$ B cells in these mice is apparent at 12 weeks because 2–32% of their anti-PC IgM express the T15 idiotype (defined by reactivity with AB1-2). This variance reflects differences in the way unresponsiveness occurs in MM-60-treated mice as compared with anti-T15-treated mice (Pollok and Kearney, 1983) and may stimulate regulatory mechanisms which occur during normal anti-PC responses because suppression of T15$^+$ idiotype B cells in MM-60-treated neonates and adults is a reversible phenomenon.

The pattern of B-cell unresponsiveness produced by administration of those MAIDs that recognize a subset of antibodies within a major idiotype family (e.g., GB4-10 and EB3-16) is largely idiotope specific. Naturally, if concomitant expression of idiotopes occurs (e.g., all GB4-10$^+$ antibodies are also AB1-2$^+$), an idiotope-specific pattern of unresponsiveness will not develop in mice treated with the MAID of the broadest specificity (in this case, AB1-2). Studies by Takemori *et al.* (K. Rajewsky, personal communication) in the NP^b system and by Marshak-Rothstein *et al.* (1981) in the Ars system showed that MAIDs specific for such private idiotopes can suppress mice when administered *in vivo*; the independent segregation in expression of certain idiotopes among serum antibodies produced by such suppressed mice was also observed.

If active suppression of B cells occurs as a result of antiidiotypic suppressor T cells in these systems, then this kind of suppression must necessarily be idiotope specific to allow idiotope-negative variants to escape from their regulatory action. In the case of neonatal treatment with GB4-10, any proposed cellular mechanism that would directly regulate GB4-10$^+$ anti-PC B-cell clones could not be directed toward those idiotopes shared by GB4-10$^+$ and GB4-10$^-$ antibodies of the T15 family, including all public, framework, and binding site-associated determinants, because the GB4-10-defined determinant is dependent on a particular D-region structure (Kearney *et al.*, 1983).

B. INDIRECT TREATMENT OF NEONATES VIA MATERNAL ROUTES

Idiotype suppression via maternal routes was first reported by Weiler *et al.* (1977) using the α1-3 dextran system. This was accomplished by immunization of SJL females with J558 prior to mating with BALB/c males. The vast majority (111 of 112) of the F_1 progeny were suppressed for anti-DEX antibody and the J558 idiotype up to 12 weeks of age. With increasing age after 12 weeks, a greater percentage of the suppressed progeny was capable of producing anti-DEX antibody. Mice that escaped suppression at 20 weeks of age were tested for expression of the J558 idiotype, and about 40% were found to lack it. It was also shown that the suppressive agent was transmitted through the milk. All F_1 mice from J558-immunized SJL mothers were suppressed when nursed by a J558-immunized SJL mother, but when members of the same litter were nursed by a normal SJL mother, only approximately 40% of the mice were found to be significantly suppressed. Maternal suppression has also been reported by Bona (1979) in the levan–inulin system and by Cosenza *et al.* (1977) in the PC system.

Administration of 100 μg of EB3-7 to BALB/c mothers 1–4 days before birth produces a pattern of B-cell unresponsiveness identical to that resulting from direct neonatal treatment with EB3-7 (Table III), although a lower total effective dose of antibody per neonate is probably realized. Administration of 100 μg of SJL18-1 to pregnant females failed to suppress specifically the M104E IdI component of the anti-DEX response. The failure of SJL18-1 to effect maternally transmitted suppression, in contrast to its efficacy when directly administered to newborn mice, is attributable to the fact that SJL18-1 is an IgM antibody and is thus unable to cross the placental barrier (Waldman and Strober, 1969).

Suppression of the J558 IdI can also be induced by administration of EB3-7 to the mother after birth of the litter. As shown (Table III), the EB3-7 idiotope is not expressed in the anti-DEX response when these mice are challenged with antigen in adult life. This suppression is probably caused by transport of EB3-7 into the milk, which after ingestion is absorbed into the blood and tissues of the suckling neonate. Evidence for this mechanism has been provided in other antigen systems (Weiler *et al.*, 1977) and also appears to be involved in the maternal transmission of T15$^+$ B-cell unresponsiveness using AB1-2 as outlined below.

A previous study on maternal transmission of idiotype-specific sup-

TABLE IIIA

DEX-Specific Antibody Levels Following
Maternal Treatment with MAIDs

		λ^+ Serum Ig (μg/ml $\pm$ SE)		
MAID	Route	Anti-DEX	EB3-7$^+$	SJL18-1$^+$
EB3-7	*In utero*	318.2 (1.6)	<0.5	48.3 (1.9)
EB3-7	Postpartum	794.0 (1.3)	<0.5	157.3 (1.5)
Control (GB4-10)	Postpartum	478.5 (1.1)	137.4 (1.3)	82.0 (1.7)

TABLE IIIB

PC-Specific Antibody Levels Following Maternal Treatment with MAIDs

		Serum IgM (μg/ml $\pm$ SE)		
MAID	Route	Anti-PC	AB1-2$^+$	GB4-10$^+$
AB1-2	*In utero*	26.9 (2.4)	<0.2	<0.2
AB1-2	Postpartum	29.7 (3.7)	1.8 (1.3)	1.7 (1.1)
Saline	*In utero*	22.5 (3.3)	21.2 (3.0)	20.4 (3.1)

pression in the PC system (Cosenza *et al.*, 1977) reported that injection of a heterologous anti-T15 idiotype antibody into the mother prior to birth did not alter the idiotypic profile of the anti-PC response among the progeny. In contrast, we found that injection of a monoclonal anti-T15 idiotype antibody (AB1-2) into the mother (ip) prior to birth permanently stifled the T15 component of the humoral anti-PC response in the progeny, in a pattern identical to that observed after direct neonatal treatment with AB1-2 (Table III). This discrepancy is resolved when it is recognized that all AB1-2 molecules that are injected (1) have the potential to cross the placenta (AB1-2 is an IgG_1 antibody) and (2) are directed at an idiotope that will mediate the regulatory effects of the antibody—properties many anti-T15 antibodies in a heterologous preparation may not possess.

Treatment of the mother with AB1-2 after birth can also prevent the dominance of the T15 component in the anti-PC response of the adult progeny; note that a substantial level of T15$^+$ B-cell responsiveness is detectable in such mice (Table III). To determine whether transfer of AB1-2 immunoglobulin from the mother to the neonate via the colostrum occurs, the stomach fluids and sera from day 3 neonates were pooled separately and assayed by ELISA for the presence of AB1-2 antibody. The presence of 572 and 156 ng/ml of anti-T15 IgG1 antibody (presumably AB1-2) was detected in stomach fluid and serum, respectively. These amounts of AB1-2 compare favorably with a dose of 250 ng of AB1-2 antibody, which if delivered intraperitoneally is sufficient to inactivate permanently the $T15^+$ B cells in neonatal mice.

IV. Mechanism of MAID-Induced Id-Specific B-Cell Unresponsiveness

The striking similarity in the pattern of B-cell unresponsiveness among mice treated as neonates with MAID, independent of the route of exposure and the antigen system used, suggests that a similar mechanism may be responsible for the maintenance of the idiotope-specific unresponsiveness observed in such adult mice. We examined this question in multiple ways: (a) B cells from EB3-7 neonatally suppressed mice were tested for functional activity in a splenic focus assay; (2) in the PC system, spleen cells from AB1-2 neonatally suppressed mice were tested for their pattern of responsiveness to PC in an adoptive transfer system; and (3) spleen cells from mice neonatally suppressed with GB4-10 were examined for expression of the GB4-10-defined idiotope before and after stimulation with lipopolysaccharide (LPS).

A. SPLENIC FOCUS OF B LYMPHOCYTES FROM EB3-7-SUPPRESSED DONORS

The splenic focus assay provides a means of comparing the functional activities of precursor B lymphocytes in MAID-exposed and normal mice. Table IV shows the predominant expression of the EB3-7 idiotope among the antibodies produced by the progeny cells of anti-DEX precursor B lymphocytes in normal BALB/c mice. When B cells from mice neonatally treated with EB3-7 are examined by identical means, there is a clear-cut lack of evidence for functional precursor B lymphocytes expressing the EB3-7 idiotope. Explanations for this observation include (1) physical deletion of idiotope-positive precursor B lymphocyte clones, (2) cotransfer of DEX- and/or idiotype-specific suppressor T cells into the irradiated recipients, and (3) permanent inactivation of idiotope-positive precursor B lymphocytes. Cotransfer of suppressor T lymphocytes is unlikely, because the

TABLE IV

Idiotope Expression among DEX-Specific
B-Cell Precursors

	Percentage of anti-DEX precursors		
Source	EB3-7[+]	SJL18-1[+]	CD3-2[+]
Control[a]	74	26	83
EB3-7 suppressed[b]	0	50	63

[a] A total of 236 anti-DEX clones was detected.
[b] A total of 8 anti-DEX clones was detected.

dilution factor used would make the probability of a specific suppressor T cell ending up in each fragment containing a complementary B cell quite small.

B. ADOPTIVE TRANSFER OF LYMPHOCYTES FROM AB1-2-SUPPRESSED DONORS

As shown in Table V, significant T15 idiotype unresponsiveness can be adoptively transferred to adult syngeneic recipients using spleen cells from AB1-2 neonatally suppressed mice. A slightly lower and more variable degree of responsiveness to PC antigen is also present in those recipients receiving cells from suppressed donors. B cells are the only detectable cell type responsible for causing the lack of T15[+] serum IgM in the humoral anti-PC response among recipients; there is no evidence for the existence of suppressor T cells when AB1-2 is

TABLE V

Adoptive Transfer of Lymphoid Cells from AB1-2 Neonatally Treated BALB/c Mice

		Recipient serum IgM (μg/ml $\pm$ SE)	
Source of spleen cells	Treatment	Anti-PC	AB1-2[+]
Normals	—	27.5 (2.1)	25.9 (2.4)
AB1-2 suppressed	—	15.8 (3.2)	1.2 (0.8)
AB1-2 suppressed	Anti-Thy-1 + C′	18.4 (2.7)	1.9 (1.1)
AB1-2 suppressed	B cell depleted	14.4 (1.9)	13.7 (1.6)
Normal + AB1-2 suppressed (1 : 1)	—	27.7 (1.6)	10.8 (1.7)

used as the suppressing agent. This finding supports the work of Kim and Hopkins (1978) and Weiler (1981), who showed that chronic idiotype unresponsiveness could be obtained by treating neonatal nude BALB/c mice with MAID. Transferring a 1 : 1 mixture of suppressed and normal spleen cells (both primed with PC) leads to a partial recovery in the proportion of the recipient's anti-PC serum IgM expressing the T15 idiotype. Consequently, active suppression of T15$^+$ B cells by regulatory B or T lymphocytes is not evident in this system.

C. ANALYSIS OF T15 Id EXPRESSION OF B CELLS FROM ANTI-T15 MAID-TREATED MICE

B cells from anti-T15 MAID neonatally suppressed BALB/c mice were examined for cell surface expression of the GB4-10 idiotope by indirect immunofluorescent staining using a GB4-10-biotin conjugate as the primary reagent, followed by an avidin-fluorescein conjugate as a detection reagent (Pohlit *et al.*, 1979). Although approximately 1.5/ 10^4 splenic lymphocytes of normal BALB/c mice express this idiotope on their surface immunoglobulin under these conditions, no GB4-10-bearing cell has yet been detected in AB1-2 or GB4-10 neonatally treated mice (resulting in a frequency of <1/10^5 spleen cells; Table VI). This finding confirms the observations made by Kohler (1975), who stated that T15$^+$ B cells as detected by immunofluorescence were absent in anti-T15 neonatally suppressed BALB/c mice.

TABLE VI

Expression of the GB4-10 Idiotope on B Cells from
Normal and MAID-Suppressed BALB/c Mice

Condition	GB4-10$^+$ B cells[a]/10^4 spleen cells
Before LPS culture	
Normal	1.8
AB1-2 suppressed	<0.1
GB4-10 suppressed	<0.1
After LPS culture	
Normal	2.6
GB4-10 suppressed	0.6

[a] B cells detected by costaining with rhodamine-labeled goat antimouse μ.

To determine whether T15$^+$ B-cell clones were physically deleted or merely lacked detectable levels of membrane immunoglobulin, spleen cells from GB4-10-suppressed mice were cultured in the presence of LPS for 4 days prior to staining with GB4-10-biotin. After LPS stimulation, a significant proportion of spleen cells from suppressed mice expressed the GB4-10-defined idiotope at approximately 25% of the frequency in similarly cultured normal BALB/c spleen cells (Table VI). It appears that idiotope-positive B cells are not physically deleted after neonatal exposure to anti-Id antibody, but remain nonfunctional in adult life because of an inability to express an antigen receptor in sufficient quantity or native form. Receptor modulation by residual anti-Id antibody cannot account for the lack of surface Ig expression, because *in vitro* culture of spleen cells from anti-T15 neonatally treated mice does not allow T15$^+$ B cells to escape from an inactive state (Strayer *et al.*, 1975). A functional immunoglobulin gene structure is obviously conserved in these inactive B cells because interaction with LPS can lead to production of Id-positive immunoglobulin; a blockade at the transcriptional or translational levels of antibody synthesis is the most probable explanation for the absence of surface Ig expression.

These and similar independent studies using anti-T15 MAIDs strongly suggest that dominance of the PC response by T15-negative B cells is the basis for T15 clonal unresponsiveness in neonatally treated mice. Studies supporting the existence of suppressor T cells after neonatal suppression regimes (DuClos and Kim, 1977) are not necessarily incompatible with these results, as heterologous anti-Id preparations may contain antibodies that stimulate regulatory T-cell sets. Taken together, the results of the cell transfer and immunofluorescence experiments presented here support the concept that establishment of clonal dominance by T15-negative B cells acts to create and/or maintain the functional unresponsiveness among T15-positive B-cell clones in mice treated neonatally with antiidiotype antibody.

The permanent nature of the T15-unresponsive state in these mice has been informally suggested by Heusser and Etlinger (in *Idiotypes: Antigens on the Inside*, 1982) to exist because establishment of an active T15$^-$ anti-PC response somehow prevents subsequent maturation of T15-positive B-cell precursors. This concept is also supported by the work of Fung and Kohler (1980), who found that T15-positive B cells were present in BALB/c mice treated neonatally with anti-T15 antibody but were in a functionally immature state. Also, Etlinger *et al.* (1982) showed that although T15$^-$ B cells from anti-T15 neonatally treated mice have a lower avidity for PC than do normal T15$^+$ B cells, the avidity of the former increases over time to become equal to that of T15$^+$ B cells, thereby establishing their selective advantage over any newly developed T15$^+$ B cells in the competition for antigen. Differences in the avidity for antigen of T15-negative and T15-positive B cells, as well as a disparity in the number of PC-reactive B cells transferred, may help to explain the observed decrease in the total PC response among mice receiving T15-negative B cells (from suppressed donors) in comparison with those receiving T15-positive B cells (from normal donors; Table V).

V. Summary

Treatment of neonatal BALB/c mice with MAIDs specific for idiotopes associated with anti-DEX or anti-PC immunoglobulins ablates the corresponding B-cell response as effectively as do heterologous antiidiotype antibody preparations. Idiotype-specific B-cell unresponsiveness can be accomplished in both antigen systems via maternal routes of MAID administration, as well as by direct treatment of neonates. Following neonatal treatment with MAIDs that distinguish among idiotope variants of a major idiotype family, the anti-DEX and anti-PC humoral responses reflect an idiotope-specific pattern of B-cell inactivation. The immunologic defect in MAID-suppressed mice is apparently at the B-cell level, because idiotope-positive B cells seemingly exist in an inactive state and suppressor T-cell activity is not detectable among lymphocytes from such mice. These findings demonstrate that a mechanism based on the dominance of idiotope-negative B cells over nonfunctional idiotope-positive B cells accounts sufficiently for the maintenance of idiotype-specific humoral unresponsiveness in mice given antiidiotype antibody early in life.

References

Augustin, A., and Cosenza, H. (1976). *Eur. J. Immunol.* **6**, 497.
Bona, C. (1979). *Prog. Allergy* **26**, 97.
Clevinger, B., Schilling, J., Hood, L., and Davie, J. (1980). *J. Exp. Med.* **51**, 1059.
Clevinger, B., Thomas, J., Davie, J., Schilling, J., Bond, M., Hood, L., and Kearney, J. (1981). *In* "Immunoglobulin Idiotypes" (C. Janeway, H. Wigzell, and E. Sercarz, eds.), p. 159. Academic Press, New York.
Cosenza, H., Julius, M., and Augustin, A. (1977). *Immunol. Rev.* **34**, 3.
DuClos, T., and Kim, B. (1977). *J. Immunol.* **119**, 1769.

Eichmann, K. (1974). *Eur. J. Immunol.* **4**, 296.

Eichmann, K. (1978). *Adv. Immunol.* **26**, 195.

Etlinger, H., Julius, M., and Heusser, C. (1982). *J. Immunol.* **128**, 1685.

Fung, J., and Köhler, H. (1980). *J. Immunol.* **125**, 1998.

"Idiotypes: Antigens on the Inside" (1982). p. 165. Editiones Roche, Basel, Switzerland.

Kearney, J., Radbruch, A., Liesgang, B., and Rajewsky, K. (1979). *J. Immunol.* **123**, 1548.

Kearney, J., Barletta, R., Quan, Z., and Quintans, J. (1981). *Eur. J. Immunol.* **11**, 877.

Kearney, J., Pollok, B., and Stohrer, R. (1984). *Ann. N.Y. Acad. Sci.* (in press).

Kelsoe, G., Reth, M., and Rajewsky, K. (1981). *Eur. J. Immunol.* **11**, 418.

Kim, B., and Hopkins, W. (1978). *Cell. Immunol.* **35**, 460.

Köhler, H. (1975). *Transplant. Rev.* **27**, 24.

Mage, M., McHugh, L., and Rothstein, T. (1977). *J. Immunol. Methods* **15**, 47.

Marshak-Rothstein, A., Margolies, M., Riblet, R., and Gefter, M. (1981). *In* "Immunoglobulin Idiotypes" (C. Janeway, H. Wigzell, and E. Sercarz, eds.), p. 739. Academic Press, New York.

Owen, F., Ju, S.-T., and Nisonoff, A. (1977). *J. Exp. Med.* **145**, 1559.

Pohlit, H., Haas, W., and von Boehmer, H. (1979). *In* "Immunological Methods" (I. Lefkovits and B. Pernis, eds.), p. 181. Academic Press, New York.

Pollok, B. A., Bhown, A., and Kearney, J. F. (1982). *Nature (London)* **299**, 447.

Pollok, B. A., and Kearney, J. F. (1984). *J. Immunol.* (in press).

Strayer, D., Lee, W., Rowley, D., and Kohler, H. (1975). *J. Immunol.* **114**, 728.

Waldmann, T., and Strober, W. (1969). *Prog. Allergy* **13**, 1.

Ward, R., and Kohler, H. (1981). *J. Immunol.* **126**, 146.

Weiler, I. (1981). *In* "Lymphocytic Regulation by Antibodies" (C. Bona and P.-A. Cazenave, eds.), p. 245. Wiley, New York.

Weiler, I., Weiler, E., Sprenger, R., and Cosenza, H. (1977). *Eur. J. Immunol.* **7**, 531.

Chapter 12

Isogeneic Antiidiotype Repertoire and Modulation of Idiotype Expression in the Antidextran System[1]

Eberhardt Weiler, Georg Lehle, Joachim Wilke, and Ivan Jeanne Weiler[2]

Fakultät für Biologie
University of Konstanz
Konstanz, Federal Republic of Germany

I. Introduction

The selection of experiments to be reported in this chapter was guided by the idiotype–antiidiotype network theory of the immune system, as first formulated by Jerne (1974) and later explored in quantitative terms with respect to both the diversification (Adam and Weiler, 1976; Adam, 1978) and the regulation (Richter, 1975; Hoffmann, 1975) of the system. A primary requirement of the theory is the

[1] This work was supported by the Deutsche Forschungsgemeinschaft, Sonderforschungsbereich 138.

[2] Present address: Institute for Cancer Research, Fox Chase Cancer Center, 7701 Burholme Avenue, Philadelphia, Pennsylvania 19111.

203

availability, within the immune system of an animal, of a set of anti-idiotypes reactive with any given idiotype from the potential repertoire of the animal. In Section II, we shall be concerned with the size of the available and potential antiidiotypic repertoires of mouse strain BALB/c. The findings in this isogeneic system will be compared with results obtained in allogeneic situations involving different strains of mice. The question of "private" versus "public" idiotypes will be addressed, as well as the relationship between the sets of paratopes, as defined by a foreign antigenic determinant, and the corresponding sets of idiotypes, as defined by oligoclonal or monoclonal isogeneic antiidiotypic reagents.

In Section III, we shall discuss the biological effects of antiidiotypic antibodies administered passively, again stressing isogeneic situations. In Section IV, some experiments will be described which bear on the question of "germline encoded" idiotypes. An incompatibility will be reported between lymphocytes which carry an idiotype family in their potential repertoire and congeneic lymphocytes which do not. In Sections III and IV, the role of the thymus in idiotype modulation will also be considered by comparing euthymic mice with their congeneic thymusless counterparts.

The work reported here is concerned with the immune response against the α1-3 glucosidic linkage, as represented by dextran B 1355 S, or by corresponding oligosaccharides.[3]

II. The Isogeneic Antiidiotypic Repertoire

A. NUMBER OF ANTIIDIOTYPIC CLONES

The first systematic investigation of isogeneic antiidiotypic diversity was performed with the idiotype of myeloma protein J558 (Schuler *et al.*, 1977). This myeloma arose in a BALB/c mouse and has the constitution λ_1, α. Its paratope is specific for α1-3 glucosidic linkages, present in dextran B 1355 S or corresponding oligosaccharides (Blomberg *et al.*, 1972; Carson and Weigert, 1973). Antiidiotypic sera had originally been raised in strain A/J against J558. Isogeneically, in strain BALB/c, they are not produced as readily as in allogeneic animals; therefore, we employed the method of Janeway *et al.* (1975): priming of mice against DNP on an unrelated carrier (ovalbumin),

[3] We are indebted to Dr. Allene Jeanes and Dr. M. W. Slodki for generous gifts of this dextran.

followed by immunization against the myeloma protein lightly conjugated with DNP (three to four groups per molecule). Tests of humoral response were carried out with the unaltered myeloma protein. More recently, we found that immunization can also be achieved without DNP-ovalbumin preimmunization and, in fact, with unsubstituted myeloma protein. All BALB/c mice so treated produce antiidiotype antibody.

By isoelectric focusing analysis, Schuler *et al.* (1977) found that any given BALB/c mouse will produce 6–16 clones reactive with the idiotype of myeloma protein J558. This result reflects the available repertoire in each mouse toward this idiotype.

In order to gain an estimate of the potential repertoire, an expansion experiment by cell transfer, following essentially the protocol of Askonas and Williamson (1972), was performed. Among 100 clones scanned, derived from five donor mice, only 2 could be called identical by the criteria applied. The potential antiidiotypic repertoire in BALB/c against myeloma protein J558 therefore contains at least 100 clonal species. The great majority of antiidiotype antibodies belonged to the IgG_1 class.

B. SPECIFICITY OF ISOGENEIC ANTIIDIOTYPE ANTIBODIES

It had been early noticed that antiidiotype sera raised against a monoclonal (myeloma) immunoglobulin cross-reacted with other related proteins (Lieberman *et al.*, 1975). Such cross-reacting reagents had been produced in mouse strains that differ in haplotype (allogeneic antiidiotypes) or belong to a foreign animal species such as the rabbit (Hansburg *et al.*, 1977). Idiotypes defined by such reagents were called cross-reacting ("IdX"), "major," or "public" idiotypes (Mäkelä and Karjalainen, 1977). Examples are the allogeneic (strain A/J) antibodies raised against the myeloma J558 (BALB/c origin). These reagents were shown to recognize a major portion of the antibody populations produced by BALB/c in the course of a physiological response toward dextran (α1-3) glucosidic linkages), as shown by Blomberg *et al.* (1972). Allogeneic antiidiotype reagents also reacted with another antidextran myeloma: MOPC104E (λ_1,μ) (Carson and Weigert, 1973). Myelomas J558 and MOPC104E differ in the variable portions of their heavy chains in positions 100 and 101: Arg-Tyr in J558 and Tyr-Asp in MOPC104E (Schilling *et al.*, 1980). Furthermore, a series of antidextran hybridomas were sequenced and used as probes for the specificity of xenogeneic (rabbit) antiidiotype sera (Schilling *et al.*, 1980). They all contained λ_1 but differed from each other in up to seven positions of V_H. Both public (IdX) and private (IdI) idiotypes could be defined by these reagents.

Isogeneic antiidiotype sera show a reaction pattern quite different from that of allogeneic ones. All antisera produced in BALB/c against myeloma protein J558 reacted only with J558 and not with myeloma protein MOPC104E. The idiotypic difference between the two proteins must be correlated with the two amino acid exchanges in V_H positions 100 and 101: Arg-Tyr versus Tyr-Asp. Their nature, however, is such that one is led to expect profound conformational differences in other parts of the V domains.

Isogeneic anti-J558 reacted only marginally with physiological antidextran sera (Schuler *et al.*, 1981). We therefore decided (Lehle, 1983) to study also antisera against protein MOPC104E. Again, cross-reactions with J558 were rarely found. In the specificity analysis, a third monoclonal antidextran protein was included: Hdex14, produced by a hybridoma cell line (Newman *et al.*, 1983).[4] It has the constitution μ,λ_1 and has the same V_H sequence as MOPC104E, except for two exchanges in positions 54 and 55: Lys-Lys instead of Asn-Asp/Asn. The reaction patterns of individual antiidiotype sera are given in Table I.

Turning again to physiological antidextran sera, Lehle (1983a) found that the MOPC104E idiotype, as defined by isogeneic sera, is present in most. However, its proportion among antidextran molecules was highly variable from animal to animal; it stayed constant for long periods in a given immunized animal. Some representative data will be given in Section III (see Fig. 1) in the discussion of idiotype suppression.

Recently, a series of eight isogeneic hybridomas was raised against protein MOPC104E and one against J558 (Wilke, 1983). Preliminary data on their specificity patterns are given in Table II. Four of eight anti-MOPC104E hybridomas (Hid104E2, -5, -6, and -8) were specific for the immunogen; so was the one anti-J558 hybridoma, HidJ558. However, two hybridomas (Hid104E1 and -7) gave cross-reactions with J558 and Hdex14, and two additional ones (Hid104E3 and -4) with Hdex14 but not with J558. Reactions were not observed with myeloma proteins TEPC183 (μ,κ), MOPC315 (α,λ_2) or RPC20 ($-,\lambda_1$).

An artificial mixture of these hybridoma proteins would show ap-

---

[4] This was kindly provided by Dr. Clevinger, St. Louis.

TABLE I

Cross-Reactions of Individual Isogeneic Antiidiotype Sera[a]

Inhibitors[b] (μg/ml)		Anti-J558 with J558-coated SRBC (serum number)					Anti-MOPC104E with 104E-coated SRBC (serum number)			
		1	2	3	4	5	1	2	3	4
None		1280	640	5120	5120	5120	640	1280	1280	320
J558	1	80	80	320	320	320	—	—	—	—
J558	100	—[c]	—	—	—	—	640	1280	640	160
104E	1	—	—	—	—	—	80	320	160	40
104E	100	1280	640	2560	5120	5120	—	—	—	—
Hdex14	1	—	—	—	—	—	320	640	160	160
Hdex14	10	—	—	—	—	—	80	320	160	80
Hdex14	100	1280	640	5120	5120	5120	—	—	—	—

[a] Hemagglutination titers using myeloma-Cr^{3+}-coated sheep erythrocytes.
[b] Concentration of inhibitor in the dilution medium.
[c] Not done.

proximately the reaction pattern of physiological antiidiotype sera (Table I) when one takes into account the fact that cross-reactions by hybridomas are generally weaker than homologous reactions.

The reactions of all hybridoma products with their homologous anti-dextran proteins could be inhibited by the haptene hepta-α1-3 gluco-pyranoside.[5] All anti-MOPC104E hybridomas were tested with a panel of eight physiologically raised antisera against dextran. In agreement with Table I, the idiotypic specificity recognized by the protein from Hid104E1 could be detected in all antisera to a consider-able extent. Additionally, the idiotope defined by Hid104E7 was also present in each antiserum, although the extent of its expression was much more heterogeneous than that defined by Hid104E1. The reac-tion of all the other hybridoma proteins with the serum antibodies exhibited great variability. Thus, for example, the Hid104E5- and Hid104E8-defined idiotopes, although present in at least trace amounts in every analyzed serum, were represented strongly only in three. It should be noted that the sera with high Hid104E5 idiotope content were in two cases not identical to those expressing the Hid104E8 idiotope. The high degree of diversity within the germline encoded anti-α1-3-dextran immune response, as shown by idiotope

[5] Kindly provided by Dr. K. Himmelspach, Freiburg.

TABLE II

Cross-Reactions of Isogeneic Antiidiotype Hybridomas[a]

Inhibitor[b]	Anti MOPC104E (Hid104E number)								Anti J558 (HidJ5581)	Sera BALB/c[c] anti-	
	1	2	3	4	5	6	7	8		104E	J558
104E	++	+++	+++	++	+++	+++	+++	+++	—	++++	—
J558	++	—	—	—	—	—	++	—	+++	—	++++
Hdex14	++	—	+	+	—	—	++	—	—	+++	—

[a] Radioimmunoassay with hybridoma proteins (or antiserum) adsorbed onto plastic wells. Concentrations of inhibitor were measured that reduce the reaction with a standardized dose of homologous ^{125}I-protein by 50%.

[b] Symbols for 50% concentrations of inhibitor in nanograms per milliliter: ++++, 5–50; +++, 51–500; ++, 501–5000; +, 5001–5 × 10^4; —, greater than 5 × 10^4.

[c] Isogeneic antisera used for comparison: see also Table I.

analysis, is in good agreement with previous data obtained through isoelectric focusing (Schuler *et al.*, 1982), as well as with the results of studies of the IdI-MOPC104E and IdI-J558 expression in antidextran antisera obtained with allogeneic anti-Id antibodies (Ward and Köhler, 1981). Experiments are underway to compare the ability of different hybridomas to modulate the immune response to dextran. One preliminary result will be mentioned in Section III.

This discussion of antiidiotype specificity and antiidiotype repertoire is useful in the interpretation of biological effects. We wish to point out especially the differences between isogeneic and allogeneic (or xenogeneic) agents and reagents, feeling that only the former can reflect a physiological state of the network. We are aware that the antidextran system may not be representative of the immune system as a whole, because it belongs to the class of germline encoded responses (Mäkelä and Karjalainen, 1977): Every mouse of strain BALB/c, or of any BALB/c derivative carrying the BALB/c chromosome 12 marked by the heavy chain allogroup a, will respond to dextran with a family of antibodies that have a high degree of sequence homology among each other in V_H, and all carry the λ_1 light chain (Schilling *et al.*, 1980). No other strain gives this response, but two germline recombinations between C_H (allotype a) and V_H (antidextran positive) have been observed (Riblet *et al.*, 1975; Kolb *et al.*, 1979). This genetic predisposition may well render BALB/c tolerant toward sets of idiotypes that are "self," but that by other strains are recognized as "foreign." This aspect will be discussed further in Section IV.

III. Idiotype Expression Manipulated by Passive Antiidiotype

A. EFFECTS IN EUTHYMIC MICE

1. Specificity

The literature on this topic is large and still expanding. We shall restrict this discussion by two criteria: (a) only those effects are considered that are chronic, that is, that demonstrate a persistent change within the system not dependent on the acute presence of the antiidiotypic agent; (b) idiotype–antiidiotype interactions should be isogeneic; no allotypes or species-specific epitopes should participate in the experiment, and all interactions should be within the potential repertoire of a given mouse haplotype (see Section I). The problems involved in the interpretation of experiments performed with xeno-geneic agents have been addressed recently by Bluestone *et al.* (1982) and by Devaux *et al.* (1982).

Chronic suppression by *allogeneic* antiidiotype is achieved readily in the newborn mouse, whether by neonatal injection of antiidiotype sera or through the milk of mothers immunized against the idiotype (Weiler *et al.*, 1977). The assay for chronic neonatally induced suppression is performed at the adult stage and shows a depression of the immune response toward a given antigen. The literature until 1980 has been reviewed by Weiler (1981). The remarkable conclusion of such experiments has been, in general, that whole families of B-cell clones, having as their common denominator paratopes reactive with the given foreign antigenic determinant, are affected in concert. In each of the cases analyzed so far, the antibody responses concerned were polyclonal: against phosphorylcholine, arsanylic acid, NIP/NP, DNP/TNP, and others. These systems will be covered in other chapters of this volume. The problem is twofold: (a) these immune responses are governed by genes on chromosome 12, the Ig heavy chain, and have therefore been called germline encoded even though they are polyclonal; (b) the polyclonal responses can be modulated *as sets* by allogeneic antiidiotype. This conceptual difficulty has been addressed recently by Siekevitz *et al.* (1982) at the level of DNA.

When we used isogeneic antiidiotype agents and reagents, the situation was different. Anti-J558 had no perceptible effect on the response to dextran B 1355 S (Schuler *et al.*, 1981), just as it essentially did not recognize antibodies from a physiological response. In a more recent set of experiments, Lehle (1983) used BALB/c antiidiotype against the antidextran myeloma MOPC104E as the agent given to newborn animals. In the adult stage the mice were immunized with dextran, and two variables were recorded: total antibodies toward dextran and the presence of the MOPC104E idiotype as detected by isogeneic reagents. The MOPC104E idiotype among antidextran molecules (already mentioned in Section II) is evident in the untreated control sets (Fig. 1).

In mice treated neonatally with anti-MOPC104E, the anti-dextran response as a whole was not depressed significantly in the experiment of Fig. 1. (In other experiments with different isogeneic antiidiotype sera, the depression of antidextran was more pronounced.) However, none of the suppressed mice had measurable amounts of the MOPC104E idiotype, nor did 17 additional animals in other experiments.

We conclude that isogeneic antiidiotype, administered neonatally,

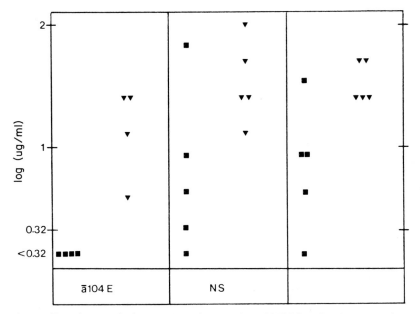

Fig. 1. Effect of neonatal administration of syngeneic anti-MOPC104E antiserum on the expression of the MOPC104E idiotype. Newborn BALB/c mice received a single ip injection of syngeneic anti-MOPC104E antiserum (ā104E) or normal serum (NS), or were left untreated. At 7 weeks of age, they were challenged with 10 μg α1-3 dextran ip. Blood was taken after 5 days. Anti-α1-3 dextran concentrations were determined by the ability of the sera to inhibit the hemagglutination reaction between α1-3 dextran and J558 myeloma protein-coated SRBC. MOPC104 idiotype concentrations were tested by inhibiting the hemagglutination reaction between a MOPC104E idiotype-specific antiserum and MOPC104E myeloma protein-coated SRBC. Standardization of both assays was done with purified MOPC104E myeloma protein. Triangles represent anti-α1-3 dextran; squares represent MOPC104E idiotype concentrations in the sera of individual mice.

affects essentially only those among antidextran clones which produce the corresponding idiotype. In that way, the biological effect of antiidiotype reflects its serological specificity (Section II).

Analogous experiments are underway using isogeneic antiidiotypic hybridomas that differ from each other in their fine-specificity patterns (Table II). Preliminary experiments show that the highly cross-reactive Hid104E1 does indeed suppress chronically a large part of the antidextran response.

2. Possible Mechanisms

Three mechanisms can be proposed to explain the effects of antiidiotype administered neonatally.

1. The antibody persists and serves with accessory mechanisms (complement, macrophages) to eliminate any clone that bears the idiotype (or block its receptors). With this possibility in mind, we stress chronic effects. The complete suppression of idiotype lasted for an observation period of up to 33 weeks after dextran challenge, never showing recovery.

In a more stringent experiment, spleen cell populations from anti-idiotypically suppressed animals were transferred to lethally irradiated BALB—Igh^b backcross mice (Lehle, 1983). (Because of the C57Bl/6-derived chromosome 12, this substrain does not give the BALB/c-type antidextran response.) Challenge by dextran after transfer produced a strongly boosted response toward dextran even when the donors had been suppressed by anti-MOPC104E. When control donors were used, the expression of the MOPC104E idiotype was also boosted strongly. But when the transferred spleen cells came from neonatally suppressed donors, their response in the hosts remained suppressed with respect to this idiotype.

Most of the isogeneic antiidiotype molecules belong to subclass IgG$_1$ (Schuler, 1977), whose half-life *in vivo* is approximately 1 week (Fahey and Sell, 1965). Taking an initial neonatal dose of 40 μg of antiidiotype per animal, one can calculate that at the time of challenge after transfer there remain at most 10 pg in each host, or about one molecule per 40 lymphocytes. We thus consider the possibility of an active interference by the injected antiidiotype to be ruled out.

2. Passive antiidiotype might eliminate the corresponding clones in the neonate, and these never again appear ("clonal elimination"). We have no direct evidence either in favor of or against this possibility. We consider it to be unlikely, however, because it is known that new lymphocyte clones emerge continuously from the undifferentiated stem cell pool, thereby presumably undergoing genetic rearrangement leading to the creation of new idiotypic clones (Osmond and Nossal, 1974). Spleen contains a full complement of precursor cells, as does bone marrow (Teale *et al.*, 1979). Experiments on the turnover of clones defined by idiotype have not yet, to our knowledge, been done.

3. If we reject possibilities 1 and 2, we are left with active antiidiotypic suppression as a result of passive antiidiotype administration. Transfers of anti-MOPC104E-suppressed cells into naive BALB/c mice to show dominant suppression have yielded only marginally positive results so far. Current experiments, with a change in protocol, appear more promising (see Section IV).

Until further experimental evidence is available, we are adopting the following working hypothesis, which has little explanatory power but at least reduces antiidiotypic phenomena to established immunological terminology: Neonatally applied antiidiotype molecules, by their very presence, eliminate or impair idiotype-bearing lymphocyte clones during the crucial period when self-tolerance becomes established. By the time passively administered antiidiotype has declined and idiotypic clones arise anew from the stem cell pool, these are identified as foreign by the then available repertoire and are suppressed by the same (not quite understood) mechanism that distinguishes self and foreign and decides on tolerance or rejection. Some suggested corroborative evidence will be presented in Section IV.

B. IDIOTYPE SUPPRESSION IN ATHYMIC ("NUDE") MICE

Dextran (α1-3 glucosidic linkages) is a thymus-independent antigen. BALB/nude mice respond as promptly as do euthymic BALB/c. [In fact, nude mice go further in their response: They readily switch to the IgG compartment, which euthymic BALB/c do not (Schuler *et al.*, 1982).] It appeared interesting to study antiidiotypic suppression in BALB/c nudes.

The experiment was done according to the same protocol as the experiments reported in Section III,A: injection of antiidiotype within 24 h after birth, followed by challenge with 10 μg dextran at 7 weeks of age. The results corresponded so closely to those obtained with euthymic mice (Fig. 1) that they need not be given here in detail (Lehle, 1983; also manuscript in preparation). In summary, 15 neonatally treated animals displayed a depressed antidextran response, as compared to 13 controls. None of the treated mice expressed any detectable molecules reacting with isogeneic anti-MOPC104E, in contrast to all of the control mice. Suppression lasted for the period of observation: 33 days after challenge. Three experiments gave the same result. We have to conclude that chronic idiotype suppression by neonatal antiidiotype injection is independent of a thymus.

For the interpretation of this result, one has to keep in mind that dextran belongs to the group of thymus-independent antigens type 2 (not mitogenic) (Mond *et al.*, 1980). Because the positive immune response occurs in thymusless mice, it may appear logical that the negative regulation, through idiotype–antiidiotype interactions, is thymus independent as well. It remains to be investigated as to which ontogenetic pathway the regulatory cells take in nude mice.

IV. Igh-Dependent Congeneic Rejection of the Antidextran Response

A. REJECTION BY Igh^b NUDES

The experiments were initiated in the expectation that BALB/c-Igh^b thymusless mice might provide an ideal environment in which to study the ontogeny of antidextran lymphocytes, because they fulfill two requirements: (1) they do not, by themselves, produce the germline-encoded antidextran response typical of BALB/c or BALB/c-*nu/nu*, from which they differ in chromosome 12, Igh; (2) they are permissive toward isogeneic or congeneic lymphocytes in adoptive transfer, whether from BALB/c or BALB-Igh^b backcross mice. This permissiveness of nudes is equal to that of lethally irradiated isogeneic or congeneic euthymic animals but is in sharp contrast to the reaction of untreated euthymic mice, which display the phenomenon called "isogeneic barrier" (Celada, 1966; Kobow and Weiler, 1975): Neither the expression of immunoglobulin in general (as marked by allotype) nor the production of specific antibodies by transferred cells is permitted (even when these came from littermates). The isogeneic barrier was effective toward memory cells as well as naive cells (C. Kolb, unpublished experiments). We had proposed (Kobow and Weiler, 1975) that individually different available repertoires of the donor and the host are responsible for the incompatibility in cell transfer, and that lymphocyte rejection by the host (or lack of permissiveness toward expression) are thymus dependent, because nude mice are permissive. All transfer experiments involving antibody production after transfer had been done with thymus-dependent antigens.

The situation was different when we turned to dextran (α1-3 glucosidic linkages), a thymus-independent antigen. Here, congeneic nudes turned out not to be permissive. This was in sharp contrast to congeneic euthymic hosts that had been irradiated lethally. Representative data are given in Fig. 2, which also shows that the rejection by nudes can be ameliorated by slight irradiation (a heavy roentgen dose is not tolerated by nudes) (Weiler *et al.*, manuscript in preparation). Internal controls for the general permissiveness of nude Igh^b hosts were (1) the expression of donor allotype and (2) the response of donor cells toward a thymus-dependent antigen (horse red blood cells); the antibody responses to HRBC were ascertained to be donor cell derived by virtue of their IgG allotype. In all controls, the nude hosts allowed a good response by the donor cells. There was no recogniz-

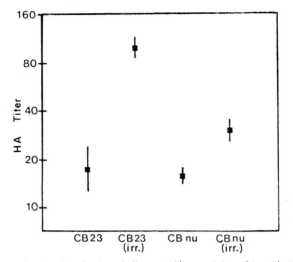

Fig. 2. Untreated or irradiated mice of allotype Igh^b were injected iv with 5×10^7 spleen cells from untreated BALB/c mice, together with 0.1 mg dextran ip. On day 7, the mice were bled and tested for serum anti-α1-3 dextran by hemagglutination assay with dextran-coated SRBC. Ordinate: hemagglutination titer. Squares give the mean titer ($\pm$SE) for 17 CB23 mice, 49 irradiated (600 rads) CB23, 59 CBnu, and 49 irradiated (200 rads) CBnu. CB23 are mice of the 23rd backcross generation, bearing allotype Igh^b on a BALB/c genetic background; CBnu mice are derived from BALB/c nudes bred into the 19th backcross generation of the same BALB/c-Igh^b line.

able difference in two sets of experiments, in which the Igh^a donors were either euthymic or nude.

If one accepts the hypothesis that donor lymphocytes are rejected (or are not permitted to function) through Igh incompatibility, and that this congeneic barrier is an active immunological transplant rejection, then one can expect that *newborn* nudes of allotype Igh^b haplotype might accept Igh^a, antidextran-positive lymphocytes, becoming tolerant. This was found to be the case in 11 out of 23 animals that had been given 3×10^7 splenic lymphocytes of the Igh^a type within 24 h of birth. When challenged as adults with dextran, they showed a fully developed response.

B. ACTIVE SUPPRESSION OF Igh^a CELLS BY Igh^b CELLS
   IN COTRANSFER

With the aim of demonstrating active suppression, the following protocol was adopted. Lethally irradiated euthymic hosts of haplotype

Igh^a or Igh^b first received untreated spleen or bone marrow cells from Igh^b nude donors. After 1 week was allowed for repopulation of the host, Igh^a spleen cells were given, and the animals were challenged with dextran.

The control recipients developed, within 1 week, the usual high antidextran response (log hemagglutination titers with dextran-coated erythrocytes = 2.13 ± 0.26 SD, 40 animals), but mice previously implanted with Igh^b cells had severely depressed responses. When pretreatment had been with Igh^b spleen cells, hemagglutination titers were log 1.25 ± 0.37 SD, 41 animals. Interestingly, Igh^b bone marrow cells were just as effective in suppression as Igh^b spleen cells; hemagglutination titers = log 1.21 ± 0.29 SD, 23 animals (I. J. Weiler, manuscript in preparation). On the average, there was 87% suppression.

In trying to interpret this type of result, we see at present no other choice but to postulate that lymphocytes of haplotype Igh^b actively reject or suppress lymphocytes of haplotype Igh^a. This rejection or suppression does not affect the expression of the constant parts of Ig molecules in general; it merely affects, in this experimental design, those clones that are concerned with the α1-3 glucosidic epitope. It has not been proved in this section (as it had been in the experiments of Section III) that the effects are mediated by idiotope–antiidiotope interactions. Because the antidextran response as a whole is concerned, such effects would be conglomerate ones, involving clones of different idiotypes.

V. Conclusions

The idiotype–antiidiotype network theory of Niels Jerne may be the kind of theory that can never be proved to be universally true. Yet, many experiments have been done under the guidance of this theory, and none have ever contradicted it.

Obviously, it is of pivotal interest to investigate the capability of the immune system to react against immunoglobulin idiotypes within its own genetic framework. Experiments showed that the isogeneic anti-idiotypic repertoire is ample.

Antiidiotype antibodies, given neonatally, have a profound effect on the lymphocyte populations of the immune system: suppression of the corresponding idiotype, with a duration that approaches the life expectancy of the animal. Specific suppression of a given idiotype did not require the presence of a thymus in the case of the thymus-independent antigen with which we were concerned.

The analysis of idiotype–antiidiotype interactions has been refined in steps: from xenogeneic to allogeneic to isogeneic to monoclonal isogeneic agents and reagents. It appears from this work, and from that of others, that the closer one gets, in specificity analysis, to single idiotopes, the less congruence one finds between idiotopes, on the one hand, and binding site populations, as defined by foreign antigen, on the other. Is there a master idiotope by which to regulate a whole immune response, such as against dextran? From present experience, this does not seem probable. Rather, each idiotope has its own regulatory circuit, and an immune response (or its suppression) is a composite of many circuits—as was implied by the term "network".

References

Adam, G. (1978). *In* "Theoretical Immunology" (G. I. Bell, A. S. Perelson, and G. H. Pimbley, eds.), pp. 603–627. Dekker, New York.

Adam, G., and Weiler, E. (1976). *In* "The Generation of Antibody Diversity" (A. J. Cunningham, ed.), pp. 1–20. Academic Press, New York.

Askonas, B. A., and Williamson, A. R. (1972). *Eur. J. Immunol.* 2, 487–493.

Blomberg, B., Geckeler, W. R., and Weigert, M. (1972). *Science* 177, 178–180.

Bluestone, J. A., Auchincloss, H., Cazenave, P.-A., Ozato, K., and Sachs, D. H. (1982). *J. Immunol.* 129, 2066–2073.

Carson, D., and Weigert, M. (1973). *Proc. Natl. Acad. Sci. U.S.A.* 70, 235–239.

Celada, F. (1966). *J. Exp. Med.* 124, 1–14.

Devaux, C., Epstein, S. L., Sachs, D. H., and Pierres, M. (1982). *J. Immunol.* 129, 2074–2081.

Fahey, J. L., and Sell, S. (1965). *J. Exp. Med.* 122, 41–58.

Hansburg, D., Briles, D. E., and Davie, J. M. (1977). *J. Immunol.* 119, 1406–1412.

Hoffmann, G. W. (1975). *Eur. J. Immunol.* 5, 638–647.

Janeway, C. A., Koren, H. S., and Paul, W. E. (1975). *Eur. J. Immunol.* 5, 17–22.

Jerne, N. K. (1974). *Ann. Immunol. (Paris)* 125C, 373–389.

Kobow, U., and Weiler, E. (1975). *Eur. J. Immunol.* 5, 628–632.

Kolb, C., Weiler, E., Sepälä, I., Eichmann K., Kaartinen, M., Pelkonen, J., Karjalainen, K., and Mäkelä, O. (1979). *Immunogenetics* 9, 455–463.

Lehle, G. (1983). Ph.D. Thesis, University of Konstanz.

Lieberman, R., Potter, M., Humphrey, W., Mushinsky, E. B., and Vrana, M. (1975). *J. Exp. Med.* 142, 106–119.

Mäkelä, O., and Karjalainen, K. (1977). *Immunol. Rev.* 34, 119–138.

Mond, J. J., Mongin, P. K. A., Sieckmann, D., and Paul, W. E. (1980). *J. Immunol.* 125, 1066–1070.

Newman, B., Sugii, S., Kabat, E. A., Torii, M., Clevinger, B. L., Schilling, J., Bond, M., Davie, J. M., and Hood, L. (1983). *J. Exp. Med.* 157, 130–140.

Osmond, D. G., and Nossal, G. J. V. (1974). *Cell. Immunol.* 13, 132–145.

Riblet, R., Weigert, M., and Mäkelä, O. (1975). *Eur. J. Immunol.* 5, 778–781.

Richter, P. H. (1975). *Eur. J. Immunol.* 5, 350–354.

Schilling, J., Clevinger, B., Davie, J. M., and Hood, L. (1980). *Nature (London)* 283, 35–40.

Schuler, W. (1977). Ph.D. Thesis, University of Konstanz.

Schuler, W., Weiler, E., and Kolb, H. (1977). *Eur. J. Immunol.* **7**, 649–654.

Schuler, W., Weiler, E., and Weiler, I. J. (1981). *Mol. Immunol.* **18**, 1095–1105.

Schuler, W., Lehle, G., Weiler, E., and Kölsch, E. (1982). *Eur. J. Immunol.* **12**, 120–125.

Siekevitz, M., Gefter, M. L., Brodeur, P., Riblet, R., and Marshak-Rothstein, A. (1982). *Eur. J. Immunol.* **12**, 1023–1032.

Teale, J. M., Layton, J. E., and Nossal, G. J. V. (1979). *J. Exp. Med.* **150**, 205–217.

Ward, R., and Köhler, H. (1981). *Cell. Immunol.* **58**, 286–292.

Weiler, I. J. (1981). *In* "Lymphocytic Regulation by Antibodies" (C. Bona and P.-A. Cazenave, eds.), pp. 245–267. Wiley, New York.

Weiler, I. J., and Sprenger, R. (1981). *Am. J. Reprod. Immunol.* **1**, 226–230.

Weiler, I. J., Weiler, E., Sprenger, R., and Cosenza, H. (1977). *Eur. J. Immunol.* **7**, 591–597.

Chapter 13

Idiotypic Manipulation of the Rabbit Immune Response against *Micrococcus luteus*

Maurice Wikler and Jacques Urbain

Laboratory of Animal Physiology
Département de Biologie Moléculaire
Université Libre de Bruxelles
Rhode-St-Genèse, Belgique

I. Introduction[1]

The role played by idiotypes, which may be of crucial importance in the regulation of the immune system, is under extensive investigation in several laboratories (see other chapters, this volume).

[1] Abbreviations: Ab1, idiotype, antibody raised against antigen; Ab1′, idiotypically cross-reactive antibody with Ab1; Ab2, antiidiotype; Ab3, anti-antiidiotype; Ab4, anti-anti-antiidiotype; CHO, carbohydrate; Pg, peptidoglycan; TMV, tobacco mosaic virus; Ab1-F_1, Ab1 produced by the offspring.

Most studies concerning idiotypic regulation have been performed using public or recurrent idiotypes. Our experimental approach has used idiotypes as originally defined by J. Oudin (Oudin and Michel, 1963) for antibodies and by H. Kunkel (Kunkel *et al.*, 1963) for myeloma proteins. These idiotypes are expressed by only a small species subset, and their expression is not inherited in a Mendelian fashion. We asked whether it was possible to elicit the synthesis of a predetermined idiotype in a randomly chosen animal. This question is related to the two main problems of immunology: the origin of antibody diversity and the regulation of the immune response. Our results suggest that a potential idiotypic repertoire is more or less the same within one species. Furthermore, an immune response does not depend only on antigenic selection but relies also on the previous idiotypic history of the animal. Although similar experiments have been performed with several antigenic systems, we shall focus here on idiotypic manipulations in the *Micrococcus* system.

II. Antigenic and Idiotypic Properties of Antibodies Induced by *Micrococcus luteus*

The immune response of rabbits to *Micrococcus luteus* is unusual in that repeated intravenous injections with bacteria stimulate a high antibody response of restricted heterogeneity to the cell wall antigens (Van Hoegaerden *et al.*, 1975).

Immunochemical studies have shown that rabbit antisera to *Micrococcus luteus* contain antibodies that precipitate strongly with soluble polysaccharide and peptidoglycan (Pg). Group-specific polysaccharide prepared by trichloroacetic acid extraction of *M. luteus* cell walls was shown to consist of a polymer composed of glucose and *N*-acetylaminomannuronic acid (Perkins, 1963). The polysaccharide precipitin reaction was strongly inhibited by maltose and D-glucose in most of the individual sera studied. In several cases, *N*-acetylmannosamine and mannosamine were strong inhibitors of the precipitin reaction. This indicates that glucose and presumably *N*-acetylmannosaminuronic acid constitute the antigenic sites of the polysaccharide (Wikler, 1975).

Several studies have shown that both the peptide moiety and the polysaccharide backbone of the Pg are antigenic determinants (Karakawa *et al.*, 1966, 1968; Schleifer and Krause, 1971). Rolicka and Park (1969) reported that *N*-acetylglucosamine is usually the immunodominant sugar of the Pg backbone polysaccharide for several bacterial cell walls. Quantitative inhibition studies revealed that in addition to N-acetylglucosamine, the immunodominant site of the glycan moiety of *M. luteus* appears to be N-acetylmuramic acid (Wikler, 1975). A difference in antigenicity of Pg of *M. luteus* origin may result from the fact that only 40% of N-acetylmuramic acid residues are substituted by peptide subunits in the polysaccharide of *M. luteus*. Moreover, after lysis of cell walls with egg lysozyme, 40–50% of the glycan is released as disaccharide and oligosaccharide fractions unsubstituted by peptide (Ghuysen, 1968).

The system also contrasts to other bacteria in that, other than the *Streptococcus* group A-variant antisera (Karakawa *et al.*, 1968), no other bacteria have yielded satisfactory amounts of antibody to Pg. It may be supposed that the low antibody response results from the possibility that the Pg is normally not exposed at the surface of the bacteria. It has been shown that lysozyme, which has no action on intact group A *Streptococcus*, is able to lyse the bacterial wall after removal of the group-specific polysaccharide (Krause and McCarty, 1961). Intact *M. luteus* cells are, however, readily attacked by lysozyme, which indicates that the Pg may be well exposed on the surface of the bacteria and therefore may constitute a potent antigen.

Because no cross-reaction was detected between the anti-Pg and the anti-CHO antibodies, the two major antibody populations could be isolated using a single immunoadsorbent column (Wikler, 1975). The immunoadsorbent was prepared with lysozyme-digested cell wall components, containing both polysaccharide and Pg antigens, which were coupled to Sepharose. Affinity chromatography permitted us to recover, from rabbit antisera, antibodies specific to the polysaccharide by the use of 5% glucose solution. Antibody to Pg, which remains bound to the immunoadsorbent after elution of the antipolysaccharide fraction, could be recovered by the use of 0.2 *M* acetic acid. For most antisera studied, this approach permitted the isolation of antibody fractions with unique electrophoretic mobility. Isoelectric focusing spectra of anti-CHO and anti-Pg antibodies often revealed restricted and nonoverlapping spectra characterized by a small number of bands demonstrating the presence in individual immune rabbit antisera of antibody of restricted clonality raised against the micrococcal antigens.

The simultaneous emergence of restricted antibodies directed against both the polysaccharide and the Pg of the bacteria offers the opportunity to study, in the same individual, structurally restricted antibodies directed against two bacterial antigens.

The restricted nature of the immune response of each animal allowed an examination of the idiotypic properties of serum antibodies. Is there an idiotypic relationship between antibodies of different specificity expressed in a single individual? Also, within a given specificity, what is the clonal origin and the idiotypic relationship between the antibody components which characterize an antibody by its electrofocusing spectrotype?

We induced antiidiotypic antibodies against a single electrofocusing band of antibody to Pg and to CHO (Wuilmart *et al.*, 1979). Specifically purified antibodies were fractionated by preparative isoelectric focusing. As an example, the focusing elution profile for (rabbit 2978) anti-CHO antibody from an individual antiserum is shown in Fig. 1. The diagram shows that the antibody was separated into six peaks. Each peak exhibited a high degree of homogeneity, as was shown by gel isoelectric focusing of individual fractions. Fraction 3 was used to produce antiidiotypic serum in allotype-matched rabbits. The antiidiotypic sera were tested for their capacity to bind homologous radiolabeled antibody. The immunizing antibody was bound to the homologous antisera to levels approaching 95%.

The specificity of the idiotypic reaction was extensively studied by immunodiffusion tests and radioimmunoassays. A frequency of 2 to 5% of cross-idiotypic reactions was observed between antibodies directed to the same antigen specificity. This result corresponds to the frequency found in other systems for which the antibodies studied were in most cases heterogeneous (Oudin, 1974; Bordenave, 1973; Urbain *et al.*, 1975). Idiotypic cross-reactions were never observed between antibodies to Pg and CHO whether or not they were present in the same immune serum. Thus, we concluded that the genetic diversity of restricted anti-CHO and anti-Pg antibodies is as large as the genetic repertoire coding for heterogeneous antibody responses in the rabbit.

The degree of idiotypic cross-reactivity among antibody subpopulations isolated by isoelectric focusing from a single antiserum was studied by binding radioimmunoassay and by inhibition of binding of the homologous idiotype–antiidiotype reaction. All antibody fractions from a given isoelectric focusing series were able to bind to a high level to the antiidiotypic reagent. Also, the amount of each antibody component required to achieve 50% inhibition of the homologous binding reaction did not vary significantly from the amount of the immunizing idiotype. The idiotypic sharing between all the fractions present in an antibody preparation was demonstrated for several other individual antibodies specific for CHO as well as for a series of 11

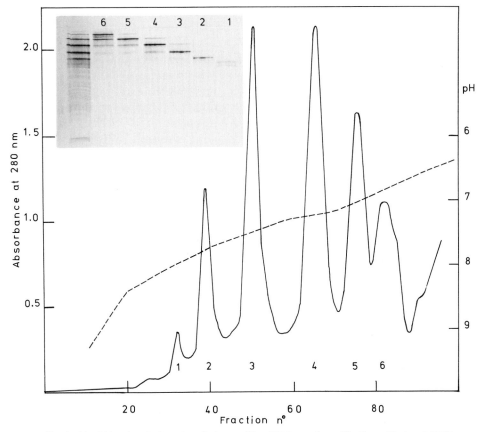

Fig..1. Liquid isoelectric focusing elution profile of 150 mg of specifically purified anti-CHO antibodies from rabbit 2978 in the pH 6–9 gradient range. ---, pH gradient. Analytical gel isoelectric focusing comparing the spectrotype of the whole antibody population prepared from antiserum 2978 to the six individual anti-CHO antibody fractions obtained by preparative isoelectric focusing. Antibody contained in fraction 3 was used to induce antiidiotypic antisera in allotype-matched rabbits.

antibody components purified by preparative isoelectric focusing and specific for the Pg (Wikler *et al.*, 1983).

We thus confirmed for immune responses of restricted clonality a sharing of idiotypic specificities between antibody components from a single immune serum (Urbain *et al.*, 1975). Antibodies produced during an immune response of any individual do possess an idiotypic relationship despite the fact that the idiotypic repertoire available to an antigen of the species can be very large.

The simultaneous occurrence of antibody subpopulations in a single individual sharing idiotypic specificities was observed in various systems. Oudin and Cazenave (1971) described a sharing of idiotypic specificities between antibody subsets from rabbits immunized with ovalbumin. Moreover, idiotypic similarities were also found between antibodies and immunoglobulins without detectable antibody activity synthesized during the response to ovalbumin (Oudin and Cazenave, 1971), peroxydase, or TMV (Urbain-Vansanten et al., 1979). Shared idiotypic properties were observed among antibody subpopulations differing in isoelectric pH from the same individual usually presenting a heterogeneous response against TMV (Urbain et al., 1975). Recently, several reports described a sharing of idiotypes among monoclonal antibodies to distinct determinants of hen lysozyme (Metzger et al., 1980) or on antibodies uniquely specific to the amino acids copolymer GAT or GLPhe and on antibodies bearing dual specificities to GAT and GLPhe (Ju et al., 1980a). Kohno et al. (1982) documented in detail a shared idiotope between two clone products derived from a single mouse, which were located within the antigen-combining sites of antibodies with distinct fine specificity for sperm whale myoglobin.

Why should antibodies share idiotypes within a given individual immune response? What is the meaning of idiotype sharing among antibodies that bind to structurally unrelated antigenic determinants or even immunoglobulins without antibody activity? The explanation we favored is based on the idiotypic network regulation but does not necessarily exclude other hypotheses (Jerne, 1974; Urbain et al., 1981).

Within an idiotypic network, clones displaying receptors with shared idiotopes are simultaneously selected. In this hypothesis, an idiotype-specific regulatory cell, for example, a helper T cell, that displays auto-antiidiotypic receptors will favor clones bearing this idiotype. This will lead to the selection of clones bearing the shared idiotype, even if the rest of the combining site of the antibody were different or devoid of any detectable antibody activity.

III. Manipulations of the Immune Response with Antiidiotypic Reagents

Antiidiotypic reagents have been used to control both idiotype expression and antibody specificity of immunized animals in various experimental systems (Binz and Wigzell, 1977; Pawlak et al., 1973). In

vivo administration of heterologous, homologous, or syngeneic purified anti-Id has been shown to suppress subsequent idiotype expression. In contrast, evidence for induction of specific idiotypes and antigen-specific cells in mice that received anti-Id antibodies in the
presence or absence of antigen has also been reported (Eichmann and
Rajewsky, 1975). In the rabbit, idiotype suppression was also obtained
with homologous anti-Id antibodies (Bordenave, 1975). The ability of
individual rabbits to synthesize antibodies directed against their own
idiotypic determinants was documented (Rodkey, 1974). The induction of auto-anti-Id antibodies in rabbits permits testing of some aspects of Jerne's network hypothesis for the regulation of the immune
response. We have studied how the induction of auto-antiidiotypic
antibodies modulates the idiotypic expression when the individual is
subsequently restimulated by the antigen.

A. AUTO-ANTIIDIOTYPE-MEDIATED REGULATION

Evidence showing the capacity of individual rabbits to synthesize
antibodies directed against their own idiotypic determinants was described (Wuilmart *et al.*, 1979). In these experiments, a single isoelectric focusing antibody fraction to Pg (Abo) was used to stimulate auto-
antiidiotypes in the rabbit. After the synthesis of auto-antiidiotypic
antibodies, a new immunization course with the original antigen was
given and new antibodies appeared (AbN). AbN were idiotypically
cross-reactive with Abo, but their affinity for the antiidiotypic antisera
directed to Abo was very low. In fact, AbN seemed to be derived from
a minor preexisting anti-Pg clone. We interpreted this result to mean
that the idiotypic shift was the consequence of induction of autoantibodies, which have by their appearance modified the state of the
immune network. Indeed, comparison of iso- and auto-antiidiotype
antisera indicates that iso-antiidiotypes seem to be more powerful
than auto-antiidiotypes in recognizing their corresponding idiotypes
(Rodkey, 1976). Auto-antiidiotypes were also shown to have a restricted specificity, which may explain why the induction of auto-
antiidiotypes modulates the idiotypic expression when the individual
is subsequently restimulated by the original antigen.

Naturally induced antiidiotype-mediated regulation of immune reactions was reported for several systems (for a review, see Urbain *et
al.*, 1981). Brown and Rodkey (1979) described a rabbit immunized
against *Micrococcus lysodeicticus* in which the production of auto-
antiidiotype could be related to the disappearance of specific antibody
clonotypes. More recently, naturally induced auto-antiidiotypic anti-

body responses specific for antimicrococcal antibody and recognizing identical idiotopes were detected in a large proportion of the rabbits in a family immunized with *M. lysodeicticus* (Binion and Rodkey, 1982). However, the natural auto-antiidiotypic response is directed to only a fraction of the total autologous antimicrococcal antibody. This result may be interpreted to mean that there is a concentration of an idiotope sufficient to trigger auto-antiidiotype synthesis or, alternatively, that not all idiotopes may be involved in the regulatory circuits and therefore do not possess the complementary auto-antiidiotype.

B. IMMUNIZATION CASCADE (Ab1, Ab2, Ab3, Ab4) WITH CARBOHYDRATE-SPECIFIC IDIOTYPE

The idiotypic network theory states that within one individual the coexistence of idiotypes and auto-antiidiotypes leads to connected systems, in which clones bearing idiotypes are interacting with clones bearing anti-Id receptors. Thus, the immune system is a web of V domains. Many data collected during the last few years clearly suggest that this could be the case. This so-called formal network has been demonstrated experimentally. The existence of such a network before immunization might be relevant to regulation of the immune responses. This has led to the notion of a functional network: As a consequence of the coexistence of Id and anti-Id, it might be predicted that any perturbation of the network could lead to profound effects on the subsequent immune response. The important question is whether a functional network is indeed operating. Available experimental data, discussed in length by a number of authors, clearly support the concept that the immune system is a functional idiotypic network.

Let us consider two outbred rabbits, X and Y. Normally, rabbits X and Y immunized with a given antigen will express the idiotypes IdX and IdY, respectively. Would it be possible to reprogram the immune repertoire of rabbit Y and to favor in this rabbit the expression of IdX? IdX may be silent because of the presence of suppressors whose receptors are able to discriminate between IdX and IdY. If we suppress the suppressors by induction of immunity against them, we would relieve the silent IdX from suppression. This hypothesis is testable and was at the origin of our development of an "immunization cascade" (Urbain *et al.*, 1977). Our results have been extended and confirmed by others (Cazenave, 1977; Bona *et al.*, 1981; Bluestone *et al.*, 1981; Pene *et al.*, 1983).

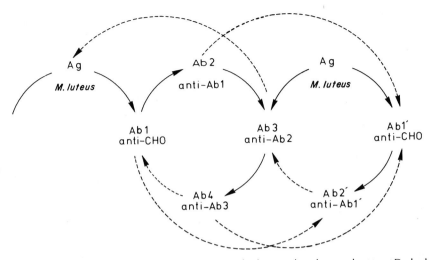

Fig. 2. Immunization cascade showing the antibodies produced at each stage. Dashed arrows indicate the peculiar reactions that are the consequence of the idiotypic manipulations.

Our approach was to obtain sequential sets of antiidiotypic antibodies in different rabbits. This experimental design allowed us to examine the properties of individual elements in a network pathway. The starting idiotype (Ab1) was prepared from rabbits immunized with *Micrococcus*. Ab1 was either an anti-CHO antibody or an anti-Pg antibody produced by individual rabbits.

We started with a randomly chosen anti-CHO antibody of restricted heterogeneity, idiotype Ab1. Allotype-matched rabbits were injected to induce antiidiotypic antibodies (Ab2). The antiidiotypic antisera were tested in immunodiffusion with a panel of sera from 60 rabbits hyperimmunized with the same antigen. Only 1 of the 60 antisera showed a precipitation line with the different Ab2. These specifically purified Ab2 were injected into a third series of rabbits, which produced anti-antiidiotypic antibodies (Ab3). Our initial experiment used five rabbits that were synthesizing Ab3 and into which antigen was injected. Anti-CHO antibodies produced were called Ab1'. We also induced antibodies Ab4 by immunization with purified Ab3 antibodies (Wikler *et al.*, 1979) (Fig. 2).

The major conclusions obtained from these experiments were as follows:

1. Purified anti-CHO antibodies Ab1' were shown to contain antibodies with shared idiotypic determinants with Ab1. Sharing of idiotypic specificities between Ab1 and Ab1' was demonstrated both

by immunodiffusion tests and by binding and inhibition of binding radioimmunoassays.

2. Because Ab4, which are antiidiotypic antibodies to Ab3, recognize Ab1 and Ab1', it may be concluded that Ab1, Ab3, and Ab1' are idiotypically cross-reactive. Despite this idiotypic similarity, the bulk of Ab3 does not react with antigen.

3. Different Ab2 (raised against the same Ab1) originating from separate rabbits are idiotypically similar. These data were confirmed by the properties of Ab2', which are anti-Id to Ab1'. Thus, the rule that any individual is making its own idiotype, Ab1, does not appear to hold at the Ab2 level. There is a striking similarity between Ab2 and Ab4. We have shown that Ab1 and Ab1' from most rabbits completely inhibit the reaction between radiolabeled Ab1 and Ab4. Ab4 appears as an "internal image" of Ab2 in the same way that Ab3 is the internal image of Ab1. Because diversity does not seem to increase along the immunization chain, we may consider that idiotypic networks are made of small interacting communities of idiotypes and antiidiotypes.

4. Antiidiotype antibodies may be of various types depending on the antigenic sites of Ab1 to which they are directed.

    a. Ab2 which recognize idiotopes of Ab1 (called by Jerne Ab2α) constitute the classical antiidiotypic antibodies. The idiotypic reaction with Ab2α may or may not be hapten inhibitable.

    b. A restricted fraction of Ab2 could occasionally be identified in different systems (Urbain et al., 1982; Bona et al., 1982). These Ab2, or homobodies, behave as the internal image of one epitope of the antigen (Lindemann, 1979). They may be induced after injection into rabbits of Ab3 antibodies which recognize both the immunogen (Ab2) and the antigen (TMV). These Ab2 behave like antigen and do not discriminate between the different Ab1 idiotypes. Because a few percent of Ab3 bind only antigen, it is probable that the antigen-like antiidiotypes do not play a significant role in the immunization cascade initiated with *Micrococcus*.

5. The final outcome of idiotypic manipulations will depend on the genetic polymorphism. Although the potential idiotypic repertoires of all rabbits appear to be more or less the same, different rabbits do not have necessarily the same V genes. The sharing of idiotypic specificities between antibodies suggests the existence of idiotypic families made up of molecules sharing some idiotypic determinants. Immunoglobulins possessing the exact combination of idiotopes capable of recognizing antigen constitute Ab1 or Ab1' antibodies. Those immunoglobulins which express only some idiotopes

behave similarly to Ab3 and eventually may bind to different antigens. A related phenomenon was probably observed on a genetic level: One of the seven genes (102) of the NP cluster seems to encode an immunoglobulin which is sharing idiotopes with the recurrent idiotype but does not bind to the hapten (Bothwell *et al.*, 1981).

6. Ab3 appears to be a heterogeneous set of immunoglobulins in which various subsets can be distinguished.

   a. One subset of Ab3 is specific only for Ab2 and behaves as an antiidiotype to Ab2 (anti-Ab2). These Ab3 may possess unique idiotopes which are different from those of Ab1.

   b. Because Ab4 has properties similar to those of Ab2 and reacts with Ab1, we can conclude that part of Ab3 shares idiotopes with Ab1. These Ab3 differ, however, from Ab1 because they do not bind antigen and therefore resemble the immunoglobulins devoid of antibody function that appear during a normal immune response. This subset of Ab3 is not really antiidiotypic antibody but rather idiotypic immunoglobulins and may be denoted Ab3 (Id^+ Ag^-).

   c. Finally, a subset of Ab3 which shares with Ab1 both idiotypic specificity and antibody activity could be characterized. These Ab3 may be similar or even identical to Ab1 and are denoted Ab3 (Id^+ Ag^+). We could detect only 5% of the total amount of Ab3 made by individual rabbits which bound to the antigen and behaved as do antibodies normally induced by immunization. Our hypothesis is that these clones are expanded by antigen stimulation and therefore are the precursors of Ab1′ antibodies. Thus, within the total amount of idiotypically cross-reactive antibodies Ab3, only a minor fraction possesses antibody activity. What is the function of the remaining Ab3, and how can a normal network function in the presence of a majority of idiotypic variants without antibody specificity? Ab3 may well be heteroclitic antibodies with a high affinity for related antigens.

C. SIMULTANEOUS EXPRESSION OF AN IDIOTYPIC COLLECTION

We showed that a given rabbit Y can be programmed to synthesize idiotypes IdX, normally expressed by a nonrelated rabbit X. If the potential idiotypic repertoire is more or less the same in different individuals, rabbit Y may not only be forced to express IdX but may also learn to make antibodies of any idiotype synthesized by rabbit N.

Because the immunization cascade can induce the expression of a silent idiotype, we attempted to provoke the simultaneous expression in a *single* individual of *several* silent clones. The simultaneous expression in a single rabbit of nonrelated idiotypes specific for CHO and originating from six different rabbits was investigated. Purified Ab2 made against Ab1a, Ab1b, Ab1c, Ab1d, Ab1e, and Ab1f were injected as a mixture into a third series of rabbits, which produced anti-antiidiotypic antibodies (Ab3) against Ab2a, Ab2b, etc. Rabbits synthesizing Ab3 received antigen in order to produce Ab1'. The analysis of Ab3 and Ab1' obtained from rabbits that received the mixture of Ab2s revealed clear-cut results. In each case, Ab3 serum contained antibodies reacting exclusively with the six different Ab2 injected. Moreover, purified anti-CHO antibodies Ab1' were reactive by immunodiffusion with three different Ab2 among those which were injected (Fig. 3). The presence of Ab1' reactive with the other Ab2s of the mixture was detected by radioimmunoassay. Thus, by idiotypic manipulations, rabbits could be forced to synthesize simultaneously a series of randomly chosen idiotypes. It was also clear from the results that each of the six idiotypes expressed within Ab1' was found on different antibody molecules. No antibody subfraction has been found to express more than one idiotypic specificity imposed.

These experiments indicate the possible presence of independent idiotypic circuits which do not interfere one with another. We may conclude that several independent silent clones were simultaneously relieved from suppression. All individuals of the species possess the potential genetic information for the synthesis of all idiotypes of the species. Recent findings suggest that the germline repertoire is largely diversified (Bothwell *et al.*, 1981). What may be the size of the repertoire for a given antibody specificity? If idiotypic cross-reactions occur with a frequency of 2 to 5%, it may be estimated that the potential idiotypic repertoire of the species encompasses 20–50 different idiotypes. The experiments described above may be extended. If a rabbit receives n distinct Ab2, it may synthesize n distinct idiotypes after stimulation with antigen. Assuming that n is the number of idiotypes of the species, such a rabbit will express the total potential repertoire of the species.

D. MATERNAL INFLUENCE ON THE IDIOTYPIC NETWORK

We investigated the possible immunoregulatory role of Ab3 by the following experimental procedure (Wikler *et al.*, 1980). Female rab-

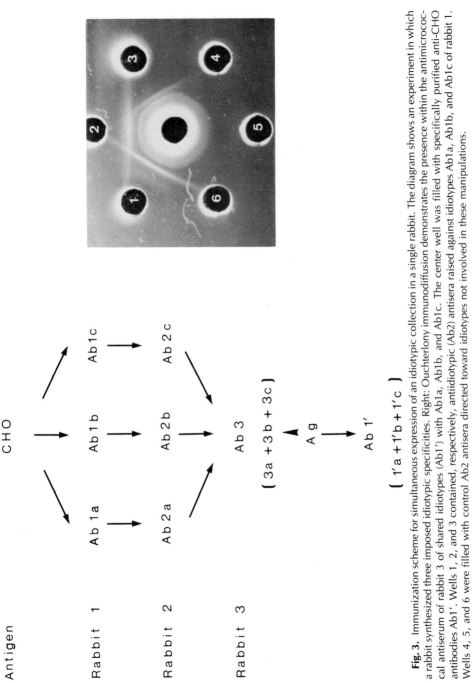

Fig. 3. Immunization scheme for simultaneous expression of an idiotypic collection in a single rabbit. The diagram shows an experiment in which a rabbit synthesized three imposed idiotypic specificities. Right: Ouchterlony immunodiffusion demonstrates the presence within the antimicrococcal antiserum of rabbit 3 of shared idiotypes (Ab1') with Ab1a, Ab1b, and Ab1c. The center well was filled with specifically purified anti-CHO antibodies Ab1'. Wells 1, 2, and 3 contained, respectively, antiidiotypic (Ab2) antisera raised against idiotypes Ab1a, Ab1b, and Ab1c of rabbit 1. Wells 4, 5, and 6 were filled with control Ab2 antisera directed toward idiotypes not involved in these manipulations.

bits were injected with Ab2. When the synthesis of Ab3 was initiated, these rabbits were crossed with naive male rabbits. Three months after the birth of their offspring, both the mothers and their progeny were immunized with the original antigen.

The starting idiotype, Ab1, directed to the Pg of *M. luteus*, was compared to idiotypes produced by five female rabbits (Ab1') and their progeny (Ab1-F_1). Our results clearly indicate that both the mothers and 40% of the offspring synthesized idiotypes cross-reactive with the starting antibody, Ab1. A rabbit can thus "learn" to make the antibodies of another rabbit, and this "learning" can be transmitted to offspring by maternal Igs of the Ab3 type. These results indicate that maternal Ab3 antibodies inhibit the suppressors of the expression of the offspring Ab1' idiotypes which are kept silent by reaction with Ab2. Hiernaux *et al.* (1981) also showed that neonatal injection of antiidiotypic antibodies specific for a silent idiotype can induce the expression of the idiotype. It should also be recalled that the imposed idiotypic specificities in Ab1' and Ab1-F_1 rabbits are long-lasting phenomena and are probably permanent. Rabbits restimulated with antigen 2 years after the initial Ab1' or Ab1-F_1 production were shown to continue to produce idiotypic cross-reactive antibodies with Ab1.

That the acquired immunological characteristics were transmitted to the progeny by maternal immunoglobulins of the Ab3 type and not by the male parent was checked by the following experiment. Instead of crossing female rabbits producing Ab3 with naive males, we crossed male Ab3 individuals with naive females and again immunized the offspring with *Micrococcus*. No idiotypic cross-reactions were found in the offspring. These findings are in contrast to the claim of Gorczynsky and Steele (1980) that an acquired immunological feature could be transmitted from the male parent to the progeny.

The next experiment was performed in order to control the restriction of the immunoregulation to the anti-Pg antibody, Ab1. Antiidiotypic serum Ab2, directed toward anti-CHO antibody isolated from the same immune serum as Ab1, was prepared. This Ab2 exclusively recognized anti-CHO antibody from rabbit 1 and failed to react with any anti-CHO idiotypes present either in Ab1'-producing rabbits or in Ab1-F_1 antisera. Thus, whatever the complexity of the initial response may be, specific idiotypes of one rabbit can be selectively induced in other rabbits. Idiotypic circuits appear normally as independent entities of lymphocytes bearing receptors of different specificities.

IV. Immunochemical Studies on Cross-Reactive Idiotypes

Immunochemical characterizations of Ab1 and Ab1' antibodies included location of the idiotypic determinants, antigen inhibition of the idiotype–antiidiotype reaction, fine antigenic specificity of antibodies, and allotype content (see Table I).

A. FINE ANTIGENIC SPECIFICITY OF Ab1 AND Ab1' ANTIBODIES

Four Ab1' specific for the CHO, all idiotypically cross-reactive with Ab1, were studied for their fine antigenic specificity. Inhibition of binding of idiotype to radiolabeled CHO was tested using sugar analogs of *Micrococcus* polysaccharide. For each system studied, significant inhibition was obtained with glucose. Inhibition of idiotype binding was, however, more efficient with disaccharides: cellobiose, gentiobiose, and maltose. Maximum inhibition (up to 68%) was observed with maltose, indicating that the series of idiotypically related antibodies may all be directed against similar or identical antigenic sites of the polysaccharide which include α-1-4 glucosidic bonds.

TABLE I

Immunochemical Studies on Cross-Reactive Idiotypes

	Ab1 (2975)	Ab1' (2281)
1. Serum anti-CHO content	15 mg/ml	7.6 mg/ml
2. Allotype content		
Binding to anti-a2	81%	85%
Binding to anti-a3	19%	13%
3. Antiidiotype (Ab2) binding to ^{125}I-labeled idiotype	85%	65%
4. Inhibition of Ab2 binding to ^{125}I-labeled idiotype		
inhibitors: *Micrococcus* CHO	56%	65%
Maltose	<5%	<5%
5. Inhibition of idiotype binding to ^{125}I-labeled CHO		
inhibitors: Antiidiotype (Ab2)	95%	100%
Glucose	24%	32%
Maltose	55%	68%

B. IDIOTYPIC DETERMINANTS OF Ab1 AND
   Ab1′ ANTIBODIES

A common feature of Ab1 and Ab1′ is the location of some of their idiotypic determinants near the antigen combining site. This was demonstrated by antigen inhibition of idiotype binding to anti-idiotype and by antiidiotype inhibition of antibody binding to cell wall antigens (Table I). The antiidiotypic serum was capable of completely inhibiting the binding of Ab1 or Ab1′ with radioiodinated CHO. Controls made with anti-Id to anti-CHO antibodies with no idiotypic cross-reactivity with Ab1 had no effect on this reaction.

To map more precisely the idiotypic sharing between Ab1 and Ab1′, we prepared hybrid molecules using various combinations of H and L chains. The specificity of reassociated H and L chains was studied by inhibition of ^{125}I-Fab Ab1 reaction with Ab2. Briefly, we observed that free H and L chains derived from Ab1 or Ab1′ were poor inhibitors; 50% inhibition required more than 100-fold molar excess as compared to homologous hybrid molecules H1-L1 and H1′-L1′. These showed the inhibitory capacity of the native Ab1 and Ab1′ or their Fab fragments. Heterologous hybrids, H1-LX and HX-L1, where LX and HX were derived from anti-CHO antibody with no idiotypic relationship to Ab1, did not inhibit the reaction significantly. Only heterologous hybrids H1-L1′ and H1′-L1 showed the inhibitory capacity of native Ab1. These observations point out the requirement of both H and L for idiotypic expression (Sirisinha and Eisen, 1971). Because the hybrids H1-L1′ and L1′-L1 both possess idiotypic specificity, it is likely that H1 and H1′, on the one side, and L1 and L1′, on the other, are idiotypically equivalent.

C. LINKAGE BETWEEN ALLOTYPES AND IDIOTYPES

All rabbits used in this study were heterozygous at the a locus; they were phenotypically a2 a3. The anti-CHO Ab1 (rabbit 2975) idiotype used to obtain Ab2 was mostly a2 (81% of radiolabeled Ab1 bound to anti-a2 serum). It is striking to note that Ab1′ (rabbit 2281) that bore idiotypic specificities similar to those of Ab1 were mainly or solely of the a2 allotype (85% of Ab1′ bound to anti-a2 serum). Therefore, the similar idiotypes detected in Ab1 and Ab1′ may be linked to the a2 allotype. Moreover, the expression of Ab3, which shares idiotypes with Ab1 but is mainly inactive toward the antigen, may be linked to the a2 allotype. Specifically purified Ab3, on an immunoadsorbent made with Ab2, possessed 70% of molecules expressing the a2 allotype. Further, 63% of radioiodinated Ab3 material was able to bind to Ab2. The strong linkage between a allotypes and idiotypes observed during idiotypic manipulations has already been described in other rabbit systems (Sogn *et al.*, 1977; Cazenave and Le Guern, 1979). The genetic origin (germline genes or somatic variants) of idiotypes is being further investigated in our laboratory by the use of monoclonal antibodies directed against subsets of a allotypes.

D. IDIOTYPIC MANIPULATIONS WITH CROSS-REACTIVE Pg-SPECIFIC IDIOTYPE

The experiments described in this section concern the fine idiotypic analysis of anti-Pg antibodies. The fine idiotypic specificity was established for anti-Pg antibodies, which shared idiotypic features with the reference antibody Ab1 (isolated from the antiserum of rabbit 2977). These were cross-reactive idiotypes of the Ab1′ type, obtained through the immunization chain (Ab1-Ab2-Ab3). Idiotypic antibodies of the Ab1-F_1 type were obtained from the offspring of female rabbits actively producing Ab3 during pregnancy (see Section III, D). Finally, cross-reactive idiotypes with Ab1 were found by screening sera from a random population of rabbits immunized with *M. luteus* that were named Ab1 CRI.

We established the existence within Ab1 molecules of three sets of idiotopes. We then studied the distribution of these idiotopes among the series of cross-reactive antibodies defined above (Fig. 4). It appeared that all of the antibodies selected shared at least one common idiotope (IdX). This idiotope was found on Ab1, Ab1′, Ab1-F_1, and Ab1 CRI antibodies and seems to be associated with anti-Pg specificity in the rabbit, as it was not detected on antibodies against the carbohydrate of *Micrococcus*. However, IdX does not seem to be directly implicated in the binding site to antigen, as Ab1 CRI binding to Ab2 is not significantly inhibited by the antigen. Although Ab1 CRI shared IdX only with Ab1, further analysis showed that this specific IdX occurred in 20% of outbred rabbits immunized with a micrococcal vaccine. However, only Ab1′ and Ab1-F_1 possess, in addition to IdX, a second idiotope in common with Ab1 (IdM). This idiotope was expressed only through idiotypic manipulations and appears to be implicated in the combining site. Finally, a private idiotope to Ab1, IdI, was never found on antibodies obtained through idiotypic manipulations or on randomly occurring Ab1 CRI antibodies.

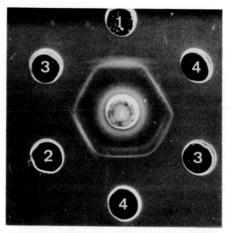

Fig. 4. Shared idiotypes among rabbit antibodies to Pg. Ouchterlony immunodiffusion demonstrates idiotypic cross-reactions among four types of anti-Pg antibodies. (1) The reference
idiotype, Ab1, was isolated from a preparative isoelectric columm as an individual antibody
fraction from rabbit 2977. (2) Anti-Pg antibody Ab1' from rabbit 76 was induced through the
immunization chain (Ab1-Ab2-Ab3) using Ab2 directed to anti-Pg Ab1. (3) Idiotypic antibodies
of the Ab1-F_1 type were obtained from the offspring of female rabbits actively producing Ab3
during pregnancy. (4) Ab1 CRI were cross-reactive anti-Pg idiotypes with Ab2 screened from
outbred rabbits immunized with *Micrococcus*. The center well contains antiidiotypic antibody
(Ab2) directed toward Ab1.

By the use of antiidiotypic antibodies, it is possible to induce a
nominated antibody idiotype on challenge with antigen. The analysis
of idiotope selection is just beginning. There are many questions to be
answered: Are some idiotypes more likely to be selected than others?
As a consequence, can we predict the emergence of some idiotypes by
idiotypic manipulations? Because shared idiotopes do not necessarily
imply shared combining sites or shared specificity, how do anti-Id and
antigen impose the production of antibodies? What is the relative
importance of both sets of regulatory requirements, specificity and
idiotype? Is there a hierarchy of idiotypic selection, and what may be
the origin and the function of "public idiotopes"?

Some idiotypic sites appear to be closely associated with the active
site of antibody. However, other idiotopes do not participate in the
active site. Moreover, dominant idiotypes may be expressed on antibody molecules with specificity for the same region of a protein antigen but differing fine specificity. In the multideterminant antilysozyme response (Benjamin *et al.*, 1980), mice belonging to eight

different strains expressed this idiotype and almost all antilysozyme bore the major idiotype.

Murine anti-PC antibodies and myeloma fall into three discrete families bearing either the T15, M603, or M511 idiotype. The three idiotypic families are known to differ in their fine specificity for the PC analogs and PC carrier conjugates, although their affinity for the PC hapten is similar. However, the predominant expression of the T15 idiotype seems to be related to its optimal protective effect against PC-containing pathogens such as *Streptococcus pneumoniae*. This suggests that the mechanisms regulating idiotype expression may play an important role in the maintenance of antibody sets that are optimally protective against various infectious agents. Moreover, these findings suggest that the T15 germline H-chain variable region gene may have been selected through evolution to code for antibody binding PC-containing pathogens (Briles *et al.*, 1982).

Network-mediated regulation implies that antibody idiotopes are capable of inducing auto-antiidiotypic responses. It may well be that the inheritance of the idiotype genes may have as a consequence the selection for germline genes coding for the immunoregulatory auto-antiidiotype (Bona *et al.*, 1981; Pierce *et al.*, 1981). We may argue that only those idiotopes capable of eliciting auto-antiidiotypic responses will be selected through evolution. Consequently, this tandem selection will be independent of whether or not the idiotopes are located in proximity to the paratope.

Cross-reactive idiotype could result from either real idiotypic similarity or the presence in Ab2 of antiidiotypic antibodies which mimic antigen. In our case, the cross-reactive idiotope of Ab1, Ab1', Ab1-F_1, and Ab1 CRI of anti-Pg antibodies described above appears to be a real idiotope, because it was not inhibitable by the antigen but was only recognized by antiidiotypic antibodies made against Ab1. Such cross-reactive idiotopes of the antimicrococcal antibodies for which naturally induced autoantiidiotypic antibodies were detected in outbred rabbits (Binion and Rodkey, 1982) support strongly the functional network concept of immunoregulation.

V. Conclusions

Sequential immunizations (Ab1-Ab2-Ab3-Ab4) were performed in rabbits in order to test various aspects of Jerne's network hypothesis. The expression of specific idiotypes was manipulated in 35 cases using antiidiotypic Ab2 antibodies directed against idiotypes Ab1 of the *Micrococcus* system. Altogether, 33 Ab1' were reactive with Ab2. On average, only 5% of Ab3 molecules were active toward the antigen. Ab3, however, shared idiotypes with Ab1 and Ab1', as was shown by the use of Ab4. A large portion of Ab4 is very similar to Ab2 and Ab2'. Anti-Id made in different rabbits are also idiotypically similar. It appears, therefore, that idiotypic networks are built up with a restricted family of clones which bear similar idiotypes that do not necessarily share a common antigenic specificity (for example, Ab1 and Ab3).

An immunization chain using a mixture made with six different Ab2 was initiated in a single rabbit. Analysis of Ab3 and Ab1' revealed that it was possible to induce in a single individual a simultaneous expression of several usually silent clones. These experiments indicate the presence of independent idiotypic circuits with no interference from one another. Silent idiotypes of expected specificity can also be revealed in the offspring of female rabbits synthesizing Ab3.

Analysis of the fine idiotypic specificity of Ab1 and Ab1' indicated that part of the common idiotypic determinants are located within or near the antigen-combining site. Both H and L chains are required for the expression of the shared idiotypic specificity between Ab1 and Ab1'. Also, a strong linkage between a allotypes and idiotypes was observed during idiotypic manipulations.

The preferential expression of some idiotypic determinants common to idiotypically related anti-Pg antibodies was revealed. These idiotopes may have a predominant regulatory function in the immunologic network.

Manipulation of the immune response with idiotypic reagents appears to be a fruitful approach in understanding both the regulatory mechanisms governing antibody synthesis and the problem of the origin of antibody diversity.

We focused our studies on idiotypes à la Oudin in the rabbit. These idiotypes occur in a frequency of 2 to 5% when the animals are confronted with the same antigen. Yet, in several idiotypic systems, using the cascade immunization methodology, we consistently forced randomly chosen rabbits to express a predetermined idiotype Ab1. The obvious conclusion is that all individuals of the species possess a more or less similar gene library of V genes. It may be assumed from the frequency of idiotypic cross-reactions that the number of idiotypes that exist in the species for a given antigen varies between 20 and 50. It is remarkable that most, if not all, of these idiotypes have an equal chance to be expressed after antigenic stimulation. In fact, cascade immunizations of individual rabbits with mixtures of anti-Id originating from non-cross-reactive idiotypes led to a simultaneous synthesis of as many as six imposed idiotypes in the same animal. Because each of these idiotypes was present on distinct antibody molecules, it is probable that the animal possessed independent genetic information for each idiotype.

That the immune response depends on the idiotypic history of the animal was shown by the maternal effect of Ab3 immunoglobulins on the idiotype expression of the offspring. Thus, idiotypic networks are setup at early ontogenetic stages of immunization. Once oriented toward a given idiotypic network, an animal appears to use for the regulation of the immune response the same set of Id–anti-Id interactions throughout a long period of its life.

It is crucial to determine the structure and genetic origin of idiotypic determinants in order to understand the various aspects of the regulatory mechanisms: regulation through idiotypes–antiidiotypes; the Ir gene control of the self anti-Id response; and cross-reactions of T-cell receptors and Ig idiotypes still unexplained at the molecular and genetic level.

Acknowledgments

Contributors to this work include Drs. C. Wuilmart, J-D Franssen, M. Francotte, C. Collignon, C. Demeur, L. Van Hamme, and G. Dewasme.

We thank all of our colleagues from the Laboratory of Animal Physiology, who provided help and discussion during this research.

This work was supported by grants from the Belgian State and Fonds de la Recherche Fondamentale Collective 2.4524-80.

References

Benjamin, C. D., Miller, A., Sercarz, E. C., and Harvey, M. A. (1980). *J. Immunol.* **125**, 1017–1025.

Binion, S. B., and Rodkey, L. S. (1982). *J. Exp. Med.* **156**, 860–872.

Binz, H., and Wigzell, H. (1977). *Contemp. Top. Immunobiol.* **7**, 113–177.

Bluestone, J. A., Epstein, S. L., Ozato, K., Sharrow, S. D., and Sachs, D. (1981). *J. Exp. Med.* **154**, 1305–1318.

Bona, C. A., Heber-Katz, E., and Paul, W. E. (1981). *J. Exp. Med.* **153**, 951–957.

Bona, C. A., Finley, S., Waters, S. and Kunkel, H. G. (1982). *J. Exp. Med.* **156**, 986–999.

Bordenave, G. R. (1973). *Eur. J. Immunol.* **3**, 718–726.

Bordenave, G. R. (1975). *Immunology* **28**, 635–651.

Bothwell, A., Paskind, M., Reth, M., Imanishi, T., Rajewsky, K., and Baltimore, D. (1981). *Cell* **24**, 625–637.

Briles, D. E., Forman, C., Hudak, S., and Claflin, J. L. (1982). *J. Exp. Med.* **156**, 1177–1185.

Brown, J. C., and Rodkey, L. S. (1979). *J. Exp. Med.* **150**, 67–85.

Cazenave, P.-A. (1977). *Proc. Natl. Acad. Sci. U.S.A.* **74**, 5122–5125.

Cazenave, P.-A., and Le Guern, C. (1979). *In* "Cells of Immunoglobulin Synthesis" (B. Pernis and H. S. Vogel, eds.), pp. 343–355. Academic Press, New York.

Eichmann, K., and Rajewsky, K. (1975). *Eur. J. Immunol.* **5**, 661–666.

Ghuysen, J. M. (1968). *Bacteriol. Rev.* **32**, 425–464.

Gorczinsky, R. M., and Steele, E. J. (1980). *Proc. Natl. Acad. Sci. U.S.A.* **77**, 2871–2875.

Hiernaux, J., Bona, C., and Baker, P. J. (1981). *J. Exp. Med.* **153**, 1004–1008.

Jerne, N. K. (1974). *Ann. Immunol. (Paris)* **125C**, 373–389.

Ju, S. T., Benacerraf, B., and Dorf, M. E. (1980a). *J. Exp. Med.* **152**, 170–182.

Ju, S. T., Pierres, M., Germain, R. N., Benacerraf, B., and Dorf, M. E. (1980b). *J. Immunol.* **125**, 1230–1236.

Karakawa, W. W., Lackland, H., and Krause, R. M. (1966). *J. Immunol.* **97**, 797–804.

Karakawa, W. W., Braun, D. G., Lackland, H., and Krause, R. M. (1968). *J. Exp. Med.* **128**, 325–340.

Kohno, Y., Berkover, I., Minna, J., and Berzofsky, J. A. (1982). *J. Immunol.* **128**, 1742–1748.

Krause, R. M., and McCarty, M. (1961). *J. Exp. Med.* **114**, 127–140.

Kunkel, H. G., Mannik, M., and Williams, R. C. (1963). *Science* **140**, 1218–1219.

Lindemann, J. (1979). *Ann. Immunol. (Paris)* **130C**, 311–319.

Metzger, D. W., Miller, A., and Sercarz, E. E. (1980). *Nature (London)* **287**, 540–542.

Oudin, J. (1974). *Antigens* **2**, 277–374.

Oudin, J., and Cazenave, P.-A. (1971). *Proc. Natl. Acad. Sci. U.S.A.* **68**, 2616–2620.

Oudin, J., and Michel, M. (1963). *C. R. Hebd. Seances Acad. Sci.* **257**, 805–808.

Pawlak, L. L., Hart, D. A., and Nisonoff, A. (1973). *J. Exp. Med.* **137**, 1442–1458.

Pène, J., Bekkhoucha, F., Desaymard, C., Zaghouani, H., and Stanislawski, M. (1983). *J. Exp. Med.* **157**, 1573–1593.

Perkins, H. R. (1963). *Biochem. J.* **86**, 475–483.

Pierce, S. K., Speck, N. A., Gleason, K., Gearhart, P. J., and Köhler, H. (1981). *J. Exp. Med.* **154**, 1178–1187.

Rodkey, L. S. (1974). *J. Exp. Med.* **139**, 712–720.

Rodkey, L. S. (1976). *J. Immunol.* **117**, 986–989.

Rolicka, M., and Park, J. T. (1969). *J. Immunol.* **103**, 196–203.

Schleifer, K. H., and Krause, R. M. (1971). *Eur. J. Biochem.* **19**, 471–478.

Sirisinha, S., and Eisen, H. N. (1971). *Proc. Natl. Acad. Sci. U.S.A.* **68**, 3130–3135.

Sogn, S. A., Coligan, J. E., and Kindt, T. J. (1977). *Fed. Proc.*, **36**, 214–220.

Urbain, J., Tasiaux, N., Leuwenkroon, R., Van Acker, A., and Mariamé, B. (1975). *Eur. J. Immunol.* **5**, 570–575.

Urbain, J., Wikler, M., Franssen, J.-D., and Collignon, C. (1977). *Proc. Natl. Acad. Sci. U.S.A.* **74**, 5126–5130.

Urbain, J., Wuilmart, C., and Cazenave, P.-A. (1981). *Contemp. Top. Immunol.* **8**, 113–148.

Urbain, J., Slaoui, M., and Leo, O. (1982). *Ann. Immunol. (Paris)* **133D**, 179–189.

Urbain-Vansanten, G., Van Acker, A., Mariamé, B., Tasiaux, N., De Vos-Cloetens, C., and Urbain, J. (1979). *Ann. Immunol. (Paris)* **130C**, 397–406.

Van Hoegaerden, M., Wikler, M., Janssens, R., and Kanarek, L. (1975). *Eur. J. Biochem.* **53**, 19–24.

Wikler, M. (1975). Z. *Immunitaets forsch., Exp. Klin. Immunol.* **149**, 193–200.
Wikler, M., Franssen, J.-D., Collignon, C., Leo, O., Mariamé, B., Van de Walle, P., De Groote, D., and Urbain, J. (1979). *J. Exp. Med.* **150**, 184–195.
Wikler, M., Demeur, C., Dewasme, G., and Urbain, J. (1980). *J. Exp. Med.* **152**, 1024–1035.
Wikler, M., Dewasme, G., and Urbain, J. (1983). In preparation.
Wuilmart, C., Wikler, M., and Urbain, J. (1979). *Mol. Immunol.* **16**, 1085–1092.

Chapter 14

Idiotypes of Anti-MHC Monoclonal Antibodies

Jeffrey A. Bluestone, Hugh Auchincloss, Jr.,
Suzanne L. Epstein, and David H. Sachs

Transplantation Biology Section, Immunology Branch
National Cancer Institute, National Institutes of Health
Bethesda, Maryland

I. Introduction[1]

Major histocompatibility complex (MHC) antigens are important in numerous immune responses involving both self-recognition and allo-reactivity. The class I antigens, encoded by the H-2K and H-2D regions in the mouse MHC, are associated with self-restricted cytotoxic T-cell recognition of foreign antigens (such as viruses and haptens) and elicit a variety of strong responses across allogeneic differences (1–3), including rapid skin graft rejection. Class II antigens, encoded

[1] *Abbreviations:* Ab3, antibodies induced by anti-Id and capable of inhibiting anti-Id binding to Id; C, complement; CFA, complete Freund's adjuvant; CML, cell-mediated lympholysis; ELISA, enzyme-linked immunosorbent assay; H and L chains, heavy and light chains of Ig; Id, idiotype; Id′, idiotype-bearing antibodies induced by anti-Id treatment; Ig, immunoglobulin; KLH, keyhole limpet hemocyanin; LPS, lipopolysaccharide; mAbs, monoclonal antibodies; MHC, major histocompatibility complex; PC, phosphorylcholine.

in the I region, play a vital role in proliferative responses to foreign antigens and are involved in cell–cell interactions in T-cell dependent antibody responses (4, 5) and in graft-versus-host responses (6). In addition, both class I and class II antigens provide a major barrier to organ transplantation (7) and are intimately involved in the generation of tolerance (8).

Fundamental to our appreciation of such MHC-related immune responses is a more precise understanding of the nature of anti-MHC receptors. One approach to the study of immune receptors has been the use of antiidiotypic antisera specific for antigenic determinants at or near the antigen-binding site of the receptor (9–12). As reported elsewhere in this volume, these reagents have been used in many systems to manipulate the repertoire of antigen-reactive cells and to regulate antigen recognition. Antibodies directed specifically at anti-MHC receptors might therefore be useful in studying the structural basis of antigen recognition and the relationship between anti-MHC receptors on T and B cells involved in self- and allorecognition, and thus might provide a greater understanding of the generation and regulation of immune responses. Of clinical importance is the fact that these reagents might provide a specific means to modify alloimmune reactivity and perhaps overcome the transplantation barrier.

Throughout the 1970s, there were many attempts to generate anti-idiotypic antisera against alloreceptors. Ramseier (13, 14), Binz *et al.* (15, 16), and others (17, 18) reported the production of antisera against both alloreactive T-cell blasts and alloantibodies. These immune sera had broad effects on *in vivo* and *in vitro* immune responses and were reported to detect public idiotypic specificities on both T and B cells (14, 15). They were used to manipulate alloresponses (13, 16) and to help elucidate the molecular structure of the alloreactive T-cell receptor (14). However, as time progressed, several criticisms were leveled at such studies. In some cases (17; N. Shinohara and D. H. Sachs, unpublished data), it has been extremely difficult to generate such antiidiotypic reagents reproducibly, perhaps because of the complex nature of anti-MHC responses. In addition, questions have been raised about the nature of the antigen-binding material used to make the alloantibody-specific anti-Id (14). Alloantibodies were clearly present in the antisera, but the possible presence of contaminating T-cell receptor material which may have served as an immunogen could not be excluded, although anti-Ig absorptions were carried out in several systems in an attempt to rule out this possibility (14). These studies were, nevertheless, quite provocative and demanded reproducible new approaches to examine their important implications.

With the generation of monoclonal antibodies (mAbs), a highly reliable, reproducible source of anti-MHC receptors became available for the production of antiidiotypic reagents (19–22). Anti-MHC antibodies purified from culture supernatant are presumably not contaminated with any mouse-derived T-cell products. In this chapter, we will summarize our attempts to study anti-MHC receptors using anti-Id produced against such anti-H-2 and anti-Ia mAbs. We have examined the prevalence of these idiotypes in conventional alloantisera and on other mAbs and employed these antiidiotypes *in vivo* to modify antibody responses to MHC antigens. Finally, in this chapter we will report our early attempts at manipulating T-cell functions and discuss possible relationships between the alloreactive T- and B-cell repertoires as revealed by these studies.

II. Production, Purification, and Specificity of Anti-MHC Antiidiotypes

Antiidiotypic antibodies have been generated against several anti-MHC mAbs directed at either class I or class II antigens. The origin of the antibodies and a summary of their characteristics are shown in Table I. Individual mAbs were directed against either public or private determinants, some of which correlate with serological specificities defined by alloantisera (20–23). Xenogeneic antiidiotypic antibodies were produced in miniature swine and rabbits immunized repeatedly at approximately monthly intervals with 200 μg (100 μg for rabbits) of protein A affinity-purified antibodies from hybridoma culture supernatants in complete Freund's adjuvant (CFA) im (24). Syngeneic and allogeneic antiidiotypes were produced by immunizing and boosting with purified mAbs coupled to solubilized keyhole limpet hemocyanin (KLH) by glutaraldehyde fixation (25). Repeated immunizations were performed, and antimouse Ig activity was monitored in xenoimmunizations by hemagglutination of sheep erythrocytes coated with a myeloma protein of the same Ig subclass (26). After the antimouse activity had plateaued, both xenogeneic and syngeneic antiidiotypes were purified by affinity chromatography (24). Sera were extensively absorbed with myeloma Ig and/or normal Ig coupled to Sepharose to remove all antinormal Ig activity. Antiidiotypic antibodies were then absorbed to and eluted from idiotype-bearing Sepharose columns.

In all systems studied, this absorption procedure has led to specific antiidiotypic antibodies, as evidenced by the loss of reactivity with

TABLE I

Summary of Anti-MHC mAbs Used to Generate Anti-Id

Hybridoma lines	Parental cells	Immunizing cells	Speci- ficity	Cross- reactions	Ig class	Reference
3-83	BALB/c	C3H/HeJ	K^k, D^k	K^b, s, p, q, r,	IgG_{2a}, κ	19
11-4.1	BALB/c	CKB	K^k	K^q, p, r	IgG_{2a}, κ	21
16-3-22	C3H.SW	C3H/HeJ	K^k	None	IgG_{2a}, κ	19
12-2-2	C3H.SW	C3H/HeJ	K^k, D^k	K^q, p, r	IgM, κ	19
36-7-5	A.TL	A.AL	K^k	None	IgG_{2a}, κ	19
142-23	BALB/c	CBA	K^k, D^k	K^b, s, q, r (p)	IgG_{2b}, κ	22
100-30	BALB/c	CBA	K^k, D^k	b, s, q, r	IgG_{2b}, κ	22
28-13-3	C3H/HeJ	C3H.SW	K^b	f	IgM, κ	20
28-14-8	C3H/HeJ	C3H.SW	D^b	L^d, D^q, L^q	IgG_{2a}, κ	20
30-5-7	BALB/c.H-2^{dm2}	BALB/c	L^d	L^q, D^q	IgG_{2a}, κ	20
23-10-1	BALB/c.H-2^{dm2}	BALB/c	L^d	L^q, D^q	IgM, κ	20
17-3-3	C3H.SW	C3H/HeJ	I-E^k	r	IgG_{2a}, κ	23
14-4-4	C3H.SW	C3H/HeJ	I-E/C^k	d, p, r	IgG_{2a}, κ	20
10-2.16	CWB	C3H	I-A^k	f, r, s	IgG_{2b}, κ	21

nòrmal Ig, but retention of very high levels of binding to the specific immunogen. Yields of purified antiidiotypes ranged from 0.05 to 0.5 mg/ml of hyperimmune serum. At least a portion of the antiidiotype activity was directed against combining site-related determinants, because these reagents were shown to inhibit the binding of homologous anti-MHC mAbs to MHC antigen-bearing lymphocytes (Fig. 1).

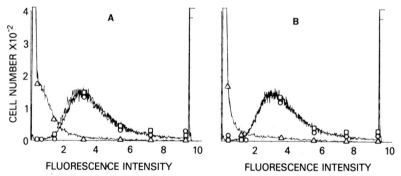

Fig. 1. Inhibition of binding of 36-7-5 to H-2K^k-bearing lymph node cells by xenogeneic and syngeneic anti-Id. (A) □——□, 36-7-5 alone; ○——○, 36-7-5 plus pig anti-3-83; △——△, 36-7-5 plus pig anti-36-7-5. (B) □——□, 36-7-5 alone; ○——○, 36-7-5 plus mouse anti-3-83; △——△, 36-7-5 plus mouse anti-36-7-5. Fluorescence-activated cell sorter (FACS) analyses are illustrated by continuous lines. Symbols have been introduced arbitrarily to facilitate profile identification.

III. Prevalence of MHC Idiotypes in Conventional Alloantisera

Although we were able to generate antiidiotypic antibodies against anti-MHC mAbs, it was unclear whether these reagents, directed to only a limited number of possible receptors, would detect determinants expressed by a significant portion of anti-MHC antibodies of similar specificities. We therefore examined the expression of idiotypes in alloantisera and on a large panel of hybridoma anti-MHC antibodies that included several mAbs with fine specificities identical to the idiotypes (27–29). Our results showed that the prevalence of Id among antibodies in alloantisera varies depending on the idiotypic system studied. The Id of the mAb 14-4-4 has been shown to be expressed widely in responses of C3H.SW mice to the I-E antigen (Fig. 2) (27). Id expression was elicited in about 90% of individuals

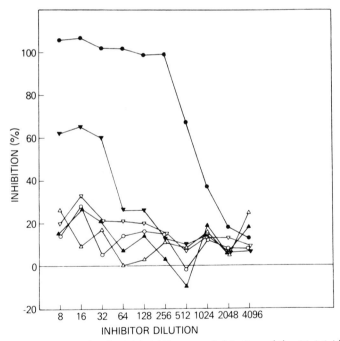

Fig. 2. Inhibition ELISA for the 14-4-4 idiotype and detection of the 14-4-4 idiotype in C3H.SW anti-C3H alloantibody. ●, purified 14-4-4; ○, purified 17-3-3; △ and ▲, C3H.SW normal serum, two different pools; ▽, LPC-1 ascites fluid; ▼, C3H.SW anti-C3H immune ascites 1080. Dilutions of antibodies purified from ascites fluids were started at 50 μg/ml. Diluent, 1 : 8 dilution of C3H.SW normal serum. Percentage of inhibition = uninhibited A492 − experimental A492/uninhibited A492 − background A492. (Reprinted from the *Journal of Immunology*.)

skin-grafted with I-E-positive tail skin, and in a pool of antibody, Id represented approximately 30–50% of the anti-I-E antibodies produced. The expressed Id could be detected both by inhibition by alloantisera of anti-Id binding to idiotype-coated plates (a noncombining site-specific assay) and by the inhibition of binding of anti-I-E antibodies to I-E-positive lipopolysaccharide (LPS)-induced B-cell blasts. Specific *in vivo* absorption of the alloantisera demonstrated that essentially all of the idiotype was expressed on anti-I-E antibodies (27).

The influence of allotype-linked genes on 14-4-4 Id expression in the response to I-E has also been investigated (27). Both the C57BL/10 and CWB (an Igh-C^b congenic of C3H.SW) strains of mice expressed extremely low levels of idiotype after immunization, much lower than that of C3H.SW and in fact not significantly above preimmune serum backgrounds. However, a few individual CWB mice expressed higher levels of Id as assessed by serological assays. These idiotype-bearing molecules, present in CWB immune sera, could be detected as discrete bands after isoelectric focusing on acrylamide gels overlaid with ^{125}I-labeled anti-Id. Thus, although allotype-linked genes clearly influence the level of Id expression, the CWB strain has the genetic capacity to express at least some of the 14-4-4-related family of idiotopes.

Predominant idiotypes were also detected in two other idiotype systems: one, an anti-H-2K^b mAb (28-13-3) (30); the other, an anti-H-2L^d mAb (23-10-1) (31). The 28-13-3 Id was expressed in all C3H mice immunized with H-2K^b tissue as assayed by an ELISA inhibition assay. The Id expression was allotype linked. C3H/HeJ and CBA/J mice expressed high levels of Id after alloimmunization, whereas B10, BALB/c, and A/J mice did not. In the 23-10-1 Id system, xenogeneic anti-Id inhibited the binding of anti-L^d antibodies produced by BALB/c.H-2^{dm2} mice hyperimmunized with BALB/c tissue. The predominant Id was present on both IgG and IgM antibodies representing approximately one-quarter to one-half of the total anti-L^d humoral response. In addition, the Id expression was limited to those alloantibodies reacting with the same serological specificity (H-2.65) as the 23-10-1 mAb. Thus, anti-Id prepared against 23-10-1 inhibited the binding of anti-L^d antibodies to B10.D2 lymph node cells, which expressed both the H-2.64 and H-2.65 determinants but did not inhibit the binding of this same alloantiserum to B10 lymph node cells expressing only the H-2.64 specificity (31, 32). This finding is illustrated in Fig. 3.

In contrast to the detection of public idiotypes in three mAb sys-

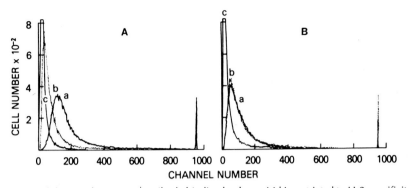

Fig. 3. Inhibition of anti-H-2L^d antibody binding by the anti-Id is restricted to H-2 specificity 65. B10.D2 (H-2.64$^+$ and H-2.65$^+$) (A) or B10 (H-2.64$^+$) (B) spleen cells were reacted with αH-2L^d sera which had been preincubated with pig Ig (a) or pig-anti-23-10-1(b). Bound antibodies were detected by FITC-goat F(ab)$_2$ antimouse IgG (Fc, γ chain specific). The profile (c) represents background fluorescence obtained by staining with F$_1$ reagent alone. (Reprinted from the *European Journal of Immunology.*)

tems, many of the anti-Id prepared against other anti-MHC mAbs detected relatively private idiotypes, as determined by either the site-specific antigen-binding inhibition assay or the non-site-specific Id-binding inhibition assay. This group included all the anti-H-2K^k mAbs studied (29, 33, 42), as well as several anti-Ia (27) and anti-L mAbs (31). The reasons for these differences remain unclear. However, one of several possible reasons for the dominance of certain idiotypes in alloantisera may be that the degree of somatic diversification away from the germline sequence differs among the mAbs used to generate anti-Ids. In two of the three Id systems in which shared Id have been detected, the mAbs used were IgM antibodies (Table I).

It has recently been shown that in several systems primary antibody responses are less diverse idiotypically then secondary responses (34, 35) and that IgM antibodies often account for the dominance of a shared idiotype. In this regard, Gearhart *et al.* (36) analyzed the amino acid and nucleotide sequences of 16 antiphosphorylcholine (PC) myeloma and hybridoma antibodies and their genes. The studies showed that the IgM antibodies were much less diverse and more closely resembled the germline anti-PC gene than either the IgG or IgA antibodies. If IgM antibodies more closely resemble germline structures, then one might expect idiotypic determinants expressed on IgM antibodies to be shared among other antibodies derived from the same or similar germline genes. On the other hand, IgG antibodies, having somatically diversified from the germline structure, may express many immunogenic determinants not shared with other antibodies of similar specificity. Thus, anti-Id made against these mAbs may more often detect determinants limited to a small number of alloreactive antibodies. It should be emphasized that the 14-4-4 mAb is an IgG_{2a}, κ, yet anti-14-4-4 Id detects a predominant Id on anti-I-E antibodies. Therefore, public idiotopes can also be found on antibodies of other Ig subclasses. One might predict that the 14-4-4 mAb sequence is close to the germline sequence, and that it therefore expresses immunodominant public idiotopes.

Another possible explanation for the differences observed among the various systems may be that they reflect the prevalence of antibodies to a given serological specificity in a given alloantiserum. For instance, Ia.7 and H-2.65, serological determinants recognized by 14-4-4 and 23-10-1, respectively, may be recognized by a significantly higher proportion of antibodies in a conventional alloantiserum than some of the specificities detected by the "private" Id systems. Idiotype-bearing antibodies which react with the H-2.5 specificity seen by the 3-83 mAb might be rarely expressed in alloantisera at a sufficient concentration to be detected by the antigen-binding inhibition assay, which requires submaximal binding of anti-MHC Abs to the MHC antigen for adequate sensitivity. To test this possibility, alloantibodies which reacted with the H-2.5 specificity were enriched from BALB/c anti-C3H antisera by successive absorptions to remove irrelevant specificities. Using the antigen-binding inhibition assay, anti-3-83 idiotype inhibited the H-2K binding of this antibody preparation >40% versus <15% inhibition of the unabsorbed alloantibodies (37), suggesting that in conventional alloantisera a significant percentage of the antibodies with similar fine specificity to 3-83 share idiotype.

A second method of examining idiotype sharing on infrequently expressed alloantibodies is the use of a large panel of hybridomas. We examined idiotype sharing among anti-MHC mAbs detecting the same or different specificities. Two representative experiments are shown in Table II. The top panel illustrates an experiment designed to examine the prevalence of the 14-4-4 idiotype among a group of anti-Ia mAbs. It is clear that only anti-I-E antibodies that detect the Ia.7 specificity and the binding of which map to epitope cluster I (see Ref. 38) share idiotype (39). Similarly, among all the anti-H-2K^k mAbs, only the anti-H-2.5 antibodies share idiotype with 3-83 (bottom panel; see Ref. 22). Considered as a whole, these findings may help to explain the difficult problems encountered when preparing anti-Id to whole alloantisera. Previous reports of anti-Id produced against al-

TABLE IIA

Inhibition of Ia Binding by Anti-Id

Hybridoma line	Specificity	Epitope cluster	Inhibition by rabbit anti-14-4-4
14-4-4	E^k	I	+
10A	E^k	I	+
10B	E^k	I	+
41A	E^k	I	+
40C	E^k	I	+
40H	E^k	I	+
40D	E^k	III	−
40K	E^k	III	−
40B	E^k, A^k	III	−
40I	E^k	III	−
9B	E^k	III	−
39D	E^k	III	−
39G	E^k	III	−

TABLE IIB

Inhibition of H-2 Binding by Anti-Id

Hybridoma line	Specificity	Epitope cluster	Inhibition by pig anti-3-83
3-83	K^k	B (H-2.5)[a]	+
12-2-2	K^k	ND	−
15-1-5	K^k	ND	−
15-3-1	K^k	A	−
16-1-2	K^k	A	−
16-1-11	K^k	A	−
16-3-1	K^k	A	−
16-3-22	K^k	Neither A nor B	−
36-7-5	K^k	A	−
142-23	K^k	B (H-2.5)	+
100-30	K^k	B (H-2.5)	+
100-5	K^k	A	−
100-27	K^k	A	−
116-22	K^k	A	−
141-11	K^k	B	−
142-45	K^k	B	−
11-4.1	K^k	A	−
20-8-4	K^b, D^b		−
27-11-13	D^b		−
28-8-6	K^b, D^b		−
28-13-3	K^b		−
28-14-8	D^b		−
30-5-7	L^d		−
34-4-20	D^d		−

[a] See Reference 22.

loantibodies may represent exceptional cases in which, for unknown reasons, the immunogen used to generate the anti-Id contained a dominant antibody species that probably had undergone less somatic diversification than the bulk population. Anti-Id generated against these rare antibodies, which expressed germline-encoded idiotopes, could then recognize cross-reactive determinants expressed on the bulk population.

One unexpected finding in our studies was the striking difference between antiidiotypes produced in xenogeneic versus syngeneic animals (37). As shown in Fig. 4, xenogeneic anti-3-83 detects shared

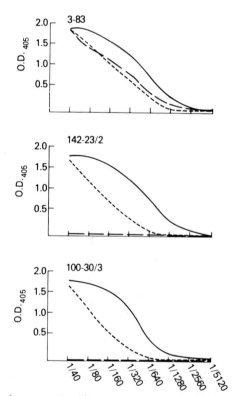

Fig. 4. Detection of cross-reactive idiotopes on anti-H-2.5 mAbs by xenogeneic and syngeneic reagents using a cross-linking ELISA assay. Microtiter plates were coated with 2 μg/ml affinity-purified mAbs. Xenogeneic or syngeneic anti-Id was incubated for 1 h at various serial dilutions. The plates were washed and incubated with an excess of FITC-coupled Id. ----, rabbit anti-3-83; ——, pig anti-3-83; –––, BALB/c anti-3-83. Alkaline phosphatase-coupled rabbit anti-FITC was used a sandwich reagent to detect bound FITC-coupled Id.

idiotopes among all three monoclonal anti-H-2.5 antibodies. However, syngeneic and allogeneic anti-3-83 demonstrate a far more restricted recognition pattern because they react with only the immunogen 3-83. Similar results have also been found in our studies of the public Id systems, 14-4-4, 23-10-1, and 28-13-3 and have also been reported by others (17; M. Pierres and T. Hansen, personal communications). It is unclear what portion of the idiotopes detected by the xenogeneic anti-Id are recognized by the syngeneic reagents. However, with one exception (40), it appears that mouse anti-Id antibodies are more "private" than xenogeneic reagents in that they detect idiotope(s) shared less broadly in the antibody population. Because mouse anti-Id that react with public determinants have been detected readily in other systems such as NP and levan (9, 12), a unique regulation of "public" idiotopes on most antibodies induced by MHC antigen may be operating. For example, the use of anti-MHC receptors sharing common idiotopes in both the allo- and self-repertoires could preclude the generation of cross-reactive antiidiotopes because of tolerance or other active suppressive mechanisms. Thus, syngeneic anti-Id induced by hyperimmunization may not accurately reflect the interactions operating in endogenous immune regulation because they may recognize idiotopes other than those involved in the network regulation of anti-MHC responses. Syngeneic anti-Ids induced in this manner may therefore be less useful as reagents for manipulating anti-MHC responses than xenogeneic anti-Ids (see Section IV,C).

IV. *In Vivo* Effects of Antiidiotypes

A. INDUCTION OF Ab3 MOLECULES

The ability to regulate immune responses to MHC antigens is of particular interest in transplantation biology. We therefore devoted considerable effort to manipulating anti-MHC responses with anti-Id reagents directed at determinants of monoclonal alloreceptors. Most of the work was done in four idiotypic systems, 3-83, 11-4.1, 36-7-5, and 14-4-4, although some studies were also performed in other systems included in Table I. In all systems studied to date, *in vivo* administration of xenogeneic anti-Id induced the expression of molecules that inhibited the binding of antiidiotype to idiotype-coated wells in an ELISA inhibition assay (33, 41, 42). The term Ab3 will be used in this chapter, as others have used it in syngeneic systems (43),

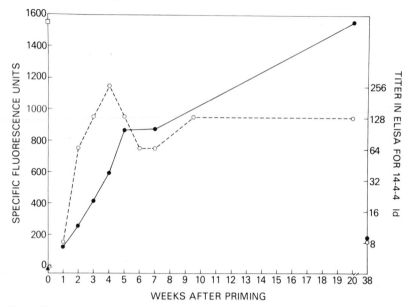

Fig. 5. Time course of the response after *in vivo* treatment with anti-14-4-4 Id. Responses are shown for an individual C3H.SW mouse primed with pig anti-14-4-4; other mice gave comparable results. ●——●, anti-I-E in specific fluorescence units, shown on the left ordinate. It was measured as the difference in staining between B10.A(2R) and B10.A(4R). ○---○, titer in an inhibition ELISA assay, shown on the right ordinate. Rabbit anti-14-4-4 Id was used in the assay. ▲, preimmune serum; □, 14-4-4; △, staining reagent alone. (Reprinted from the *Journal of Experimental Medicine*.)

to describe all anti-Id-induced molecules that inhibit the binding of antiidiotype to idiotype. These molecules include anti-antiidiotypic antibodies, as well as idiotype-bearing molecules that have structural similarities to the original Id but may or may not bind the relevant MHC antigen. An example of the effects of anti-Id treatment is shown in Fig. 5. Small amounts (20 µg per dose) of pig anti-14-4-4, injected in saline ip on days 0 and 3, led to the production of idiotype which could be detected in sera as early as day 10 and as late as 9 months postinoculation. In several systems (11-4.1, 36-7-5, 14-4-4), the idiotype produced was specific in that it did not cross-react with other anti-Id, could not be induced by normal pig Ig, pig antimouse Ig, or irrelevant anti-Id, and reacted with both rabbit and syngeneic anti-Id. Similarly, rabbit (and in one case goat) anti-Ids have also been found to induce Ab3 antibodies detectable by the various anti-Id reagents.

The ability to express Ab3 antibodies after antiidiotype treatment was found in some systems to be influenced by *Igh-V* region genes but

TABLE III

Genetic Analysis of Id Expression in Allotype Congenic Mice
Treated with Pig Anti-11-4.1 Anti-Id

Sample (serum pool)	Allotype		H-2 type	Id (HAI[a] titer $\log_2$)
	V_H	C_H		
BALB/c	a	a	d	5–7
BAB.14	a	b	d	5
BC.8	a	a	b	5–6
BALB.B	a	a	b	7
BALB.K	a	a	k	5
C.B20	b	b	d	<1
C57BL/6	b	b	b	<1
A.TL	e	e	d	<1

[a] Hemagglutination inhibition assay (see Reference 42).

not MHC genes (Table III). In the 11-4.1 (Igh-V^a) system, Igh allotype congenic mice and backcross animals that expressed the *Igh-V^a* genes produced significantly higher levels of Ab3 than Igh-V^b animals (42). Within the different strains of Igh-V^a mice, the H-2 haplotype did not appear to affect Ab3 levels. In the 14-4-4 system, however, anti-Id treatment induced significant levels of Ab3 even in strains such as B10 and CWB that did not express idiotype upon immunization with I-E antigen (41).

B. NATURE OF Ab3 MOLECULES INDUCED BY ANTI-Id

Understanding the nature of the molecules induced in response to anti-Id might help to clarify the idiotypic network involved in anti-MHC responses. Our first approach to analyzing these molecules was to examine the antigen-binding activity of Ab3 induced by anti-Id (33, 41, 42). Using flow microfluorometry, sera from anti-Id-treated mice were examined for binding to lymphocytes of the appropriate or inappropriate H-2 haplotype. Although the mice had never been exposed to MHC antigens, sera from some anti-Id-treated mice demonstrated specific antigen-binding activity to the same MHC antigen as that bound by the monoclonal Id. For example, anti-H-2K^k antibodies were detected in the sera of about 20% of BALB/c mice treated with rabbit anti-3-83 or pig anti-11-4.1 (Fig. 6).

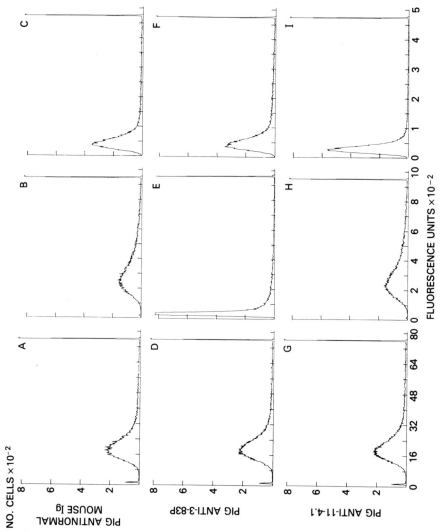

The binding activity could be specifically inhibited by either the relevant pig or the relevant rabbit antiidiotype but not by normal Ig or irrelevant anti-Id. In addition, anti-H-2 mAbs that bound to the same epitope cluster on the K^k molecule as the original Id inhibited binding of the induced anti-H-2 activity. These results suggest that antibodies with a specificity similar to that of the original Id are induced by anti-Id treatment. The MHC-binding Ab3 antibodies induced by anti-Id remained detectable for several months (Fig. 5). MHC-binding Ab3 molecules were predominantly of the IgG_1 subclass and represented only a small portion (<10%) of the total Ab3 induced by anti-Id.

Although antigen-binding Ab3 antibodies have been found in all the systems studied, the level of penetrance varied among the different Id systems. In some very private systems such as 36-7-5 and 17-3-3, few anti-Id-treated mice were found to express anti-MHC activity in their sera. In other relatively private systems such as 11-4.1 and 3-83, only 15–25% of mice treated with antiidiotype expressed anti-H-2 activity in their sera. In contrast, in the predominant idiotype system, 14-4-4, all C3H.SW mice treated with anti-Id produced anti-I-E antibodies in readily detectable amounts. The differences between the various systems may be caused by the relative prevalence of the idiotype in the B-cell repertoires but may also reflect regulatory events as yet not understood.

The finding that anti-MHC antibodies could be induced by anti-Id, although in some cases these idiotypes were rare in the normal response, indicates that the relevant V genes must be present in mice of the appropriate Igh allotype. However, unlike the induction of total levels of Ab3 molecules in the 14-4-4 system, which is approximately equal in mice of both appropriate and inappropriate allotypes, the expression of Ab3 with anti-MHC reactivity seemed to be more strictly allotype linked. For example, C3H.SW mice produced anti-I-E

Fig. 6. Anti-H-2K^k antibodies from alloimmunized and antiidiotype-treated mice were examined for idiotype expression by a binding inhibition assay. Serum (25 μl) from treated mice was mixed with either 25 μl of antiidiotype (100 μg/ml) or 25 μl of antinormal pig immunoglobulin (100 μg/ml). After incubation for 1 h, the test sera plus inhibitor were incubated with C3H lymph node cells and the binding was assessed. Binding of conventional pooled alloantisera to C3H cells was not appreciably inhibited by pig antinormal mouse IgG (A), pig anti-3-83 (D), or pig anti-11-4.1 (G). Columns 2 (profiles B, E, and H) and 3 (profiles C, F, and I) illustrate the inhibitory ability of the same pig antibodies on the binding of anti-H-2K^k antibodies induced in mice treated with rabbit anti-3-83 (1529) or pig anti-11-4.1 (1505), respectively. As the fluorescence units (FU) in each set of profiles differ, the level of inhibition must be compared with the reactivity of the serum with the congenic H-2K^d cells. Such comparisons indicated that <10% of the anti-H-2K^k binding activity in mice treated with antiidiotype remained after inhibition with the appropriate antiidiotype (profiles E and I). (Reprinted from *Nature*.)

antibody with 100% penetrance, as mentioned above, but C57Bl/10 mice expressed no anti-I-E activity after anti-Id treatment. In fact, with one exception (see below), in all systems studied allotype congenic mice of an inappropriate allotype expressed little, if any, detectable anti-MHC activity. These results support the hypothesis that mice of different allotypes may possess genes expressing certain individual idiotopes expressed on an array of Ab3 molecules induced by anti-Id. However, the ability to express all the idiotopes together on one Ab3 molecule having anti-MHC binding activity may be limited to specific *Igh-V* genotypes.

An anomaly has recently been noted in the 14-4-4 system. The allotype congenic strain CWB, which carries the *Igh-C* genes from C57BL/10 on the C3H.SW background, expresses very little Id when immunized to I-E. However, when treated with anti-Id, it expresses high levels of Id' and just as much specific anti-I-E activity as does C3H.SW following similar treatment (41). One explanation for these results may be that the CWB strain represents a recombinant which carries some but not all of the 14-4-4-related *Igh-V* genes. Alternatively, in addition to the 14-4-4-related genes, these mice may carry additional *Igh-V* genes that are preferentially expressed in the response to antigen. Finally, other regulatory genes may be present in the CWB which regulate idiotype expression after I-E antigen exposure. Anti-Id treatment, however, selectively triggers those clones that do share idiotopes with 14-4-4. Independent evidence of allotype-linked control of the induction of I-E binding Ab3 by anti-14-4-4 has recently been obtained using allotype congenics on a different background (S. L. Epstein, unpublished observations). Thus, the 14-4-4 system may provide an interesting model with which to study the genetic basis of idiotypy in an anti-MHC system.

Because the majority of Ab3 molecules induced by anti-Id did not bind MHC antigens, it was of interest to characterize these MHC antigen-nonbinding Ab3 molecules. The common characteristic of all of these molecules was their ability to inhibit the binding of anti-Id to Id. The inhibitory activity might have been caused by the induction of antipig Ig antibodies. However, this possibility seems unlikely because neither normal pig Ig nor pig antimouse Ig, each of which is capable of eliciting a potent antipig Ig response, induced these molecules. In addition, all assays were performed in the presence of excess normal pig Ig to absorb antipig Ig activity. Finally, rabbit and syngeneic anti-Id, which would not be expected to react with mouse antipig Ig antibodies, were inhibited specifically by the Ab3 molecules (44).

The nature of the Ab3 molecules induced by anti-Id treatment has been evaluated using Ab3 mAbs generated from mice treated with anti-Id (45). Four monoclonal Ab3 were generated from a BALB/c mouse treated *in vivo* with pig anti-11-4.1. None of the four mAbs induced bound to H-2K^k antigen or to antigens from a series of other H-2 haplotypes examined. At least two different classes of Ab3 molecules could be distinguished. The first class, represented by three of the four monoclonal antibodies, reacted with several different xenogeneic anti-11-4.1 reagents, including pig, rabbit, and goat, but did not react with syngeneic anti-11-4.1. When examined structurally, all three of these monoclonal Ab3 were found to differ extensively from the original Id in their H chain N-terminal sequences. Although we expect to find sequence homologies responsible for the shared idiotypes (e.g., in the hypervariable regions or in the L chain sequences), such structural correlations may not be apparent until much more of the Ab3 amino acid sequences has been determined. It is possible that these Ab3 are, in fact, anti-anti-Id. This possibility seems unlikely because such molecules, in general, would not be expected to bear any resemblance to the original idiotype, and they would bind to unique determinants on anti-Id molecules. In addition, since three monoclonal Ab3 bound rabbit, pig, and goat anti-Id, which would not be expected to express similar V regions, it seems more likely that the anti-Id induces antibodies that express shared idiotopes similar in nature to those of the original immunogen. Mechanistically, anti-Id may trigger B cells by interacting with antigenic determinants of idiotope-bearing receptors. This interaction would result in the induction of Id-bearing molecules that would not necessarily bind the original antigen. This interpretation is consistent with the finding that the induction of the Ab3 molecules is allotype linked and suggests that Ab3 induction might be an immunoregulatory event rather than an immunization to the xenogeneic anti-Id.

The second class of Ab3 identified among these mAbs exhibited extensive homology to the original Id. The H chain N-terminal amino acid sequence of an mAb, J1-8-1, was identical to that of 11-4.1 through the 39th residue. Although neither the native Ig nor the isolated H chains of the mAb bound detectably to H-2K^k antigen, the reassociation of Ab3 H chains with 11-4.1 L chains (which did not themselves bind antigen) resulted in the recovery of significant H-2K^k antigen-binding activity (45). These results suggest that anti-Id may trigger Id-bearing molecules through H chain-encoded structures either directly on B cells or perhaps on T-cell receptor structures. This suggestion is consistent with the findings of other studies on the 11-4.1 idiotype system in which the predominant idiotope(s) detected by the xenogeneic reagents were expressed on the native Ig as well as on isolated H chains of the idiotype (46). Finally, this monoclonal Ab3 was found to react with syngeneic anti-11-4.1. This confirms results found with sera from xenogeneic anti-Id-treated mice in which the syngeneic anti-Id reacted with a small subpopulation of the non-antigen-binding Ab3 (44).

C. MECHANISM OF INDUCTION OF Ab3

The previous results clearly suggested that treatment of mice with xenogeneic anti-Id had a profound effect on both Id expression and humoral anti-MHC responses. A better understanding of the mechanism of Ab3 induction might help to clarify the precise nature of the idiotypic network in these animals. To this end, we examined the requirements for the induction of the Ab3. The first approach was to determine whether anti-Id directed at either public or private idiotopes could induce Ab3. As demonstrated above, a significant portion of rabbit anti-3-83 cross-reacted with another anti-H-2.5 mAb, 142-23 (37). Rabbit anti-3-83 was therefore fractionated by affinity chromatography on a 142-23-coupled-Sepharose column. Mice were then treated with either the anti-Id which detected private determinants on 3-83 or anti-Id eluted from the 142-23 column which detected cross-reactive idiotopes. Both reagents were found to induce Ab3 with equal efficiency.

Another approach to analyzing the mechanism of Ab3 induction was the alteration of the anti-Id molecules. It is widely thought that the Fc moiety of immunoglobulin plays an important role in some immune responses. Macrophages and B cells, which may both be involved in the *in vivo* induction of Ab3, are known to express Fc receptors capable of binding antigen–antibody complexes. To examine the role of Fc in the induction of Ab3, $F(ab')_2$ fragments of rabbit anti-11-4.1 were generated and administered *in vivo*. Although the anti-Id probably binds to Id-bearing receptors via its combining sites, $F(ab')_2$ fragments of rabbit anti-11-4.1 did not lead to Ab3 induction (Fig. 7). The differences could not easily be attributed to different rates of clearance of the various reagents because $F(ab')_2$ fragments were able to induce an amount of antirabbit antibody equal to that induced by the whole molecule. These results suggest that the Fc portion of the xenogeneic anti-Id antibodies may be involved in Ab3 induction perhaps by interacting with Fc receptor-bearing cells (e.g., macrophages and B

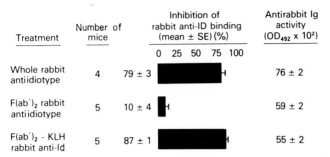

Treatment	Number of mice	Inhibition of rabbit anti-ID binding (mean ± SE) (%)					Antirabbit Ig activity (OD_{492} × 10^2)
		0	25	50	75	100	
Whole rabbit antiidiotype	4	79 ± 3					76 ± 2
F(ab')₂ rabbit antiidiotype	5	10 ± 4					59 ± 2
F(ab')₂ - KLH rabbit anti-Id	5	87 ± 1					55 ± 2

Fig. 7. The presence of the Fc moiety on the xenogeneic anti-Id influences the Ab3 response to antiidiotype treatment. Mice were treated with 30 µg of pig antiidiotype in saline on days 0 and 3. After 3 weeks, sera from individual mice were tested for their ability to inhibit the binding of rabbit antiidiotype to idiotype-coated ELISA plates. Data are presented as the mean inhibition for each group ± SEM.

cells). However, these same fragments, when coupled to KLH, induced levels of Ab3 equivalent to those induced by the whole anti-Id molecule. Therefore, the effect of xenogeneic Fc determinants may be to act as carrier determinants recognized by T helper cells required in the induction of Ab3 molecules.

Finally, attempts were made in several of the anti-H-2K systems to induce Ab3 by treatment *in vivo* with syngeneic or allogeneic anti-Id. To date, we have been unable to reproduce the *in vivo* effects of xenogeneic anti-Id using the mouse reagents. One possible reason for this difficulty may be the lack of sufficient foreign carrier determinants on the mouse Fc moiety. However, in preliminary experiments, KLH-coupled syngeneic anti-Id also failed to induce the Ab3. Another possible reason for the different effects of syngeneic and xenogeneic anti-Id involves the specificity of the reagents. As discussed above, syngeneic anti-Id did not detect the cross-reactive idiotypes expressed in conventional alloantisera and detected only a small portion of the Ab3 induced by the xenogeneic reagents. These results suggest the possibility that the induction of Ab3 depends on the recognition of specific idiotopes which are detected by the xenogeneic anti-Id but not by the syngeneic anti-Id produced by hyperimmunization. This restricted class of idiotopes, perhaps similar to what have been termed "regulatory idiotopes" (12), may play an important role in the ongoing regulation of immune responses to alloantigens. Thus, any attempts to generate syngeneic reagents specific for such regulatory idiotopes by exogenous administration of Id may be blocked by ongoing regulatory networks.

D. ROLE OF T CELLS IN Ab3 INDUCTION

The possibility that T cells might be involved in the induction of Ab3 was suggested by the findings that the majority of the Ab3 molecules were of the IgG_1 subclass [a particularly thymus-dependent isotype (47)] and that carrier determinants were required for Ab3 induction. Formal analysis of the role of T cells in the induction of Ab3 was performed using BALB/c nude mice. The results showed that after treatment with pig anti-11-4.1, the degree of inhibition of antiidiotype binding was significantly greater using sera from the euthymic group of mice than the nude group. Thus, a major portion of the Ab3 response appeared to be T cell dependent. These findings were confirmed in T-cell reconstitution experiments in which anti-Id-treated nude mice previously given purified T cells or engrafted with thymuses expressed amounts of Ab3 equivalents to those expressed by euthymic mice. Analysis of the T cells involved revealed that T cells from normal or anti-Id-treated mice reconstituted equally well. In addition, the pretreatment of the T cells with either Id plus C or anti-Id plus C failed to abrogate the ability to reconstitute nude mice. Taken together, these studies suggested that much of the Ab3 response by B cells might depend on carrier-specific rather than idiotype-specific helper T cells (48).

V. Modification of the Expressed Anti-MHC Repertoire by *in Vivo* Treatment with Anti-Id

As discussed above, in several of the more private Id systems such as 36-7-5 and 11-4.1 the alloantibodies present in sera of conventionally immunized mice rarely express detectable levels of Id-bearing anti-H-2 antibodies. However, mice treated with xenogeneic anti-Id and subsequently grafted with skin bearing the original MHC antigen developed a significantly higher percentage of Id-positive alloantibodies than were detected in the immune sera of untreated mice (42, 48). These results suggested that the anti-Id treatment had a profound effect on the expressed anti-H-2 antibody repertoire in these animals. This effect, like the induction of Ab3, was found to be under *Igh-V* region gene control and was idiotype specific in nature. These findings thus provided an alternative model with which to investigate the involvement of Id-specific T cells in the expression of anti-H-2 B-cell idiotypes. To this end, adoptive transfer experiments were performed in which purified primed T cells from either BALB/c or C.B20 mice

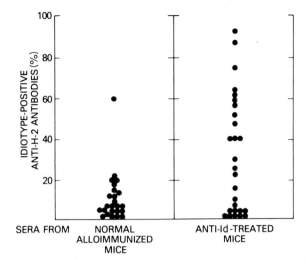

Fig. 8. Adoptive transfer of T cells from antiidiotype-treated mice can induce the expression of idiotope-positive anti-K^k antibodies after antigen exposure. BALB/c mice were irradiated with 200 rads and then $1-5 \times 10^6$ T cells purified from lymph nodes and spleens of donor animals. After 1–2 days, mice were skin grafted with BALB.K tail skin. Subsequent anti-K^k antibodies were tested by FACS analysis for the ability of antiidiotype to inhibit their binding to B10.A lymph node targets. Data represent the percentage of inhibition obtained for antibodies of individual animals. Control T cells came from mice that had been previously treated with either normal pig immunoglobulin or an irrelevant pig antiidiotype. Primed T cells came from mice which had been treated with pig anti-11-4.1 1–2 months previously. (Reprinted from the *Journal of Experimental Medicine*.)

were transferred into lightly irradiated (200 rads) BALB/c mice. The mice were skin grafted with H-2K^k-bearing tail skin, and alloantibodies were assessed for idiotypy. The results of such experiments are shown in Fig. 8. T cells from anti-Id-primed BALB/c mice, but not from normal pig Ig-treated mice, altered the expressed detectable idiotypic repertoire of B cells which responded to the H-2K^k antigen. Surprisingly, C.B20 T cells were also able to convert the BALB/c B-cell anti-H-2K^k repertoire from Id$^-$ to Id$^+$ (48). Because anti-Id-primed C.B20 mice never expressed detectable idiotype-positive anti-K^k antibodies, the idiotype conversion upon transferral of either BALB/c or C.B20 T cells could not be attributed to contaminating anti-Id-primed B cells in the inoculum. It therefore does not appear that the priming of T cells is determined by the same *Igh-V*-linked genes which control the antibody response.

The most likely explanation for this finding is that the idiotype-specific T cells are antiidiotypic in nature. Because the B cells of

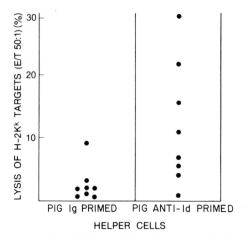

Fig. 9. *In vivo* treatment with anti-Id primed T$_H$ cells for anti-H-2K^k CML. A.TL mice were treated with 50 μg of pig anti-36-7-5 in saline on days 0, 3, and 21. Two weeks later, spleen cells from individual mice were tested for their ability to help an A.TL thymocyte response to a K^k only difference in a 5-day CML.

C.B20 do make a small amount of antigen non-binding, idiotope-bearing molecules in response to treatment with anti-Id, these Id-positive molecules could induce Id-recognizing T cells in primed animals. This possibility links our studies with the recent work of Nutt *et al.* (49) and L'age-Stehr (50), which suggested that the T cells that regulate idiotype expression may actually be primed by the idiotype initially expressed by B cells. Alternatively, T cells may exist in anti-Id-primed C.B20 mice that express individual idiotopes similar to those expressed by the small population of Id-expressing C.B20 B cells. These Id$^+$ T cells may, in turn, induce idiotype-recognizing T cells or, when transferred to subsequent BALB/c adoptive hosts, these Id-bearing T cells may be able to collaborate in an antigen-specific manner with the BALB/c cells which can express idiotope-positive antigen-binding molecules.

Although this is a significant step toward modifying T-cell immune responses to alloantigens, the functional T cells identified have so far been limited to those regulating B-cell responses. It therefore remains unclear whether antiidiotypes against B-cell products can have any effect on T-cell alloreactive responses to MHC antigens. Efforts to manipulate transplantation immunity, as judged by altered skin graft rejection, changes in mixed lymphocyte reactions, and graft-versus-host or cell-mediated lympholysis, have been uniformly unsuccessful to date (48). However, preliminary results suggesting an effect on cell-mediated immunity have been obtained using a helper T cell-limited cell-mediated lympholysis (CML) assay (J. A. Bluestone, unpublished observations). The rationale for such experiments stemmed from the finding that the idiotype-specific T cells observed in anti-Id-treated mice function as T helper cells for antibody production. Thus, any effects in CML might be at the helper rather than the effector level. Thymocytes devoid of T-helper-cell activity were cultured in a class I-only different CML assay in the presence of irradiated (850 rads) spleen cells from normal pig Ig or pig anti-Id-treated mice. As seen in Fig. 9, a significant percentage of anti-Id-treated mice provided helper activity, whereas spleen cells from only one of the normal Ig-treated mice augmented the thymocyte response. The nature and specificity of the helper T cells are currently under investigation.

VI. Conclusions and Future Approaches

Antireceptor antibodies specific for the effector cells involved in transplantation immunity could be a useful tool for modulating alloresponses. We have generated antiidiotypes against anti-MHC mAbs which, in some cases, detect predominant idiotypes in conventional alloantisera. Treatment of mice with these antiidiotypic reagents has been shown to have a profound effect on humoral anti-MHC antibody responses. We would like to suggest a hypothetical model which may account for the observed effects of xenogeneic antiidiotype treatment:

1. Xenogeneic antiidiotype treatment *in vivo* triggers those B cells that express idiotopes in common with the original anti-H-2 mAb. The number of B-cell clones and their ability to bind the original H-2 antigen depend on the nature and number of the structural V_H genes encoding the idiotope-bearing molecules.

2. Three types of T cells might also be triggered in response to the exogenous anti-Id. First, T cells that recognize xenogeneic constant region carrier determinants are induced. These cells provide helper factors involved in the expansion of idiotype-positive B-cell clones. Second, idiotope-bearing T helper cells are triggered independently of the Igh V region of the animal. Third, idiotope-recognizing T helper cells are induced by the idiotope-positive Ab3 molecules.

3. The latter two T-cell types function in the presence of an additional antigen challenge to alter the expressed anti-MHC repertoire of the resulting B-cell antibody response. Experiments are currently in progress to test various aspects of this model.

In light of the profound effects of these anti-Ids on the expressed B-cell allorepertoire, it was perhaps surprising that with the possible exception of the T helper cell, no significant effect on alloreactive T-cell function was observed. Recently, it has become evident that in many systems T cells recognize different antigenic determinants than do B cells. In addition, there is no solid evidence at the molecular level to suggest that T and B cells share a common receptor gene pool. Therefore, it is possible that, with the exception of an occasional clone, T and B cells may express different sets of idiotopes.

Studies of alloreactive T-cell receptors may thus require new reagents, perhaps produced against T-cell clones. However, the studies of antibody Id described herein have revealed a great deal about the alloantibody repertoire and the regulation of its expression. In addition, it appears that anti-MHC responses, although complex, can be analyzed in certain systems in which predominant idiotypes are expressed in conventional antisera. Thus, these reagents provide powerful tools with which to dissect the anti-MHC response and perhaps to modify the humoral responses involved in the transplantation reaction.

References

1. Zinkernagel, R. M. (1978). Thymus and lymphohemopoietic cells: Their role in T cell maturation in selection of T cells' H-2-restriction specificity and in H-2 linked Ir gene control. *Immunol. Rev.* **42**, 224.
2. Cerottini, J.-C., and Brunner, K. T. (1974). Cell mediated cytotoxicity, allograft rejection and tumor immunity. *Adv. Immunol.* **18**, 67.
3. Bevan, M. J. (1975). Allo immune cytotoxic T cells: Evidence that they recognize serologically defined antigens and bear clonally restricted receptors. *J. Immunol.* **114**, 316.
4. Rosenthal, A. S., and Shevach, E. M. (1973). Function of macrophages in antigen recognition by guinea pig T lymphocytes. *J. Exp. Med.* **138**, 1194.
5. Hodes, R. J., Hathcock, K. S., and Singer, A. (1980). Major histocompatibility complex restricted self recognition. A monoclonal anti-I-A^k reagent blocks helper T cell recognition of self major histocompatibility complex determinants. *J. Exp. Med.* **152**, 1779.
6. Davies, D. A. L., and Staines, N. A. (1976). A cardinal role for I region antigens (I-a) in immunological enhancement and the clinical implications. *Transplant. Rev.* **30**, 18.
7. Billingham, R. E., Brent, L., and Medawar, P. B. (1953). "Actively acquired tolerance" of foreign cells. *Nature (London)* **172**, 603.
8. Streilein, J. W., and Gruchalla, R. S. (1981). Analysis of neonatally induced tolerance of H-2 alloantigens. I. Adoptive transfer indicates that tolerance of class I and class II antigens is maintained by distinct mechanisms. *Immunogenetics* **12**, 161.

9. Kelsoe, G., Reth, M., and Rajewsky, K. (1980). Control of idiotype expression by monoclonal anti-idiotypic antibodies. *Immunol. Rev.* **52**, 75.

10. Hart, D. A., Wang, A. L., Pawlak, L. L., and Nisonoff, A. (1972). Suppression of idiotypic specificities in adult mice by administration of anti-idiotypic antibody. *J. Exp. Med.* **135**, 1293.

11. Eichmann, K., and Rajewsky, K. (1975). Induction of T and B cell immunity by anti-idiotypic antibody. *Eur. J. Immunol.* **5**, 661.

12. Bona, C. A., Heber-Katz, E., and Paul, W. E. (1981). Idiotype-anti-idiotype regulation. I. Immunization with a levan-binding myeloma protein leads to the appearance of auto-anti-(anti-idiotype) antibodies and to the activation of silent clones. *J. Exp. Med.* **153**, 951.

13. Ramseier, H. (1979). Anti-idiotypic antibodies induce formation of anti-H-2 sera and of idiotype. *Exp. Cell Biol.* **47**, 107.

14. Ramseier, H., Aguet, M., and Lindemann, J. (1977). Similarity of idiotypic determinants of T- and B-lymphocytes receptors for alloantigens. *Immunol. Rev.* **34**, 50.

15. Binz, H., and Wigzell, H. (1975). Shared idiotypic determinants on B and T lymphocytes reactive against the same antigenic determinants. I. Demonstration of similar or identical idiotypes on IgG molecules and T-cell receptors with specificity for the same alloantigens. *J. Exp. Med.* **142**, 197.

16. Frischknecht, H., Binz, H., and Wigzell, H. (1978). Induction of specific transplantation immune reactions using anti-idiotypic antibodies. *J. Exp. Med.* **147**, 500.

17. Krammer, P. H. (1981). The T cell receptor problem. *Curr. Top. Microbiol. Immunol.* **91**, 179.

18. McKearn, T. J. (1974). Anti-receptor antiserum causes specific inhibition of reactivity to rat histocompatibility antigens. *Science* **183**, 94.

19. Ozato, K., Mayer, N., and Sachs, D. H. (1980). Hybridoma cell lines secreting monoclonal antibodies to mouse H-2 and Ia antigens. *J. Immunol.* **124**, 533.

20. Sachs, D. H., Mayer, N., and Ozato, K. (1981). Hybridoma antibodies directed toward murine H-2 and Ia antigens. *In* "Monoclonal Antibodies and T Cell Hybridomas" (G. J. Hämmerling, U. Hämmerling, and J. F. Kearney, eds.), pp. 95–101. Elsevier/North-Holland Biomedical Press, Amsterdam.

21. Oi, V. T., Jones, P. P., Goding, L. A., Herzenberg, L. A., and Herzenberg, L. A. (1978). Properties of monoclonal antibodies to mouse allotypes, H-2 and Ia antigens. *Curr. Top. Microbiol. Immunol.* **81**, 115.

22. Lemke, H., and Hämmerling, G. J. (1981). Topographic arrangement of H-2 determinants defined by monoclonal hybridoma antibodies. *In* "Monoclonal Antibodies and T Cell Hybridomas" (G. J. Hämmerling, U. Hämmerling, and J. F. Kearney, eds.), p. 109. Elsevier/North-Holland Biomedical Press, Amsterdam.

23. Sachs, D. H., El-Gamil, M., Arn, J. S., and Ozato, K. (1981). Complementation between I region genes is revealed by a hybridoma anti-Ia antibody. *Transplantation* **31**, 308.

24. Cuatrecasas, P. (1970). Protein purification by affinity chromatography. Derivatization of agarose and polyacrylamide beads. *J. Biol. Chem.* **245**, 3059.

25. Buttin, G., LeGuern, G., Phalente, L., Lin, E. C. C., Medrano, L., and Cazenave, P.-A. (1978). Production of hybrid lines secreting monoclonal anti-idiotypic antibodies by cell fusion on membrane filters. *Curr. Top. Microbiol. Immunol.* **81**, 27.

26. Sachs, D. H., El-Gamil, M., and Miller, G. (1981). Genetic control of the immune response to staphylococcal nuclease. XI. Effects of in vivo administration of anti-idiotypic antibodies. *Eur. J. Immunol.* **11**, 509.

27. Epstein, S. L., Ozato, K., Bluestone, J. A., and Sachs, D. H. (1981). Idiotypes of anti-

Ia antibodies. I. Expression of the 14-4-4S idiotype in humoral immune responses. *J. Exp. Med.* **154**, 397.

28. Sachs, D. H., Bluestone, J. A., Epstein, S. L., and Ozato, K. (1981). Anti-idiotypes to monoclonal anti-H-2 and anti-Ia hybridoma antibodies. *Transplant. Proc.* **13**, 953.

29. Sachs, D. H., Bluestone, J. A., Epstein, S. L., Kiszkiss, P., Knode, M., and Ozato, K. (1981). Idiotypes of anti-MHC monoclonal antibodies. *ICN-UCLA Symp. Mol. Cell. Biol.* **20**, 751–758.

30. Bluestone, J. A., Sunshine, J. L., and Sachs, D. H. (1983). Idiotypes on anti-MHC antibodies: Detection of a public idiotype on anti-H-2K^b antibodies. In (Y. Yamamura and T. Tada, eds.). Progress in Immunology, Vol. V. Academic Press, Tokyo.

31. Ozato, K., Epstein, S. L., Bluestone, J. A., Sharrow, S. O., Hansen, T., and Sachs, D. H. (1983). The presence of a common idiotype in anti-H-2 immune sera as detected by anti-idiotype to a monoclonal anti-H-2 antibody. *Eur. J. Immunol.* **13**, 13–18.

32. Hansen, T. H., and Sachs, D. H. (1978). Isolation and antigenic characterization of the product of a third polymorphic H-2 locus, H-2L *J. Immunol.* **121**, 1469.

33. Bluestone, J. A., Sharrow, S. O., Epstein, S. L., Ozato, K., and Sachs, D. H. (1981). Induction of anti-H-2 antibodies in the absence of alloantigen exposure by in vivo administration of anti-idiotype. *Nature (London)* **291**, 233.

34. Imanishi-Kari, T., Rajnavolgyi, E., Takemori, T., Jack, R. S., and Rajewsky, K. (1977). *Eur. J. Immunol.* **9**, 324.

35. Conger, J. D., Lewis, G. K., and Goodman, J. A. (1981). Idiotype profile of an immune response. I. Contrasts in idiotypic dominance between primary and secondary responses and between IgM and IgG plaque-forming cells. *J. Exp. Med.* **153**, 1173.

36. Gearhart, P. J., Johnson, N. D., Douglas, R., and Hood, L. (1981). IgG antibodies to phosphorylcholine exhibit more diversity then their IgM counterparts. *Nature (London)* **291**, 29.

37. Bluestone, J. A., Auchincloss, H., Jr., Sachs, D. H., Fibi, M., and Hämmerling, G. J. (1983). Anti-idiotypes against monoclonal anti-H-2 antibodies. VI. Detection of shared idiotypes among monoclonal anti-H-2 antibodies. *Eur. J. Immunol.* **13**, 489–495.

38. Pierres, M., Devaux, C., Dosseto, M., and Marchetto, S. (1981). Clonal analysis of B and T cell responses to Ia antigens. 1. Topography of epitope regions of I-A^k and I-E$^\kappa$ molecules analysed with 35 monoclonal alloantibodies. *Immunogenetics* **14**, 481.

39. Devaux, C., Epstein, S. L., Sachs, D. H., and Pierres, M. (1982). Cross-reactive idiotypes of monoclonal anti-Ia antibodies: Characterization with xenogeneic anti-idiotypic reagents and expression in anti-H-2 humoral responses. *J. Immunol.* **129**, 2074.

40. Grützman, R., and Hämmerling, G. J. (1982). Idiotypic relationship of anti-Ia.2 antibodies. *Eur. J. Immunol.* **12**, 307.

41. Epstein, S. L., Masakowski, V. R., Bluestone, J. A., Ozato, K., and Sachs, D. H. (1982). Idiotypes of anti-Ia antibodies. II. Effects of in vivo treatment with xenogeneic anti-idiotypes. *J. Immunol.* **129**, 1545.

42. Bluestone, J. A., Epstein, S. L., Ozato, K., Sharrow, S. O., and Sachs, D. H. (1981). Anti-idiotypes to monoclonal anti-H-2 antibodies. II. Expression of anti-H-2K^k idiotypes on antibodies induced by anti-idiotype or H-2K^k antigen. *J. Exp. Med.* **145**, 1305.

43. Cazenave, P.-A. (1977). Idiotypic-anti-idiotypic regulation of antibody synthesis in rabbits. *Proc. Natl. Acad. Sci. U.S.A.* **74**, 5122.

44. Bluestone, J. A., Auchincloss, H., Jr., Cazenave, P.-A., Ozato, K., and Sachs, D. H. (1982). Anti-idiotypes to monoclonal anti-H-2 antibodies. III. Syngeneic anti-idiotypes detect idiotopes on antibodies induced by in vivo administration of xenogeneic anti-idiotypes. *J. Immunol.* **129**, 2066.
45. Bluestone, J. A., Krutzsch, H. C., Auchincloss, H., Jr., Cazenave, P.-A., and Sachs, D. H. (1982). Comparative analysis of monoclonal anti-H-2K^k idiotype and idiotype-positive molecules induced by in vivo anti-idiotype treatment. *Proc. Natl. Acad. Sci. U.S.A.* **79**, 7847–7851.
46. Bluestone, J. A., Metzger, J.-J., Knode, M. C., Ozato, K., and Sachs, D. H. (1982). Anti-idiotypes to monoclonal anti-H-2 antibodies. I. Contribution of isolated heavy and light chains to idiotype expression. *Mol. Immunol.* **19**, 515.
47. Bankhurst, A. D., Lambert, P. H., and Miescher, P. A. (1975). Studies on the thymic dependence of the immunoglobulin classes of the mouse. *Proc. Soc. Exp. Biol. Med.* **148**, 501.
48. Auchincloss, H., Jr., Bluestone, J. A., and Sachs, D. H. (1983). Anti-idiotypes against anti-H-2 monoclonal antibodies. V. In vivo anti-idiotype treatment induces idiotype-specific helper T cells. *J. Exp. Med.* **157**, 1273–1286
49. Nutt, N., Haber, J., and Wortis, H. H. (1981). Influence of Igh-linked genes products on the generation of T helper cells in response to sheep erythrocytes. *J. Exp. Med.* **153**, 1225.
50. L'age-Stehr, J. (1981). Priming of T helper cells by antigen-activated B cells. B cell-primed Lyt-1$^+$ helper cells are restricted to cooperate with B cells expressing the Ig V_H phenotype of the priming B cells. *J. Exp. Med.* **153**, 1236.

Idiotypes in Other Biological Systems

Chapter 15

Production of Monoclonal Antibodies to Integral Membrane Transport and Receptor Proteins and Their Use in Structural Elucidation

J. Craig Venter, Barbara Eddy, Ursina Schmidt,
and Claire M. Fraser

Department of Molecular Immunology
Roswell Park Memorial Institute
New York State Department of Health
Buffalo, New York

I. Introduction

The isolation and molecular characterization of neurotransmitter receptors and ion and substrate transport proteins have lapsed far behind the elucidation of the biochemistry of many other important cellular proteins. The reasons for this lag are twofold. First, these macromolecules are integral membrane proteins and therefore require detergent to remove them from the membrane milieu and to maintain their solubility in aqueous solutions. Consequently, biological responses such as hormone activation of membrane enzymes (e.g., adenylate cyclase) or ion transport across the membrane are lost as a result of detergent solubilization. Reconstitution of these soluble biomolecules into lipid vesicles or native membranes is usually required in order to demonstrate their characteristic biological functions (Klausner *et al.*, 1983). Second, because of signal amplification from biological cascades such as cyclic AMP formation and cation movement, receptor and transport proteins can exist on the surface of cells at extremely low densities. For example, in the heart, β-adrenergic receptors and slow inward calcium channels exist at a density of one or less per square micrometer of membrane surface area (Venter *et al.*, 1983b). Such low concentrations of cell protein have provided one of the biggest obstacles to a detailed structural analysis of receptor proteins.

However, two technical approaches—the first using monoclonal antibodies and the second using radiation inactivation–target size analysis—provide the means of overcoming the above limitations on structural analysis (Venter, 1983; Fraser and Venter, 1982; Venter *et al.*, 1983b) of minor membrane proteins. The key advantage of each of these techniques is that neither requires purified material. As this chapter will illustrate, monoclonal antibodies to minor membrane proteins can be produced in abundance even when the starting material is intact cells or membranes (Fraser *et al.*, 1983; Venter *et al.*, 1983a).

Our laboratory has been successful in producing monoclonal antibodies to a number of integral membrane proteins (Table I), including adrenergic and cholinergic receptors, cell-specific markers, and transport proteins. The antibodies were produced as a means of purifying and characterizing the membrane protein in question and/or as a means of isolating specific cells by electronic cell sorting (Fraser *et al.*, 1983). The exact details of monoclonal antibody production, cell cloning, and antibody purification are the subject of many reviews and articles (e.g., see Fraser and Lindström, 1983, for a comprehensive

TABLE I

Monoclonal Antibodies Produced to Functional Membrane Proteins

Monoclonal antibody[a]	Antigen	Specificity
FV-101	Partially purified TEβR (isoelectric focusing)	β-Adrenergic receptor
FV-103		β-Adrenergic receptor
FV-104		β-Adrenergic receptor
M.6	Purified muscarinic receptor	Muscarinic cholinergic receptor
M.30		Muscarinic cholinergic receptor
M.42		Muscarinic cholinergic receptor
M.43		Muscarinic cholinergic receptor
M.44		Muscarinic cholinergic receptor
α1D8	Rat liver plasma membrane	α_1-Adrenergic receptor
α1F9		α_1-Adrenergic receptor
α3E3	Purified α_1-receptor	α_1-Adrenergic receptor
α3F3		α_1-Adrenergic receptor
α4C2		α_1-Adrenergic receptor
DA.18	Purified D_2-dopamine receptor	D_2-Dopamine receptor
DA.28		D_2-Dopamine receptor
RBC 4.5.5	Purified band 4.5	RBC-glucose carrier
RBC 4.5.21		RBC-glucose carrier
RBC 4.5.22		RBC-glucose carrier
RBC 4.5.23		RBC-glucose carrier
RBD 4.5.24		RBC-glucose carrier
RBC 4.5.25		RBC-glucose carrier
RBC 4.5.26		RBC-glucose carrier
RBC 4.5.27		RBC-glucose carrier
RBC 4.5.28		RBC-glucose carrier
RBC 4.5.29		RBC-glucose carrier
RBC 4.5.30		RBC-glucose carrier
RBC 4.5.31		RBC-glucose carrier
RBC 4.5.32		RBC-glucose carrier
RBC 4.5.33		RBC-glucose carrier
RBC 4.5.34		RBC-glucose carrier
RBC 4.5.35		RBC-glucose carrier
RBC 4.5.36		RBC-glucose carrier
C 1.26	Guinea pig ileal membranes	Ca^{2+} channel
C 1.32		Ca^{2+} channel
C 1.47		Ca^{2+} channel
C 1.65		Ca^{2+} channel
C 1.69		Ca^{2+} channel
C 1.76		Ca^{2+} channel
C 1.99		Ca^{2+} channel
C 1.130		Ca^{2+} channel
C 1.136		Ca^{2+} channel
C 1.145		Ca^{2+} channel

(continued)

TABLE I (continued)

Monoclonal antibody[a]	Antigen	Specificity
C 1.151		Ca^{2+}.channel
C 1.152		Ca^{2+} channel
C 1.156		Ca^{2+} channel
P 1.3	Type II pneumocyte membranes	Type II pneumocyte membranes
P 1.24		Type II pneumocyte membranes
P 1.40		Type II pneumocyte membranes
P 1.42		Type II pneumocyte membranes
P 1.44		Type II pneumocyte membranes
P 1.49		Type II pneumocyte membranes
P 1.56		Type II pneumocyte membranes
P 1.63		Type II pneumocyte membranes
P 1.83		Type II pneumocyte membranes
P 1.84		Type II pneumocyte membranes
P 1.88		Type II pneumocyte membranes
P 1.92		Type II pneumocyte membranes
P 1.97		Type II pneumocyte membranes
P 1.105		Type II pneumocyte membranes
P 1.106		Type II pneumocyte membranes
P 1.114		Type II pneumocyte membranes
P 1.117		Type II pneumocyte membranes
P 1.119		Type II pneumocyte membranes
P 1.124		Type II pneumocyte membranes
P 1.125		Type II pneumocyte membranes
P 1.128		Type II pneumocyte membranes
P 1.129		Type II pneumocyte membranes
P 1.139		Type II pneumocyte membranes
P 1.141		Type II pneumocyte membranes
P 1.152		Type II pneumocyte membranes
P 1.194		Type II pneumocyte membranes
IM.1	Brush-border membranes	Brush-border membranes
IM.2		Brush-border membranes
IM.7		Brush-border membranes
IM.8		Na^+-dependent glucose carrier
IM.9		Brush-border membranes
IM.10		Brush-border membranes
IM.11		Na^+-dependent glucose carrier
IM.18		Brush-border membranes
IM.24		Na^+-dependent glucose carrier
IM.25		Brush-border membranes
IM.30		Na^+-dependent glucose carrier
IM.31		Brush-border membranes
IM.32		Brush-border membranes
IM.34		Na^+-dependent glucose carrier
IM.35		Brush-border membranes
IM.36		Brush-border membranes

TABLE I (continued)

Monoclonal antibody[a]	Antigen	Specificity
IM.38		Brush-border membranes
IM.39		Brush-border membranes
IM.41		Brush-border membranes
IM.42		Na^+-dependent glucose carrier
IM.46		Brush-border membranes
IM.55		Brush-border membranes
IM.56		Brush-border membranes
IM.57		Brush-border membranes
IM.59		Brush-border membranes
IM.60		Brush-border membranes
IM.62		Brush-border membranes
IM.63		Brush-border membranes
IM.66		Na^+-dependent glucose carrier

[a] Antibodies were produced by Fraser, Eddy, and Venter.

discussion) and will not be reported here. This chapter will cover the approaches we have used for immunization protocols and in screening for antibodies to functional proteins that exist in minute quantities in the cell membrane. We will also describe the purification and characterization of some of these proteins with monoclonal antibody affinity columns.

II. Production of Monoclonal Antibodies to Membranes

Immunization of BALB/c mice with intact cells or isolated plasma membranes is one of the best approaches we have found for obtaining monoclonal antibodies to cell membrane proteins (Fig. 1). For example, if intact type II pneumocytes or membranes isolated from these lung cells are used as a source of antigen for monoclonal antibody production, antimembrane antibodies are found in a high percentage of the clones derived from cell fusion (Fraser et al., 1983). Similar results have been obtained when intestinal brush-border membranes are used as antigen (Schmidt et al., 1983). As will be described below, the antibodies obtained are to membrane proteins ranging from the major proteins to proteins such as adrenergic receptors, which exist in

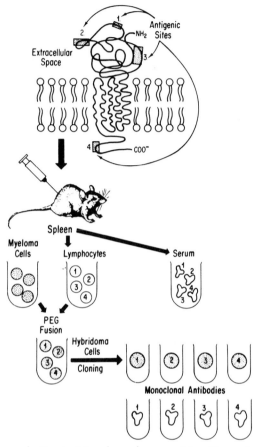

Fig. 1. Antibody production to integral membrane proteins. Comparison of monoclonal antibodies to conventional serum antibodies. (Venter *et al.*, 1983a.)

such minute amounts as to be present in only a few hundred to a few thousand copies per cell. This finding emphasizes the tremendous importance of the screening protocols used for identification of monoclonal antibodies to specific cell membrane proteins.

When membranes are used as antigen, our first screening assay is either an ELISA or a radioimmunoassay for antibodies against membrane antigens. The results of a typical assay are illustrated in Fig. 2. This figure illustrates the results of a first screening of hybridomas from a cell fusion of splenic lymphocytes from BALB/c mice which were immunized twice at 4-week intervals with rabbit intestinal

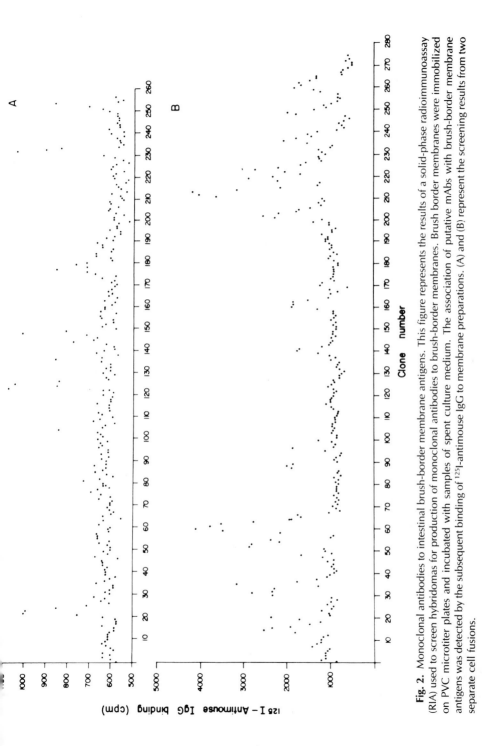

Fig. 2. Monoclonal antibodies to intestinal brush-border membrane antigens. This figure represents the results of a solid-phase radioimmunoassay (RIA) used to screen hybridomas for production of monoclonal antibodies to brush-border membranes. Brush border membranes were immobilized on PVC microtiter plates and incubated with samples of spent culture medium. The association of putative mAbs with brush-border membrane antigens was detected by the subsequent binding of ^{125}I-antimouse IgG to membrane preparations. (A) and (B) represent the screening results from two separate cell fusions.

brush-border membranes with SP2/0 myeloma cells. The cell fusion was performed 4 days subsequent to the second immunization. Hybrid cells were plated into 300-microtiter wells and sampled for putative antibodies on the 10th day following cell fusion. For the assay, brush-border membranes were immobilized on microtiter plates to create a solid-phase assay. Culture medium from wells containing hybridomas was incubated with the membranes, and the presence of monoclonal antibodies specific for the brush border was detected with ^{125}I-labeled antimouse IgG. As can be seen in Fig. 2, approximately one-third of the wells were positive for anti-brush-border antibodies.

The ultimate purpose of the brush-border membrane study was to obtain monoclonal antibodies with specificity for the sodium-dependent glucose transporter. The number of positive clones (~100) identified in the first screening assay was still too large for a second functional screening assay. Therefore, to reduce the number of functional assays required, the 66 most positive wells were selected. The cells in these wells were subcultured and grown in larger cultures. Figure 3 illustrates the results of a second radioimmunoassay (RIA) screening of the initial 66 clones. On rescreening with the ^{125}I-labeled antimouse IgG solid-phase assay, ~50% of the hybridoma clones were still positive.

The technique of an initial screening followed by subculture of positive clones and rescreening effectively reduces the number of clones to be screened in a functional assay by 10-fold (Fig. 3). Admittedly, this is a "survival of the fittest" approach, but it has a number of advantages. The screening assays used up to this point are extremely simple and rapid, and assure relatively high-affinity antibodies that are stable to subculturing, cloning, and expansion. Although we had ~50% attrition from the early stages, the surviving positive cells are very stable. It is a rare event to lose clones after the second stage of screening.

For studies in which the desired end product of cell fusion is a monoclonal antibody suitable for use as a cell surface marker for drug targeting, electronic cell sorting, etc., the initial two steps are of even greater importance. For example, in studies designed to produce monoclonal antibodies specific for rabbit type II pneumocytes (Fraser et al., 1983), the initial screening assays were performed as described above. Subsequent to recloning and rescreening, assays were performed in order to detect major antibody cross-reactivity with other cell types (Table II).

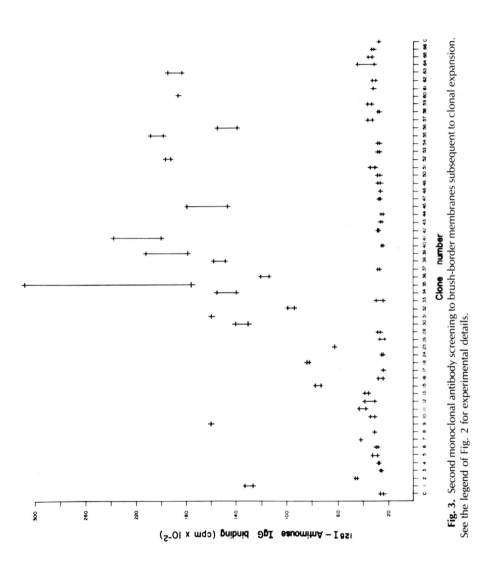

Fig. 3. Second monoclonal antibody screening to brush-border membranes subsequent to clonal expansion. See the legend of Fig. 2 for experimental details.

TABLE II

Screening of Monoclonal Antibodies Produced to Adult Rabbit Type II Pneumocyte Membranes

Clone number	Freshly isolated type II pneumocytes	Type II pneumocytes: cell culture	Rabbit lung fibroblasts: cell culture	Human fibroblasts (foreskin): cell culture	Rat hepatocytes: cell culture	Turkey erythrocyte membranes	Human erythrocyte membranes	Dog lung membranes	Rat brain membranes	Rat heart membranes
3	+	+	+	0	0	+	0	+	+	0
24	+	+	+	+	0	+	0	+	+	+
40	+	0	0	0	0	+	0	0	+	+
42	+	+	+	+	0	+	0	+	+	+
44	+	0	+	0	0	+	+	+	+	0
49	+	+	0	+	0	0	0	+	0	+
56	+	+	+	0	0	0	0	+	0	0
63	+	0	0	0	0	+	0	+	+	0
83	+	0	0	0	0	0	0	+	+	+
84	+	0	+	+	0	+	0	+	+	0
88	+	0	+	0	0	0	0	+	0	0
92	+	0	0	0	0	+	+	+	0	0
97	+	+	+	+	0	+	0	+	+	+
105	+	+	+	0	0	0	0	0	0	0
106	+	0	0	0	0	0	0	0	0	0
116	+	0	0	0	0	0	0	+	0	0
117	+	+	+	0	0	+	0	+	0	0
119	+	0	0	0	0	0	0	+	+	0
124	+	0	+	+	0	0	0	+	+	0
125	+	+	+	+	0	0	0	+	0	0
128	+	+	+	0	0	0	+	+	0	0
129	+	0	0	0	0	0	0	0	0	0
139	+	0	+	0	0	0	0	0	0	0
141	+	0	0	0	0	0	0	+	0	0
152	+	+	+	+	0	0	+	+	0	0
194	+	+	+	+	0	0	0	+	0	0

III. Antibody Assays for Functional Proteins (Receptors and Transport)

The use of functional assays as a means of screening for monoclonal antibodies from samples of culture medium is one of the least desirable forms of antibody screening because of the multitude of potential artifacts possible with functional assays of various types. For example, ligand-binding assays for cell surface receptors are phenomenological in nature, and any means of reducing ligand binding (such as nonspecific adsorption of the ligand by proteins present in culture medium) might, without appropriate controls, be interpreted to represent an antibody effect on a receptor molecule. In a case in which a direct or indirect immunoprecipitation assay is not available (see below) and a functional assay is needed, as with a membrane transport protein of unknown molecular structure, ligand binding can be the first functional screening procedure as long as it is followed with other assays, for example, transport or enzyme measurements. This permits the development of a number of lines of evidence for identification of monoclonal antibodies to particular proteins.

A. Na^+-DEPENDENT GLUCOSE TRANSPORT

The antibodies identified as positive in the screening assay illustrated in Fig. 3 were further screened for possible specificity for the brush-border Na^+-dependent glucose transporter by a ligand-binding inhibition assay. [^3H]Phlorizin, a competitive antagonist of glucose transport, binds to brush-border membranes in a manner consistent with binding to the glucose carrier (Toggenburger et al., 1982). Spent culture medium from the clones to be screened was tested at various dilutions for the ability to block Na^+-dependent phlorizin binding to brush-border vesicles. Five antibodies that were positive in this assay were then further screened for their ability to block glucose transport in kinetic studies. Figure 4 illustrates the data on ligand inhibition, and Fig. 5 illustrates a typical glucose transport experiment.

B. RECEPTOR ASSAYS

Although we have performed functional assays with receptors, they were utilized not as a primary screening tool but as a means of characterizing epitope specificity of known antireceptor antibodies from immunoprecipitation assays (Fraser and Venter, 1980; Venter and Fraser, 1981, 1983) (see Section IV,A,B).

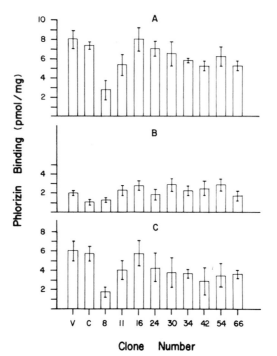

Fig. 4. Inhibition of phlorizin binding to the Na^+-dependent glucose carrier of the brush border by monoclonal antibodies. Na^+-dependent [^3H]phlorizin binding to brush-border vesicles was assayed in the presence and absence of anti-brush-border mAbs; mAb from clone No. 8 demonstrated significant inhibition of the Na^+-dependent binding, suggesting possible specificity for the glucose carrier. (A), total (Na^+); (B), nonspecific (K^+); (C), specific (Na^+ dependent).

IV. Indirect Immunoprecipitation Assays

A. AFFINITY-LABELED PROTEINS

We have utilized three types of indirect immunoprecipitation assays for identification and characterization of monoclonal antibodies to detergent-solubilized receptor proteins. The first assay is straightforward and is applicable to situations in which a covalent affinity label or photoaffinity label is available for the receptor in question or in which the receptor can be isolated to isotopic purity subsequent to the incorporation of a radiolabel [as with direct iodination (Fraser and Venter, 1980)]. Obviously, the affinity-label approach permits the detection of receptors in the nonpurified state. An example of this type of assay, the indirect immunoprecipitation of muscarinic cholinergic re-

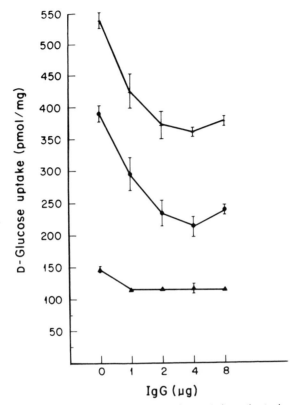

Fig. 5. Monoclonal antibody inhibition of specific (Na^+-dependent) glucose transport in brush-border vesicles. Specific Na-dependent D-glucose uptake (●) was measured under tracer equilibrium conditions as the difference between total (Na^+) (-) and nonspecific (K^+, ▲) D-glucose uptake. The inhibition of this specific Na^+-dependent D-glucose uptake was assayed with different amounts of an immunoaffinity-purified IgG fraction of ascites fluid, IM-24.

ceptors with monoclonal antibodies, is illustrated in Fig. 6. These data demonstrate that in mixtures containing affinity-labeled, detergent-solubilized muscarinic receptors, antireceptor monoclonal antibodies, and antimouse IgG, the disappearance of receptors from the supernate correlates with the quantitative appearance of receptor–antibody complexes in the immunoprecipitate.

B. DIRECT ASSAY OF SOLUBLE RECEPTORS

When receptors are stable to detergent solubilization in the absence of covalent reagents, as with turkey erythrocyte β-adrenergic recep-

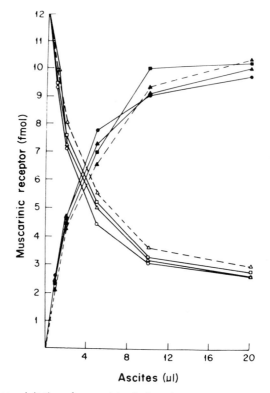

Fig. 6. Immunoprecipitation of muscarinic cholinergic receptors with monoclonal antibodies. The open symbols indicate supernate muscarinic receptors; the closed symbols indicate the appearance of receptors in the pellet.

tors (Fraser and Venter, 1980), a different approach can be used. For example, β-adrenergic receptors can be solubilized from turkey erythrocyte ghosts with 0.5% digitonin and partially purified by preparative isoelectric focusing (Venter and Fraser, 1981) (Fig. 7). Fractions from isoelectric focusing columns are assayed for β-adrenergic receptors by labeling receptors with [^{125}I]iodohydroxybenzylpindolol (IHYP), a high-affinity β-receptor antagonist, in the presence and absence of 10 μM L-propranolol, followed by precipitation of labeled receptors with polyethylene glycol (PEG), as described by Fraser and Venter (1980) and Venter and Fraser (1981).

Hybridomas secreting antibodies to β-adrenergic receptors are identified using an indirect immunoprecipitation assay as follows. A sample of spent culture medium from each hybridoma is incubated with an aliquot of soluble, partially purified turkey erythrocyte β-adrenergic receptors for 18 h at 4°C. Precipitation of receptor–mono-

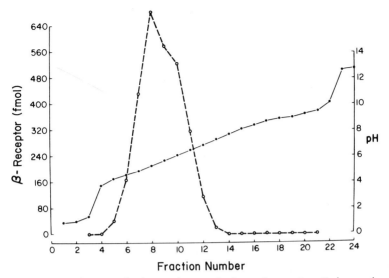

Fig. 7. Isoelectric focusing of turkey erythrocyte β-adrenergic receptors. Turkey erythrocyte β-adrenergic receptors were solubilized from erythrocyte ghosts by treatment with 0.5% digitonin for 12 h at 4°C. Soluble β-receptors were added to sucrose density gradients (0–50%) containing 1% ampholines (pH 3–10) for isoelectric focusing (110-ml column) for 16 h at 4°C (constant power, 15 W; maximum voltage, 1600 V). Fractions from isoelectric focusing columns were assayed for β-adrenergic receptors. The open circles represent the concentration of β-adrenergic receptors present in each fraction (4 ml) from the isoelectric focusing column; the closed circles represent the pH gradient. [Venter, J. C., and Fraser, C. M. (1981). *In* "Monoclonal Antibodies in Endocrinology Research" (G. Eisenbarth and R. Fellows, eds.). With permission from Raven Press, New York.]

clonal antibody complexes is accomplished by addition of an excess of rabbit antimouse IgG. An appropriate volume of medium serves as a control. A significant loss of β-receptors (as determined by a loss in IHYP specific binding) from the sample supernates following immunoprecipitation was used as the criterion for determining the presence of monoclonal antibodies to β-adrenergic receptors (Fraser and Venter, 1980).

Using the indirect immunoprecipitation assay described for hybridoma screening, ascites fluid containing monoclonal antibodies FV-103 or FV-104 was found to precipitate partially purified turkey erythrocyte β-adrenergic receptors in a concentration-dependent fashion, as illustrated in Fig. 8. In order to validate the receptor precipitation assay, we demonstrated that the loss of β-receptors from solution as a consequence of antibody binding resulted in the appearance of β-receptors in the immunoprecipitate. In addition, with the use of biosynthetically labeled monoclonal antibodies, we demonstrated com-

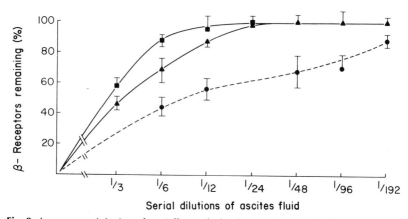

Fig. 8. Immunoprecipitation of partially purified turkey erythrocyte β-adrenergic receptors. Soluble, partially purified turkey erythrocyte β-adrenergic receptors were incubated with serial dilutions of ascites fluid containing mAb 101 (squares), mAb 103 (circles), or mAb 104 (triangles) for 18 h at 4°C, followed by precipitation of receptor-antibody complexes by addition of rabbit antimouse IgG. Supernates were assayed for the loss of β-adrenergic receptors from immunoprecipitation. (Fraser and Venter, 1980.)

plete precipitation of monoclonal antibodies by antimouse IgG at each antibody dilution employed (Fraser and Venter, 1980). These data indicate that quantitation of receptors remaining in solution is not complicated by residual monoclonal antibody inhibiting ligand binding. The titers and shapes of the immunoprecipitation curves suggest that two monoclonal antibodies differ in their affinity for turkey erythrocyte β-receptors (Fraser and Venter, 1980; Venter and Fraser, 1981).

C. IMMUNOPRECIPITATION AND ASSAY OF UNSTABLE RECEPTORS

Because of problems of mammalian β-receptor stability on solubilization from membranes (Strauss *et al.*, 1979), the assay of human lung β-adrenergic receptors necessitated a somewhat different approach from that employed in the assay of turkey erythrocyte β-receptors. Lung membranes were prepared as described in Strauss *et al.*, 1979.

β-Adrenergic receptors in calf lung membranes were specifically labeled with IHYP; membranes were treated with Triton X-100 for 15 min at 30°C and then centrifuged for 30 min at 48,000 Xg. The supernatant after solubilization and centrifugation at 48,000 Xg was considered to be the solubilized receptor fraction, because no additional material sedimented at 100,000 Xg during a further 2-h centrifugation.

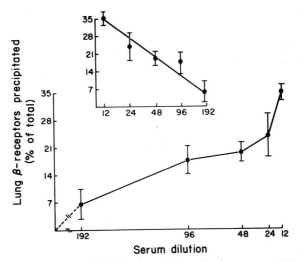

Fig. 9. Immunoprecipitation of solubilized canine lung β_2-adrenergic receptors with autoantibodies. Triton X-100 solubilized canine lung β_2-adrenergic receptors specifically labeled with an ^{125}I β-adrenergic antagonist (IHYP) were incubated for 18 h at 4°C with dilutions of serum from a patient with allergic rhinitis shown to have autoantibodies to β_2-receptors. Immunoprecipitation of β_2-receptor-autoantibody complexes was accomplished by addition of sheep anti-human IgG. Precipitates were counted for the presence of radiolabeled β_2-receptors. [Venter, J. C., Fraser, C. M., and Harrison, L. C. (1980). *Science* **207**, 1361–1366. Copyright 1980 AAAS; with permission.]

In addition, the detergent-extracted receptor–ligand complexes were retained by ultrafilters with a 10,000-dalton retention size (Pellicon type PT, Millipore Corp.), but not by filters with a 0.45-μm filtration size, unless the complexes were first precipitated by 15% polyethylene glycol. The solubilized receptors were retained in a Sepharose 6B column with a calculated Stokes radius of 5.8 nm (Strauss *et al.*, 1979).

Aliquots of soluble receptor complexes that had been labeled with IHYP in the presence and absence of 10 μM L-propranolol were incubated with spent culture medium for 18 h at 4°C, and precipitation of IHYP–receptor complexes was accomplished by addition of antiserum to mouse IgG. The concentration of soluble β-receptors precipitated under these conditions was calculated as the difference between the amount of IHYP precipitated in samples initially labeled in the absence of 10 μM L-propranolol, followed by incubation with identical dilutions of medium, and the amount precipitated in the presence of propranolol. Incubation of IHYP with medium alone did not result in precipitable IHYP on the subsequent addition of antimouse IgG.

An example of this last assay is illustrated in Fig. 9 with autoimmune receptor antibodies specific for β_2-receptors (Venter *et al.*, 1980;

Fraser *et al.*, 1981). Although some of these assays are complex, we believe that the screening data obtained are more reliable than binding inhibition data alone and permit the detection of antibodies to the majority of the receptor molecule, not just the ligand-binding site.

V. Immunoaffinity Chromatography of β-Adrenergic Receptors Using Monoclonal Antibodies

Monoclonal antibody FV-104, which is specific for some portion of the β-adrenergic ligand-binding site (Fraser and Venter, 1980), cross-reacts equally well with both β_1- and β_2-adrenergic receptors from a number of sources (Fraser and Venter, 1980; Venter and Fraser, 1981). Antibody FV-104 was purified from ascites fluid by 45% ammonium sulfate precipitation, followed by preparative isoelectric focusing. For preparative isoelectric focusing, ascites fluid was added to sucrose density gradients (0–50%) containing 1% ampholines (pH 3–10) for 16 h at 4°C (constant power, 15 W; maximum voltage, 1600 V). Both procedures were followed by dialysis against 10 mM sodium phosphate buffer (pH 8). Fractions from isoelectric focusing columns containing monoclonal antibody FV-104 were identified by double immunodiffusion against rabbit antimouse IgG. Purified monoclonal antibody FV-104 IgG and control mouse IgG were coupled to cyanogen bromide-activated Sepharose 4B (5 mg protein/ml gel). Affinity columns have ranged from 400 μl of Sepharose 4B in Eppendorf pipette tips to 20 ml of Sepharose 4B in a 2.4-cm-diameter column (Fraser and Venter, 1980; Venter and Fraser, 1981, 1983).

Monoclonal antibody FV-104 coupled to Sepharose 4B specifically adsorbs turkey erythrocyte β-receptors that have been partially purified by isoelectric focusing. The specificity of this receptor adsorption was demonstrated by comparing the binding of β-receptors to FV-104-Sepharose 4B or to control mouse IgG-Sepharose 4B. β-Receptor binding to control IgG was consistently less than 20% of the total concentration of β-receptors applied to the columns, whereas greater than 95% of applied receptor was retained on FV-104 columns. Prior receptor occupation by adrenergic ligands reduced the β-receptor binding to monoclonal antibody FV-104 columns to values with control IgG columns. Binding of β-receptors to control mouse IgG columns was not affected by receptor occupation.

That the determinant recognized by monoclonal antibody FV-104 is within the adrenergic ligand-binding site of the receptor and is common to both β_1- and β_2-receptor subclasses provides a unique situation with regard to receptor purification. In addition, the relatively low affinity of monoclonal antibody FV-104 for the β-receptor makes this antibody well suited for affinity purification procedures. The most significant characteristic, however, of the monoclonal antibody FV-104–β-receptor interaction is the ability of adrenergic receptor antagonists to compete directly with the antibody for the ligand-binding site on the receptor. We capitalized on these properties of monoclonal antibody FV-104 by binding both β_1- and β_2-receptor subclasses to monoclonal antibody FV-104 immunoaffinity columns and eluting receptors from the columns with low concentrations of the β-adrenergic receptor antagonist, L-propranolol (Venter and Fraser, 1983). This procedure adds selectivity to the immunoaffinity chromatography procedure, providing a clear link between ligand-specific affinity chromatography procedures and immunoaffinity chromatography. The elution of receptors with receptor-specific ligands provides pure, nondenatured receptor molecules (see below) which can be recovered for ligand-binding characterization and reconstitution studies. We have successfully applied these procedures to the purification of turkey erythrocyte β_1-adrenergic receptors (Fraser and Venter, 1980; Venter and Fraser, 1981, 1983) and, more recently, to the purification of human lung β_2-adrenergic receptors (Fraser and Venter, 1982).

The results of the turkey erythrocyte β_1-receptor purification are as follows. Turkey erythrocyte β-receptors were labeled in the erythrocyte membrane with ^{131}I and partially purified by isoelectric focusing. The partially purified receptors were applied to immunoaffinity columns, eluted with NaDodSO$_4$ and mercaptoethanol, and analyzed by NaDodSO$_4$ polyacrylamide gel electrophoresis. Three major components were identified at 70,000, 31,000, and 22,000 daltons. When the specificity of immunoaffinity purification was increased by utilizing 10 μM L-propranolol for elution of turkey erythrocyte B-receptors, only a single protein with a molecular weight of 70,000 was found on NaDodSO$_4$–polyacrylamide gels as determined by iodination of the eluate with ^{125}I (Fig. 10).

Additional evidence supporting the identity of the eluate as the turkey erythrocyte β-receptor is derived from its ability to bind adrenergic ligands both in the pure soluble state and subsequent to reconstitution in human erythrocyte membranes. The fact that iodination of the material eluted from monoclonal antibody FV—104 immunoaffinity columns reveals a single labeled protein on NaDodSO$_4$–polyacrylamide gels strongly suggests that the receptor eluted from the monoclonal antibody column is pure.

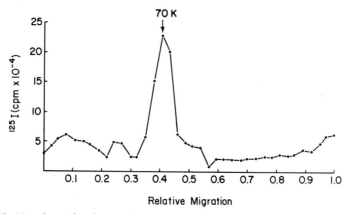

Fig. 10. Ligand-specific elution of turkey erythrocyte β-adrenergic receptors from monoclonal antibody immunoaffinity columns. Partially purified turkey erythrocyte β-receptors were applied to immunoaffinity columns composed of mAb 104–Sepharose 4B. Columns were washed extensively with buffer, and adsorbed β-receptors were eluted with 10 μM L-propranolol. The eluate was radiolabeled with Na ^{125}I and analyzed on SDS–polyacrylamide gels which were sliced and counted for radioactivity. [Venter, J. C., and Fraser, C. M. (1981). *In* "Monoclonal Antibodies in Endocrinology Research" (G. Eisenbarth and R. Fellows, eds.). With permission from Raven Press, New York.]

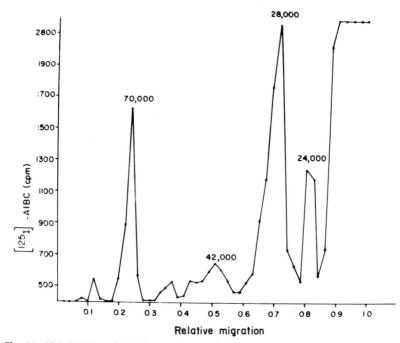

Fig. 11. SDS–PAGE analysis of canine heart β₁-adrenergic receptors labeled with [^{125}I]azidoiodobenzylcarazolol. Canine heart β₁-receptors were irreversibly labeled with AIBC, a β-adrenergic photoaffinity reagent, solubilized from membranes with 10% SDS, and analyzed on SDS–polyacrylamide gels which were sliced and counted for radioactivity. Specific receptor

TABLE III

Cross-Reactivity of Monoclonal Antibodies (mAb) to Turkey Erythrocyte B_1-Adrenergic Receptors

Monoclonal antibody binding to purified membranes		
	mAb 103	mAb 104
Turkey erythrocytes (β_1)	−	+
Canine heart (β_1)	−	+
Canine lung (β_2)	−	+
Indirect immunoprecipitation of solubilized β-receptors		
	mAb 103	mAb 104
AIBC-labeled turkey erythrocyte β_1-receptors	+	−
AIBC-labeled canine heart β_1-receptors	+	−

The monoclonal antibodies made against the turkey erythrocyte β-receptor effectively immunoprecipitate photoaffinity-labeled cardiac β_1-receptors (Fig. 11). However, as Table III illustrates, antibody FV-104 to the ligand-binding site will not precipitate the heart β_1-receptor while it is occupied by the affinity ligand.

VI. Elucidation of Receptor Structure and Function

A. NICOTINIC ACETYLCHOLINE RECEPTOR STRUCTURE

Cholinergic receptors were originally subclassified as nicotinic and muscarinic based on the effects of nicotine and muscarine. Although these receptors have been classified under the same name, "cholinergic," their main and perhaps only commonality is their shared neurotransmitter, acetylcholine.

The nicotinic cholinergic receptor is the best-characterized receptor to date. It was the first neurotransmitter receptor to be purified (see Venter, 1982, for a review), and some of the receptor subunits have been sequenced (Raftery et al., 1980).

The receptor is composed of five interacting subunits: two α units (each containing one ligand-binding site), 40,000 daltons; one β subunit, 50,000 daltons; one δ subunit, 64,000 daltons; and one γ subunit, 57,000 daltons, to give an overall mass approximating 250,000–270,000 daltons (Karlin, 1980). The nicotinic acetylcholine receptor also contains a sodium ion transport system or channel which opens on the binding of acetylcholine to the ligand-binding sites. Significant advances in the elucidation of the nicotinic acetylcholine receptor

---

labeling in the presence and absence of L-propranolol indicated that the 70,000-, 42,000-, and 28,000-dalton proteins were associated with the β-receptor, whereas the 24,000-dalton protein represented a protein labeled nonspecifically by AIBC.

structure have been made by Lindström and co-workers (Tzartos and Lindström, 1980; Tzartos *et al.*, 1981), who have produced more than 200 monoclonal antibodies to the nicotinic receptor. The antibodies have been used to determine the structural homology between receptors from different species as well as between the five receptor subunits. The 200 antibodies recognize only a small number of epitopes and structural domains on the receptor, which probably represent the main immunogenic portions of the receptor protein.

Lindström and co-workers utilized their substantial library of monoclonal antibodies generated against purified nicotinic acetylcholine receptors to investigate the antibody specificities from sera of patients with myasthenia gravis (Lindström *et al.*, 1976; Tzartos *et al.*, 1982). The monoclonal antibodies inhibited serum autoantibody binding to the human muscle nicotinic receptor. Autoantibodies from human sera were able to recognize the "main immunogenic region" located on the extracellular surface of the α subunit of the receptor distinct from the acetylcholine binding site. Regions on the β and γ subunits near the main immunogenic site were also found to be significantly antigenic in humans. Therefore, humans with myasthenia gravis expressed antibodies to the immunogenic sites that were detected with monoclonal antibodies to the receptor and in experimental myasthenia gravis. There were no apparent correlations between antibody specificity and clinical state. This is consistent with the observation that antiidiotypic antibodies which recognize the neurotransmitter-binding site can produce symptoms in animals similar to those produced by antibodies with specificity for the main immunogenic region (Wasserman *et al.*, 1982; Tzartos *et al.*, 1982).

B. MUSCARINIC ACETYLCHOLINE RECEPTOR STRUCTURE

The structure of the skeletal muscle nicotinic receptor contrasts markedly to the muscarinic cholinergic receptor from the autonomic and central nervous systems (Venter, 1983). Figure 12 illustrates that the muscarinic receptor from a number of tissues and species is a single polypeptide of 80,000 daltons. Radiation inactivation of muscarinic receptors (Venter, 1983) demonstrates that the 80,000-dalton protein is the complete functional receptor as it exists in the intact membrane. Table IV summarizes the molecular weights of muscarinic receptors from a wide variety of species ranging from human to frog brain.

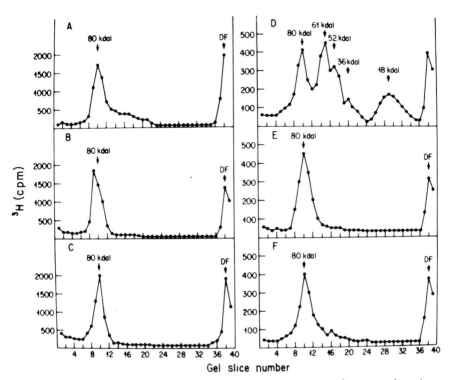

Fig. 12. SDS–PAGE analysis of muscarinic receptors from a variety of tissues and species. Muscarinic receptors were labeled with [³H]propylbenzyilylcholine mustard, solubilized from membranes with 2% SDS, and analyzed on SDS–polyacrylamide gels which were sliced and counted for radioactivity. Tissues in A–C, E, and F were isolated in the presence of protease inhibitors. (A) Human brain; (B) canine brain; (C) rat brain; (D) guinea pig ileum, smooth muscle; (E) rat heart; (F) canine heart. (Venter, 1983.)

Limited proteolysis studies on muscarinic receptors from diverse tissues and species indicate the absence of any major phylogenetic structural diversity among muscarinic receptors (Venter, 1983). The apparent structural identity of the various muscarinic receptors is in part confirmed by cross-reactivity studies with a series of monoclonal antibodies to muscarinic receptors which demonstrate specificity for all muscarinic receptors studied to date.

Monoclonal antibody studies have also demonstrated an apparent lack of molecular identity between the muscarinic receptor and any of the nicotinic receptor subunits. A total of 160 monoclonal antibodies to the nicotinic acetylcholine receptor (Tzartos and Lindström, 1980; Tzartos et al., 1981) displayed no cross-reactivity with muscarinic receptors as assayed by immunoprecipitation (Venter, 1983).

TABLE IV

Muscarinic Cholinergic Receptor Molecular Weights from Different
Species and Tissues[a]

Tissue	Method	Molecular weight
Human		
Brain	NaDodSO$_4$–PAGE[b]	78,000 ± 1200
Brain	Radiation inactivation	82,000
Canine		
Brain	NaDodSO$_4$–PAGE	82,000 ± 1800
Heart	NaDodSO$_4$–PAGE	81,000 ± 3000
Rat		
Brain	Radiation inactivation	82,000
Brain	Hydrodynamic	86,000
Brain	NaDodSO$_4$–PAGE	80,000 ± 2000
Brain	NaDodSO$_4$–PAGE	83,200 ± 2500
Heart	NaDodSO$_4$–PAGE	78,000 ± 1800
Guinea pig		
Ileum smooth muscle	Radiation inactivation	78,000
Ileum smooth muscle	NaDodSO$_4$–PAGE	79,000 ± 4200
Ileum smooth muscle	NaDodSO$_4$–PAGE	77,600 ± 2000
Brain	NaDodSO$_4$–PAGE	83,200 ± 6000
Frog		
Brain	NaDodSO$_4$–PAGE	80,000

[a] From Venter (1983).

[b] NaDODSO$_4$–PAGE: sodium dodecyl sulfate polyacrylamide gel electrophoresis.

Analysis of muscarinic receptor structure indicates that a considerable portion of the receptor molecular protrudes into the extracellular space from the plasma membrane. These results are not unlike those found for other integral membrane proteins, for example, the nicotinic acetylcholine receptor, in which 50% of the receptor mass protrudes from the membrane surface into the extracellular space and approximately 14% protrudes from the cytoplasmic side of the membrane (Kistler *et al.*, 1982).

Limited proteolysis of affinity-labeled, membrane-bound muscarinic receptors released a water-soluble receptor fragment of 42,000 daltons (Venter, 1983). Tryptic digestion of muscarinic receptors also suggests the presence of a 16,000-dalton receptor "tail" that may protrude into the cytoplasm. Studies are currently underway in our laboratory to determine if this tail is responsible for receptor coupling to other membrane proteins (Venter, 1983).

C. α_1-ADRENERGIC RECEPTOR STRUCTURE

The α-receptor antagonist, phenoxybenzamine, has been demonstrated to have a high selectivity for α_1-adrenergic receptors (Kunos *et al.*, 1983). We have utilized a high-specific-activity [^{3}H]phenoxybenzamine to affinity-label α_1-adrenergic receptors from rat liver membranes (Kunos *et al.*, 1983). In our initial study, an SDS-PAGE subunit of 85,000 daltons was determined for the liver α_1-receptor, along with either a proteolytic fragment or a receptor subunit of 60,000 daltons (Kunos *et al.*, 1983). Further labeling studies done in the presence of high concentrations of protease inhibitors demonstrated that the α_1-adrenergic receptor monomer had a molecular mass of 85,000 and that the 60,000-dalton protein probably represented a proteolytic fragment of the receptor (Venter *et al.*, 1983c).

Radiation inactivation analysis of the α_1-adrenergic receptor was also performed. When receptor inactivation was quantitated by the loss of [^{3}H]phenoxybenzamine-labeled protein (85,000 daltons) on SDS–polyacrylamide gels, it was found that this subunit derives from a 160,000-dalton complex in the intact membrane. These data suggest that the functional α_1-adrenergic receptor structure in the membrane may be a dimer of 85,000-dalton proteins, each of which contains an α_1-adrenergic ligand-binding site.

Limited proteolysis of the α_1-receptor monomer (85,000 daltons) reveals a marked structural similarity to the muscarinic cholinergic receptor. Detailed studies are currently underway to map receptor determinants recognized by monoclonal antibodies to specific proteolytic fragments from both muscarinic and α_1-adrenergic receptors to examine the homology between these receptor classes in more detail.

D. D_2-DOPAMINE RECEPTOR STRUCTURE

The least characterized neurotransmitter of those under study in our laboratory is the dopamine receptor. However, with the recent development of monoclonal antibodies to this receptor, we expect more rapid progress. Data derived from radiation inactivation studies indicate a molecular size of 123,000 for the D_2-dopamine receptor from dog and human striatal membranes (Lilly *et al.*, 1983).

Monoclonal antibodies specific for the D_2-dopamine receptor also recognize and immunoprecipitate the serotonin receptor from frontal cortex. This suggests a possible common ancestor for the serotonin and dopamine receptors (Fraser *et al.*, 1983).

E. THYROTROPIN RECEPTOR FUNCTION

In a study by Kohn and co-workers (Valente *et al.*, 1982), human monoclonal antibodies were developed with specificity for the thyrotropin receptor by fusing peripheral lymphocytes from Graves' disease patients with mouse myeloma (NS1) cells. Two of the hybridomas produced antibodies that are representative of the autoimmune stimulating antibodies in Graves' disease, and two other antibodies were "blocking" antibodies that had no stimulating activity on thyroid function but inhibited thyrotropin function. These data help to establish that patients with Graves' disease contain a spectrum of antibodies, not all of which mimic hormone action.

F. INSULIN RECEPTOR STRUCTURE

The first report on a monoclonal antibody with specificity for the human insulin receptor appeared in 1982 (Kull *et al.*, 1982). The monoclonal antibody α-IR-1 immunoprecipitates the human insulin receptor but has no effect on insulin binding to the receptor. The α-IR-1 recognized the human placental receptor, the IM-9 cell human monocyte receptor, and about 60% of the human erythrocyte receptor. There was little or no recognition of the rat or horse insulin receptor (Kull *et al.*, 1982).

G. LDL RECEPTOR STRUCTURE

LDL receptors were isolated using an LDL receptor-specific monoclonal antibody and found to be single proteins with a molecular mass of 164,000 (Schneider *et al.*, 1982). This is the same molecular weight obtained by ligand-specific affinity chromatography (Schneider *et al.*, 1982).

VII. Antiidiotypic Antibodies and Receptors

In 1980, Strosberg and co-workers reported on the production of antiidiotypic antibodies with specificity of β-adrenergic receptors (Schreiber *et al.*, 1980). This was achieved by immunizing rabbits with a β-receptor antagonist, alprenolol, followed by immunization of allotype-matched rabbits with the antialprenolol antibodies (Schreiber *et al.*, 1980). The antiidiotypic antibodies were produced in four out of five injected rabbits but varied in properties from β-receptor antagonist to receptor agonist which stimulated adenylate cyclase activity (Schreiber *et al.*, 1980). Similar results have now been reported by another group (Homcy *et al.*, 1982).

Shechter *et al.* (1982) similarly demonstrated that mice immunized with insulin spontaneously developed antibodies against their insulin receptors. The antiidiotypic antibodies were able to block insulin binding to its receptor and to mimic insulin action at the receptor level. It was suggested that spontaneously produced antiidiotypic antibodies might be associated with the development of autoimmune receptor disease (Shechter *et al.*, 1982). Such diseases involving autoantibodies to hormone and neurotransmitter receptors include myasthenia gravis (nicotinic acetylcholine receptor), Graves' disease (TSH receptor), allergic respiratory disease (β_2-adrenergic receptor), and type B insulin-resistant diabetes (insulin receptors; Evered and Whelan, 1982).

The first direct evidence that antiidiotypic antibodies directed against a cell-surface receptor can be associated with disease symptomology was presented in 1982. Erlanger and co-workers (Wasserman *et al.*, 1982) produced a rabbit antibody against a rigid but potent agonist of the nicotinic acetylcholine receptor. Antiidiotypic antibodies produced from immunization of rabbits with the antiligand antibodies were specific for the nicotinic receptor. The immunized rabbits displayed muscle weakness and other signs of experimental myasthenia gravis. The symptoms produced with immunization of the antiligand antibody were equivalent to those produced by direct immunization with purified acetylcholine receptor.

VIII. Conclusions

Although the major potential of monoclonal and antiidiotypic antibodies in receptor research is yet to be realized, substantial progress has clearly been made on many fronts. It is expected that antireceptor antibodies will become the primary reagents in receptor studies. Monoclonal and antiidiotypic antibodies will allow investigators to utilize standardized reagents of remarkable specificity in a diverse range of biochemical and physical research.

References

Evered, D., and Whelan, J. (1982). *In* "Receptors, Antibodies and Disease" (D. Evered and J. Whelan, eds.). Pitman, London.

Fraser, C. M., and Lindström, J. (1983). *In* "Receptor Biochemistry and Methodology" (J. C. Venter and L. Harrison, eds.). Alan R. Liss, Inc., New York (in press).

Fraser, C. M., and Venter, J. C. (1980). *Proc. Natl. Acad. Sci. U.S.A.* **77**, 7034.

Fraser, C. M., and Venter, J. C. (1982). *Biochem. Biophys. Res. Commun.* **109**, 329.

Fraser, C. M., Venter, J. C., and Kaliner, M. (1981). *N. Engl. J. Med.* **305**, 1165.

Fraser, C. M., Venter, J. C., Finkelstein, J. N., and Shapiro, D. L. (1983). Submitted for publication.

Homcy, C. J., Rockson, S. G., and Haber, E. (1982). *J. Clin. Invest.* **69**, 1147.

Karlin, A. (1980). *In* "The Cell Surface and Neuronal Function" (G. Poste, G. Nicolson, and C. W. Cotman, eds.), p. 191. Elsevier/North-Holland, Amsterdam.

Kistler, J., Stroud, R. M., Klymkowsky, M. W., Lalancette, R. A., and Fairclough, R. H. (1982). *Biophys. J.* **37**, 371.

Klausner, R., van Renswovde, J., Blumenthal, R., and Rivnay, B. (1983). *In* "Receptor Biochemistry and Methodology" (J. C. Venter and L. Harrison, eds.). Alan R. Liss, Inc., New York (in press).

Kull, F. C., Jacobs, S., Su, Y.-F., and Cuatrecasas, P. (1982). *Biochem. Biophys. Res. Commun.* **106**, 1019.

Kunos, G., Kan, W., Greguski, R., and Venter, J. C. (1983). *J. Biol. Chem.* **258**, 326.

Lilly, L., Fraser, C. M., Jung, C. Y., Seeman, P., and Venter, J. C. (1983). *Mol. Pharmacol.* **24**, 10.

Lindström, J. M., Seybold, M. E., Lennon, V. A., Wittingham, S., and Duane, D. (1976). *Neurology* **26**, 1054.

Raftery, M., Hunkapiller, M. W., Strader, C. D., and Hood, L. E. (1980). *Science* **208**, 1454.

Schmidt, U., Eddy, B., Fraser, C. M., Venter, J. C., and Semenza, G. (1983). *FEBS Lett.* **161**, 279.

Schneider, W. J., Beisiegel, U., Goldstein, J. L., and Brown, M. S. (1982). *J. Biol. Chem.* **257**, 2664.

Schreiber, A. B., Couraud, P. O., Andre, C., Vray, B., and Strosberg, A. D. (1980). *Proc. Natl. Acad. Sci. U.S.A.* **77**, 7385.

Shechter, Y., Maron, R., Elias, D., and Cohen, I. R. (1982). *Science* **216**, 542.

Strauss, W. L., Ghai, G., Fraser, C. M., and Venter, J. C. (1979). *Arch. Biochem. Biophys.* **196**, 566.

Toggenburger, G., Kessler, M., and Semenza, G. (1982). *Biochim. Biophys. Acta* **688**, 557.

Tzartos, S. J., and Lindstrom, J. M. (1980). *Proc. Natl. Acad. Sci. U.S.A.* **77**, 755.

Tzartos, S. J., Rand, D. E., Einarson, B. L., and Lindström, J. M. (1981). *J. Biol. Chem.* **256**, 8635.

Tzartos, S. J., Seybold, M. E., and Lindstrom, J. M. (1982). *Proc. Natl. Acad. Sci. U.S.A.* **79**, 188.

Valente, W. A., Vitti, P., Yavin, Z., Yavin, E., Rotella, C. M., Grollman, E. F., Toccafondi, R. S., and Kohn, L. D. (1982). *Proc. Natl. Acad. Sci. U.S.A.* **79**, 6680.

Venter, J. C. (1982). *Pharmacol. Rev.* **34**, 153.

Venter, J. C. (1983). *J. Biol. Chem.* **258**, 4842.

Venter, J. C., and Fraser, C. M. (1981). *In* "Monoclonal Antibodies in Endocrinology Research" (G. Eisenbarth and R. Fellows, eds.), p. 119. Raven Press, New York.

Venter, J. C., and Fraser, C. M. (1983). *Fed. Proc., Fed. Am. Soc. Exp. Biol.* **42**, 273.

Venter, J. C., Fraser, C. M., and Harrison, L. C. (1980). *Science* **207**, 1361.

Venter, J. C., Eddy, B., Schaber, J. S., Lilly, L., and Fraser, C. M. (1983a). *In* "Developmental Pharmacology (S. Macleod, ed.), p. 183. Alan R. Liss, Inc., New York.

Venter, J. C., Fraser, C. M., Schaber, J. S., Jung, C. Y., Bolger, G., and Triggle, D. J. (1983b). *J. Biol. Chem.* **258**, 9344.

Venter, J. C., Horne, P., Eddy, B., Gregoski, R., and Fraser, C. M. (1983c). Submitted for publication.

Wasserman, N. H., Penn, A. S., Freimuth, P. I., Treptow, N., Wentzel, S., Cleveland, W. L., and Erlanger, B. F. (1982). *Proc. Natl. Acad. Sci. U.S.A.* **79**, 4810.

Chapter 16

Studies on Idiotypes Shared by Neuronal and Lymphoid Cells

John H. Noseworthy and Mark I. Greene

Department of Pathology
Harvard Medical School
Boston, Massachusetts

I. Introduction

Binding of such varied ligands as hormones, neurotransmitters, toxins, drugs, and viruses is determined by cell-surface structures of limited and often single specificity. The nature of such cell-surface receptors in many cases is poorly understood, because receptor isolation and purification are frequently difficult. There has been substantial clarification of the recognition of antigen by the immune system in the case of the B-cell receptor for antigen. It is now known that antigen recognition by B cells is determined by the specific amino acid sequences of the hypervariable regions at the antigen-combining site of an immunoglobulin molecule. The hypervariable regions are encoded in part by germline V-region genes and in part by hypermutation and rearrangement of these V-region genes (Kim *et al.*, 1981). Both the amino acid sequences of entire immunoglobulin molecules and the DNA sequences of the appropriate V-region genes are known for a number of antibodies. Although the nature of the T-cell receptor remains unclear, evidence suggests that V_H-like gene products may contribute in part to the antigen recognition structure. B and T cells that share antigen specificity have been shown to share common idiotypes on their antigen receptors (Binz and Wigzell, 1975; Eichman *et al.*, 1980; Hetzelberger and Eichman, 1978).

In some cases, such as insulin and other hormones, highly specific interactions occur when ligand binds to a membrane receptor. The highly specific recognition and binding of ligand by somatic cells are reminiscent of the highly selective binding of antigen by the immune system. In experimental systems in which an antigen is recognized by both immune and nonimmune elements, an interesting question emerges; Are antigen recognition structures (and the genes that encode them) shared between immune and nonimmune cells, or do the respective populations recognize ligand with structurally similar but genetically unrelated receptors?

In collaboration with Dr. B. N. Fields' laboratory, we have begun a series of studies utilizing the mammalian reovirus as a model to determine if structures responsible for virus binding and recognition in the immune system are shared by nonimmune cell surface receptors for reovirus. It was postulated that if immune and somatic cells share such virus-binding determinants, antibody to these structures could serve as a probe for the reovirus receptor. It was hoped that such studies would give further insight into the nature of antigen recognition and idiotype expression by B and T cells and the nature of the gene families utilized by immune cells to build these receptors.

II. Role of the Reovirus Sigma 1 Protein

The mammalian reoviruses are icosahedral viruses containing double-stranded, segmented RNA. They can be divided by neutralization and hemagglutination studies into three serotypes (S1, S2, and S3). Each of the 10 genomic segments transcribes a single messenger RNA which encodes a single polypeptide. In this chapter, we will concentrate on the sigma 1 protein (viral hemagglutinin, HA), encoded by the S1 dsRNA genomic segment. This protein, one of the three structural proteins located on the outer capsid of the virus, was shown in a large number of studies to specify several interesting properties of the reovirus. The sigma 1 protein determines the cell and tissue tropism of reovirus, a number of types of interactions of reovirus with cells and cell surface structures, and the specificity of the host immune response to virus. These studies are the subject of an in-depth recent review (Sharpe and Fields, 1982). Here we will summarize only the findings most pertinent to our studies.

As mentioned, the genome of the reovirus is segmented. Coinfection *in vitro* of mammalian cells by viruses of different serotypes results in the exchange of nucleic acid segments between parental viruses. In this manner, recombinant strains are generated consisting of genomic segments derived from both parental viruses. Utilizing these recombinant strains, it was possible to map a number of viral properties to the polypeptide products of single segments of the viral genome.

Stated briefly, the sigma 1 protein (HA) determines the characteristic cellular and neural tropism of reovirus. Intracerebral inoculation of suckling mice with reovirus type 3 results in a highly lethal, necrotizing encephalitis in which neurons are diffusely infected and ependymal cells are spared. Intracerebral inoculation with reovirus type 1 results in a nonlethal ependymitis that frequently results in hydrocephalus. Neurons are characteristically not involved by infection with reovirus type 1. Using a series of recombinant strains, it was demonstrated that this tropism mapped to the S1 gene product, the viral HA. A recombinant virus containing nine viral genomic segments of reovirus 1 and the HA gene of reovirus 3 (1 HA 3) was shown to induce encephalitis in a manner indistinguishable from that of wild-type reovirus 3 (Dearing strain). Intracerebral inoculation of neonatal mice with a recombinant virus possessing nine genomic segments of reovirus 3 and also the HA gene of reovirus 1 (3HA1) resulted in ependymitis typical of reovirus type 1 (Weiner *et al.*, 1977, 1980c).

In a recent study, Spriggs and Fields showed that variant viruses, selected by growing virus under conditions of excess monoclonal neutralizing antibody (G5, see Section III), encode an HA of different antigen specificity; these variants are no longer neutralized by the neutralizing monoclonal antibody (Spriggs and Fields, 1982). In addition, these variant viruses with an antigenically altered HA are markedly less virulent and show a strikingly altered neurotropism following *in vivo* administration. Similarly, reovirus tropism for cells of the pituitary appears to be determined by the sigma 1 protein (Onodera *et al.*, 1981). In these studies, infection with virus containing the type 1 HA resulted in anterior pituitary damage; the type 3 HA results in minimal involvement of the intermediate lobe and posterior pituitary, with sparing of the anterior pituitary. In addition, reoviruses with different sigma 1 genes differ in their binding to nonimmune lymphoid cells (Weiner *et al.*, 1980a). Reovirus type 3 binds murine and human lymphocytes via the surface HA. These studies indicate that

the sigma 1 protein determines the binding of reovirus to cell surfaces. *In vitro* studies have shown that the sigma 1 protein also mediates the binding to microtubules by reovirus 1 (Babiss *et al.*, 1979) and
the inhibition of cellular DNA synthesis characteristically seen in
reovirus 3-infected cells (Sharpe and Fields, 1981).

In addition to these findings, which suggest that both tropism and
viral attachment to cells are mediated by the sigma 1 protein, a large
number of studies have demonstrated that both the cellular and the
humoral response to reovirus are directed against by the sigma 1 protein. Once again, recombinant strains were useful in showing that
both neutralization and hemagglutination inhibition antibodies, the
characteristic anti-viral antibody responses, were directed to the
sigma 1 protein. Burstin *et al.* (1982) extended the observation that
hemagglutination-inhibiting and neutralizing antibodies are directed
to the sigma 1 protein. Using monoclonal antibodies, they defined at
least three functionally distinct epitopes on the sigma 1 protein. One
epitope mediates neutralization, a second site blocks hemagglutination inhibition, and a third site reacts with neither neutralizing nor
hemagglutination-inhibiting antibodies.

In a similar manner, the fine specificity of the thymus-dependent
response to reovirus was investigated. An interesting conclusion from
these studies is that the cellular immune response to reovirus is also
serotype specific. Recombinant strains have been used to demonstrate
that the serospecificity of cytotoxic T cells (Finberg *et al.*, 1979), DTH
cells (Weiner *et al.*, 1980b), and suppressor cells (Greene and Weiner,
1980) maps to the sigma 1 gene product.

From these observations, it is clear that the sigma 1 gene product is
uniquely important both in directing the tropism and cellular attachment of the reovirus and in determining the host response to viral
infection. With these observations in mind, we attempted to identify
an HA-binding recognition structure shared by reovirus-binding cells
and antibodies (Nepom *et al.*, 1982a)

III. Identification of the Id3 Determinant

A. SEROLOGICAL DEFINITION OF THE Id3
DETERMINANT BY A XENOGENIC ANTIIDIOTYPE

To prepare HA-specific antisera, mice were repeatedly inoculated
intraperitoneally with 10^9 particles of purified reovirus type 1 or type
3. Immune serum was twice precipitated with ammonium sulfate and

purified by gel filtration on a Sephacryl-200 column. To enrich for anti-HA antibodies and to remove antibodies directed at viral determinants other than the HA, the serum was absorbed three times on 10^{11} particles of reovirus of the opposite serotype. Specifically, antireovirus 3 antiserum was serially absorbed on either reovirus 1 or the recombinant 3HA1 strain. As mentioned previously, the 3HA1 strain is a recombinant strain differing from the background 3 strain only in the gene encoding the HA surface protein. Antireovirus 1 antiserum was similarly absorbed on reovirus 3 or 1HA3. Although absolute HA specificity was not obtained, it was determined in a series of binding assays that such absorption resulted in antisera with an HA-specific binding titer 2^4 times higher on the relevant viral serotype than on serotypes bearing the opposite HA. These absorbed antireovirus antibodies exhibited limited heterogeneity by isoelectric focusing. Both antireovirus 1 and antireovirus 3 antisera were predominantly of the IgG_{2a} isotype.

The absorbed antireovirus antibodies were used to prepare rabbit antisera to antireovirus immunoglobulin (designated rabbit anti-anti-1 for antisera directed against HA 1-specific antibody and anti-anti-3 for antisera directed against HA 3-specific antibody). A competitive binding RIA was developed to measure the ability of test antisera to inhibit the binding of radiolabeled antireovirus antisera to the rabbit antianti-3 antisera. In this assay, it was possible to identify a distinct antireovirus 3 determinant common to both antireovirus 3 antisera and a hybridoma antibody directed at the reovirus 3 HA. As shown in the first two lines of Table I, the binding of the rabbit anti-anti-3 antisera by the radiolabeled antireovirus 3 antibody was inhibited to a similar degree by both the absorbed mouse antireovirus 1 and antireovirus 3 antisera, indicating a considerable amount of cross-reactivity between the antireovirus antisera in this type of competitive binding assay.

To determine if the rabbit antiserum recognized an HA-binding structure, six monoclonals to the reovirus type 3 HA and four monoclonals to the reovirus type 1 HA were tested for inhibition. Four antireovirus 1 HA monoclonals and five of the six antireovirus 3 HA monoclonals did not inhibit significantly. One antireovirus 3 HA monoclonal, designated G5, did inhibit the binding of the antireovirus 3 antibody by the rabbit antiserum. This inhibition by the G5 monoclonal does not appear to be caused by nonspecific binding of mouse immunoglobulin by the rabbit antisera, as none of the other nine reovirus HA 1 or HA 3 monoclonals inhibited to a comparable, or even significant, degree. This inhibition by an antireovirus 3 HA mono-

TABLE I

Identification of a Distinct Antireovirus 3 Determinant Shared between
Antisera to Reovirus 3 and Hybridoma Ab to the Reovirus 3 HA[a]

Rabbit antisera	^{125}I-labeled antireovirus Ab	Inhibiting Ab	Ab concentration at 50% inhibition (μg/ml)	Percentage of inhibition at 200 μg/ml
Anti-anti-3[b]	III	III	12	92
		I	15	90
		F4[c]	>200	38
		A2	>200	46
		B2	>200	34
		D2	175	55
		G5	35	83
		F7	>200	40

[a] Adapted from Nepom et al. (1982a).
[b] Rabbit antisera to mouse anti-reovirus 3 HA.
[c] F4, A2, B2, D2, G5, and F7 are monoclonal antibodies to reovirus 3 HA (Burstin et al., 1982).

clonal suggests recognition by the rabbit antisera of a major determinant shared between the hybridoma and the absorbed antireovirus 3 HA antisera.

Both the G5 and A2 monoclonals were shown to have neutralizing but not hemagglutination inhibiting activity against reovirus 3 and were used to define the functional domains for neutralization of the reovirus 3 HA. Binding studies showed that the A2 and G5 appear to recognize the same site on the reovirus 3 HA, as both compete for binding to reovirus 3. The failure of the A2 monoclonal to inhibit binding by the rabbit antisera indicates that the binding of the G5 antibody by the rabbit antisera is probably not simply an example of antigenic mimicry by the rabbit antiserum but rather is caused by a true idiotype–antiidiotype interaction. The implications of these findings will be elaborated later.

In a competition binding RIA using the rabbit antisera to antireovirus 1 antibody, it was possible to demonstrate that the inhibition by G5 was specific for the rabbit anti-anti-3 (Nepom et al., 1982a, data not shown). A threefold higher concentration of G5 was required for 50% inhibition of the binding of antireovirus 1 antisera by the rabbit anti-anti-1 antisera than was needed for the inhibition of the anti-type 3 by rabbit anti-anti-3. In addition, G5 and anti-type 3 immunoglobulin inhibited the binding of anti-type 1 by rabbit anti-anti-1 to a similar

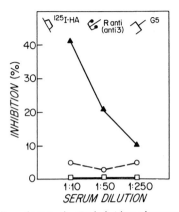

Fig. 1. Inhibition of binding of HA to the G5 hybridoma by test antisera was assessed in this indirect radioimmunoassay (RIA). After 250 ng of partially purified G5 was adsorbed onto the bottoms of polyvinyl microtiter plates, test rabbit sera were added to each well for 1 h. After washing, 10 ng (3000 cpm/ng) of purified HA was added to each well. The binding of purified HA to G5 is specifically inhibited by the affinity-purified rabbit anti-anti-3 antiserum. O———O, rabbit anti-anti-1; ▲———▲, rabbit anti-anti-3; □———□, normal rabbit serum. (Adapted from Nepom et al., 1982b.)

degree, and each was fourfold less able to inhibit this binding than was anti-type 1 immunoglobulin. As the G5 monoclonal has specificity for the reovirus 3 HA and the antisera used in the inhibition studies have been enriched for HA-binding activity, these studies appear to demonstrate a major HA 3 binding determinant shared by the absorbed antisera and the G5 hybridoma.

Further studies were necessary, however, to confirm this hypothesis and show that this determinant was HA specific. For these and further studies, rabbit anti-anti-3 antisera were affinity purified for binding to the G5 idiotype by acid elution from a Sepharose 4B column to which 2 μg/ml of partially purified G5 monoclonal had been coupled. To establish that the affinity-purified rabbit antisera (rabbit antiidiotype) recognized a determinant on the antigen-combining site of the G5 monoclonal, a competition RIA was developed to measure the ability of the rabbit antisera to inhibit the binding of the G5 antibody to the radiolabeled, purified reovirus 3 HA polypeptide. As illustrated in Fig. 1, affinity-purified rabbit anti-anti-3, but not rabbit anti-anti-1, significantly inhibited the binding of purified HA by the G5 hybridoma when compared with control values for normal rabbit sera.

Having established that the affinity-purified rabbit anti-anti-3 binds to the antigen-combining site of the G5 monoclonal, a highly sensitive

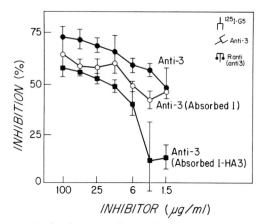

Fig. 2. In this competitive binding RIA, selective absorption on the HA of reovirus 3 removed the inhibition by mouse antireovirus 3 antiserum of the binding of radiolabeled G5 hybridoma to affinity-purified rabbit anti-anti-3 antiserum. The Id3 determinant was specific for the reovirus 3 HA. (Adapted from Nepom *et al.*, 1982a.)

competition RIA using the affinity-purified rabbit anti-anti-3 antiserum and radiolabeled G5 hybridoma immunoglobulin was developed to assay for the presence of a major HA-binding determinant in the absorbed antisera. Anti-3 antisera were found to inhibit the binding of G5 by the rabbit antisera much more than anti-1 antisera (data not shown). As illustrated in Fig. 2, the inhibition by anti-3 antiserum of binding of the G5 hybridoma to the affinity-purified rabbit antisera was almost totally removed by absorption on a recombinant strain containing the reovirus 3 HA (1HA3), but not after absorption on reovirus type 1. This is very strong evidence that there is a reovirus 3 HA-binding idiotypic determinant, designated Id3, shared by the G5 hybridoma and the HA-selected antireovirus 3 antisera.

B. DISTRIBUTION OF THE Id3 DETERMINANT ON CELL POPULATIONS

Having serologically defined the Id3 determinant on antisera to reovirus 3 and on an antireovirus 3 HA hybridoma (G5), we next used indirect cell-surface immunofluorescence to study a number of cell populations known to bind reovirus 3 to determine if they express the Id3 determinant on their cell surface. The R1.1 thymoma cell line binds reovirus 3 and not reovirus 1. As depicted in the fluorescence-activated cell sorter (FACS) tracing in Fig. 3A, R1.1 stains brightly

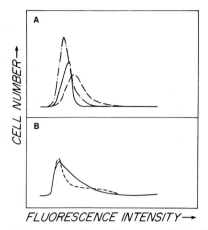

Fig. 3. FACS tracings of the staining of R1.1 thymoma cells by the affinity-purified rabbit anti-anti-3 antiserum. In (A), 50,000 R1.1. cells were stained with normal rabbit serum (–.–) rabbit anti-anti-1 (solid line), or rabbit anti-anti-3 antiserum (dashed line) followed by FITC-coupled protein A. Staining with the rabbit anti-anti-3 antiserum caused a marked shift in fluorescence intensity. (B) The fraction of rabbit anti-anti-3 antiserum enriched for ID3 binding by acid elution from a G5 affinity column stained the R1.1 cell line. (Adapted from Nepom et al., 1982a.)

with rabbit anti-anti-3 antisera. As shown in Fig. 3B, the majority of the staining was derived from the acid eluate of the G5 affinity column, indicating that the fraction of rabbit antiidiotypic serum that binds to G5 corresponds to the fraction that stains the R1.1 cell surface. These findings paralleled the serological data and suggested that the R1.1 cell line expresses the Id3 determinant on its cell surface; this presumably accounts in part for its ability to bind reovirus 3. The YAC lymphoma line is both unable to bind reovirus 3 and is Id3 negative by this form of cell-surface analysis (data not shown).

These findings encouraged us to pursue the tissue distribution of the Id3 determinant. As indicated earlier, the characteristic neurotropism of the mammalian reovirus maps to the HA. As noted, murine neurons but not ependymal cells bind and are susceptible to reovirus 3 infection in the neonatal murine host, as well as in tissue culture. Indirect immunofluorescence on explanted cells from rat and mouse nervous system is shown in Fig. 4. Previous correlative studies utilizing tetanus toxoid binding and intracellular microelectrode recordings permitted Dr. M. A. Dichter to identify cells as neurons by their characteristic morphology. Both the cell bodies and the dendritic processes of cells identified by such parameters as neurons stain brightly

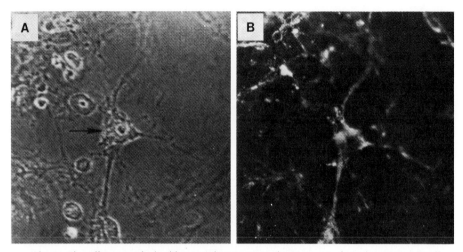

Fig. 4. The affinity-purified rabbit antiidiotype stained mouse spinal cord neurons in cell culture. Cells identified morphologically as multipolar neurons by phase contrast microscopy (A) show bright immunofluorescence (B) of both their cell bodies and processes when incubated with rabbit antiidiotypic antiserum followed by FITC-coupled protein A. Glial elements were repeatedly negative in these preparations. Neurons did not stain with the rabbit anti-anti-1 antiserum or with the fraction of rabbit anti-anti-3 antiserum that did not bind to the G5 affinity column. Magnification 344×. (Data from Nepom *et al.*, 1982a.)

with the rabbit anti-anti-3 acid eluate from the G5 affinity column. As has been shown for the R1.1 cell line, neurons did not stain with the unbound fraction (filtrate) from the affinity column or with rabbit anti-anti-1 or normal rabbit serum. Single-cell preparations of ciliated ependymal cells did not stain with the rabbit antiserum, a finding that parallels the failure of ependymal cells to bind reovirus 3. These studies suggest that murine neurons may express the cell surface Id3 determinant and that this determinant may account, in part, for their susceptibility to reovirus 3 infection.

It was shown previously that murine nonimmune lymphoid cells bind reovirus 3. Studies done in collaboration with Howard Weiner, Marc Tardieu, and Rochelle Epstein comparing the binding of reovirus 3 and the rabbit antiidiotypic antisera as determined by indirect immunofluorescence are depicted in Fig. 5. In these studies (Nepom *et al.*, 1982b), a plate adherence technique was used to enrich for cells that bind reovirus 3. As noted, there is a striking similarity in the percentage of cells that bind reovirus and stain with the rabbit antiidiotypic antisera. Double-labeling experiments (data not shown) indicated that all T cells that stain with the rabbit antiidiotype also bind

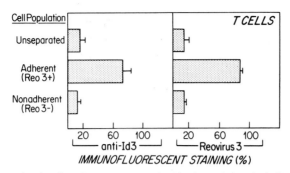

Fig. 5. Reovirus-binding lymphocytes express the Id3 determinant. A similar percentage of unseparated T cells bind reovirus 3 and the rabbit antiidiotypic antisera. Approximately 70% of reovirus-binding T cells stain with the antiidiotype following a plate adherence procedure. (Adapted from Nepom et al., 1982b.)

reovirus 3, implying that this subset of T cells expresses a common HA-recognizing determinant that cross-reacts with the rabbit anti-idiotype.

Thus, the studies that have been completed indicate that there exists an idiotypic determinant, Id3, which is shared by reovirus HA 3-binding antibodies and neuronal and lymphoid cells that bind to reovirus HA 3. This determinant can be recognized by a xenogenic antiidiotype serum raised against antireovirus HA 3 antisera and affinity purified on an antireovirus HA 3 immunoadsorbent column. These preliminary findings supported the hypothesis that antiviral receptors on somatic cells may share idiotypic determinants with antibodies to virus.

C. MONOCLONAL ANTIIDOTYPE CHARACTERIZATION OF THE Id3 DETERMINANT

Having identified an idiotype linked to HA recognition on both reovirus-binding immunoglobulins and several different somatic cell types, we proceeded to generate a monoclonal antibody directed against this idiotype (Noseworthy et al., 1983). This monoclonal anti-idiotype, 87.92.6, shares many of the characteristics of the rabbit anti-idiotype and has proven to be a useful tool in understanding reovirus 3 recognition.

Briefly, syngeneic BALB/c mice were repeatedly immunized with irradiated G5 cells. Immune spleen cells were then fused with the nonsecreting myeloma line P3 X 63-AG8.653 (653), according to standard procedures (Köhler and Milstein, 1975). Fused cells were initially grown in HAT media, and supernatants were tested for G5 recognition in a direct-binding RIA. Positive wells were expanded, cloned, retested, and recloned. One line, 87.92.6, was repeatedly found to specifically bind G5 and was used for further study. The 87.92.6 line secretes an IgM, κ product in relatively low amounts. Despite repeated recloning, a stable high-producing line could not be established. Monoclonal immunoglobulin was partially purified from culture supernatant and ascites preparations by serial 50% ammonium sulfate precipitations at 4°C. Normal mouse serum, culture supernatant, and ascites preparations from the parent 653 line and hybridomas of the same IgM isotype (anti-Thy-1.1 and an antiazobenzenearsonate monoclonal, GP1) were used for controls in the studies outlined below.

As the 87.92.6 line was generated against the G5 hybridoma in a syngeneic host, we anticipated that the specificity of this monoclonal would be strictly antiidiotypic for the G5 idiotype. To confirm this, an indirect competition RIA was developed that measured the ability of the monoclonal 87.92.6 to inhibit the binding of radiolabeled purified HA polypeptide by the G5 immunoglobulin. As shown in Fig. 6, 87.92.6 effectively inhibits the binding of the HA protein by the G5 monoclonal at a concentration of the G5 determined to be limiting for binding to the HA peptide. The anti-Thy-1.1 monoclonal antibody, 22.1, of the same IgM isotype did not inhibit significantly.

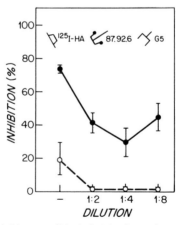

Fig. 6. The 87.92.6 hybridoma (solid circles) is directed to an idiotype on or near the antigen-combining site of the G5 monoclonal. In this competitive binding RIA, 87.92.6 but not the anti-Thy-1.1 (22.1) monoclonal (open circles) of the same isotype (IgM) inhibits the binding of radiolabeled purified reovirus 3 HA by 0.8 μg/ml G5.

Further evidence that the 87.92.6 line is G5 specific was provided by the interesting observation that this monoclonal antiidiotype-producing hybridoma expresses a G5-binding determinant, presumably the membrane form of IgM, on its cell surface. As illustrated in Fig. 7 in the direct immunofluorescence study, FITC-labeled G5 shows definite staining of the 87.92.6 cell line. The cytofluorographic pattern is admittedly less striking than the staining of the reovirus 3-infected P815 cells, but was consistently positive when compared with the repeatedly negative 653 myeloma line used to generate the monoclonal antiidiotype. The observation that the 87.92.6 cell line expresses antiidiotype on its cell surface suggests that this hybridoma is actually an immature B-cell hybrid, and is consistent with the finding that this cell line secretes very little immunoglobulin.

A series of cell surface immunofluorescence studies confirmed that the 87.92.6 product recognized the previously described Id3 determinant. As depicted in Fig. 8A, the R1.1 thymoma line stained brightly with the 87.92.6 immunoglobulin in a manner similar to the previously discussed rabbit anti-anti-3 antiserum. Staining with the antiidiotype was always found to be as bright as or brighter than staining of H-2 surface structures on the R1.1 line, as determined by studies with the 11.4.4 anti-K^k monoclonal (Ozato et al., 1980). Figure 8B shows that the determinant recognized by 87.92.6 is not the H-2 surface antigen. In this preparation, the R1.E thymoma line was used. This C58-derived thymoma line differs from the R1.1 cell of origin in that it no longer expresses H-2^k surface antigens. R1.E, like R1.1, binds reovirus 3 and stains brightly with the 87.92.6 hybridoma but is repeatedly negative for staining with the anti-H-2 monoclonal.

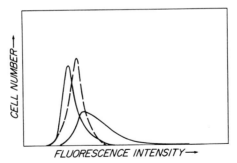

Fig. 7. Fluorescence-activated cell sorter tracings of direct staining by FITC-labeled G5 of reovirus 3-infected P815 cells (P815-3) (solid line), the monoclonal antiidiotype 87.92.6 (dashed line), and the 653 myeloma (peak on left) used to generate the antiidiotypic hybridoma. 87.92.6 expresses antiidiotypic determinants on its cell surface. ●———●, P815 reovirus 3 infected; △———△, 87.92.6 (antiidiotypic hybrid).

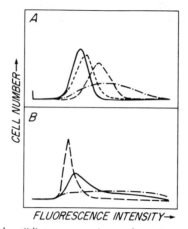

Fig. 8. The monoclonal antiidiotype recognizes a determinant on thymoma cells distinct from H-2. (A) Cytofluorographic profiles of R1.1 thymoma cells stained with the anti-H-2K$^\kappa$ (——) hybridoma (11.4.1; Ozato et al., 1980), with 87.92.6 (–·–) grown in ascites (undiluted) and diluted 1/200 (– – –) and stained with 653 culture supernatant (control, solid line). The staining by 87.92.6 is qualitatively different from that of the anti-H-2 monoclonal. (B) The H-2-negative R1.E cell line stains brightly with 87.92.6, indicating that the Id3 determinant is not H-2 (anti-theta, solid line).

A further observation that indicated that 87.92.6 recognized the same Id3 determinant on the R1.1 cell line and the G5 hybridoma is illustrated in Fig. 9. In this direct RIA, binding of the G5 immunoglobulin by 87.92.6 was completely removed by prior absorption of the monoclonal antiidiotype on 5×10^6 R1.1 cells. By FACS criteria, this cell line does not express Fc receptors. Loss of activity in such absorption studies indicates that the antiidiotypic antibody binds spe-

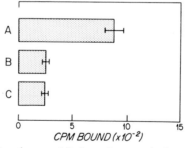

Fig. 9. 87.92.6 recognizes the same Id3 determinant on the R1.1 thymoma cell line and the G5 hybridoma (A). Absorption on R1.1 cells removes the binding of the monoclonal antiidiotype to the G5 idiotype, as measured in a direct RIA (B). The monoclonal antiidiotype does not bind the IgG$_{2a}$ isotype control hybridoma 14.4.4S (C) (anti-I-E^k; Oi et al., 1978).

TABLE II

Reovirus 3 and Antiidiotypic Ab Binding as Determined by
Cell Surface Immunofluorescence

Cell	Theta	H-2[a]	Reovirus 3	Reovirus 1	Rabbit anti-anti-3	87.92.6
R1.1 thymoma	1.2	H-2^k	+	−	+	+
R1.E thymoma	1.2	H-2 neg	+	−	+	+
BW 5147 thymoma	1.1	H-2^k	+	−	ND	+
YAC lymphoma	1.2	H-2$^{k/d}$	−	−	−	−
EL-4 lymphoma	1.2	H-2^b	+	±	ND	±
P815 mastocytoma	—	H-2^d	+	±	ND	±
Murine neurons			+	−	+	+
Ependymal cells			−	+	−	−
Murine T cells						
Unseparated						7%
Lyt-1$^+$,2$^-$,3$^-$						10%
Lyt-1$^-$,2$^+$,3$^+$						20%
Human T cells[b]						5–10%

[a] The expression of theta and H-2 antigens was confirmed by FACS analysis using the HO 13.4 (anti-theta-1.2), HO 22.1 (anti-theta-1.1), and 11.4.1 (anti-H-2^k; Ozato et al., 1980) hybridomas. Standard alloantisera were used to confirm the H-2^b an H-2^d haplotypes.

[b] Prepared as per Mendes et al. (1973) and English and Anderson (1974).

cifically to a cell surface determinant—presumably the Id3. Together, these studies strongly suggested that the 87.92.6 hybridoma was indeed antiidiotypic, with specificity for the Id3 determinant on both the reovirus 3-binding immunoglobulin and cell surfaces.

A series of cell surface immunofluorescence studies was undertaken to determine the presence of the Id3 determinant in a number of cell populations. The results of a large number of such studies are summarized in Table II. In the studies on lymphoid cell lines, the staining of cells with the monoclonal antiidiotype paralleled closely, but not absolutely, the previously demonstrated reovirus 3-binding studies. As discussed, R1.1 and R1.E stain brightly with both the xenogenic and the monoclonal antiidiotype; both also bind reovirus 3. BW5147 binds both reovirus 3 and 87.92.6. The YAC lymphoma line binds neither reovirus nor either antiidiotype. Immunofluorescence studies with EL-4 and P815 suggest that each cell line may bind the monoclonal antiidiotype, but staining has been weak in all cases and may indicate either low-affinity binding or possibly a virus-binding structure related to but differing in some way from the Id3 determinant.

Studies on murine CNS cells, done in collaboration with Drs. Dichter and Weiner, corroborated the previously described pattern found with the rabbit anti-anti-3. Neurons in both tissue sections and suspension cultures stain brightly with the monoclonal antiidiotype. Ependymal cell preparations have always been uniformly negative. The monoclonal antiidiotype also stains approximately 7–10% of purified murine T cells and 5–12% of human peripheral blood T cells. Studies of T-cell subsets are currently in progress. Preliminary results suggest, as indicated in Table II, that the Ly2,3$^+$ subset stains preferentially with the monoclonal antiidiotype.

Studies are underway to isolate and purify the Id3 receptor. Initial studies investigated the susceptibility of the Id3 determinant on the R1.1 cell line to treatment with the antibiotic tunicamycin (which inhibits addition of carbohydrate residues to glycoproteins) and the proteolytic enzymes pronase and trypsin. Briefly, 1×10^7 R1.1 cells were incubated for 30 min with 1.5 μg of either pronase or trypsin or were grown in suspension culture for 48 h with 0.05–1.0 μg/ml of tunicamycin as described. The cells then were washed extensively in media containing fetal calf serum and prepared for immunofluorescence analysis. FACS analysis showed that R1.1 cells no longer bound the anti-H-2 monoclonal, 11.4.1 (anti-H-2^k), after incubation for 48 h with even very low concentrations (0.05 μg/ml) of tunicamycin. Binding of 87.92.6 was initially unaltered at low concentrations (0.05–0.1 μg/ml) of tunicamycin but was slightly diminished at a high concentration (1.0 μg/ml) of tunicamycin. As tunicamycin inhibits the glycosylation of glycoproteins by blocking the formation of N-acetylglucosamine-lipid intermediates (Takatsuki and Tamura, 1971; Takatsuki et al., 1975), these findings suggest that the Id3 determinant may require a carbohydrate moiety for binding to the antiidiotype but that this requirement may be quantitatively less than or qualitatively different from the glycosylation of the H-2 structure. There is published evidence that bovine erythrocytes pretreated with neuraminidase are no longer agglutinated by reovirus 3, suggesting that sialic acid groups are important for HA binding (Gomatos and Tamm, 1962). On the other hand, binding of 87.92.6 was almost completely abolished by prior treatment of R1.1 cells with trypsin or pronase. These observations are consistent with the finding that the reovirus receptor on erythrocytes is trypsin sensitive, and suggest that the Id3 determinant on erythrocytes and reovirus-recognizing T cells is a protein with possibly only a minor carbohydrate component that is important for the Id3 configuration. Further biochemical analysis of the Id3 determinant is currently underway.

IV. Expression of HA-Specific Idiotype on Tc Cells

In the studies outlined to date, the binding of the antiidiotypic preparations to reovirus HA 3-recognizing determinants closely paralleled reovirus 3 binding to these determinants. As mentioned, Tc cells directed against reovirus-infected cells are specific for the sigma 1 gene product. The observation that the 87.92.6 cell line expresses a significant amount of antiidiotype on its cell surface (Section III,C) provided us with the opportunity to see if reovirus-specific Tc cells could lyse the antiidiotypic B-cell hybridoma. Such an observation would suggest that Tc cells may express an idiotype on their cell surface which is shared by B cells of the same antigenic specificity. A number of investigators have convincingly shown that T helper cells and T suppressor cells express hapten-related idiotypic determinants. To date, however, it has proven to be more difficult to determine if Tc cells express idiotypic determinants. Sherman *et al.* (1978) concluded that Tc cells do not express idiotypic determinants after failing to block Tc cell activity or stain ABA-specific Tc lymphocytes with antiidiotypic antibody. On the other hand, recent studies by Krammer *et al.* (1980) and Kees (1981) suggested that Tc cells may express idiotype.

A series of studies by Ertl, Nepom, Spriggs, Fields, and Finberg in collaboration with our laboratory demonstrated that reovirus 3-specific Tc cells effectively lyse the 87.92.6 B cell hybridoma in an H-2-restricted manner. This recognition is inhibited by free G5 immunoglobulin. These results strongly suggest that Tc cells express surface antiidiotype-recognizing structures and indeed may share these idiotypes with B cells. These studies will be briefly summarized (Ertl *et al.*, 1982).

For these experiments, Sendai virus-specific cytolytic T cells were used as virus-specificity controls. As illustrated in Fig. 10, reovirus 3-specific Tc cells but not Sendai virus-specific Tc cells effectively lyse the uninfected B-cell hybridoma line 87.92.6. Uninfected P815 target cells and the G5 hybridoma cell line were not lysed. Prior treatment of the Tc cells with antitheta serum and complement but not complement alone completely abolished lysis of the antiidiotypic cell line, as illustrated in Fig. 11. This suggests that lysis is T cell mediated and is not caused by natural killer cell activity or antibody-dependent cytolytic cells (ADCC). The Tc lysis of 87.92.6 is H-2 restricted, as illustrated in Fig. 12. B10.BR T cells (H-2^k) did not lyse the 87.92.6 (H-2^d) line, whereas the H-2^d-matched B10.D2 Tc cells did effectively lyse the hybridoma. This indicates that reovirus 3 Tc cells recognize the

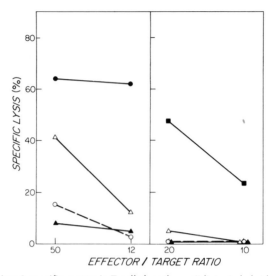

Fig. 10. Reovirus 3-specific cytotoxic T cells lyse the antiidiotypic hybridoma cell line. (A) Cytotoxic T cells to reovirus 3 prepared by *in vitro* restimulation of spleen cells from primed BALB/c mice were tested at different effector-to-target-cell ratios in a 6-h ^{51}Cr-release assay. (B) A Sendai virus-specific Tc cell line (2H-11) of B10.D2 origin was used as a virus-specific Tc-cell control. O——O, P815 uninfected; ●——●, P815 reovirus 3 infected; △——△, 87.92.6 (antiidiotypic hybrid); ▲——▲, G5 idiotypic hybrid; ■——■, P815 Sendai virus infected. (Adapted from Ertl *et al.,* 1982.)

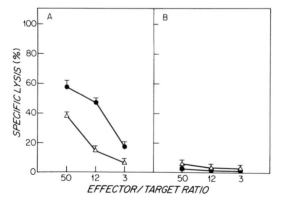

Fig. 11. Reovirus 3-specific Tc cells (A) treated for 30 min with anti-Thy-1.2 antibody and rabbit complement (B) no longer lyse the uninfected monoclonal antiidiotypic cell line in a 6-h ^{51}Cr-release assay (B). ●——●, P815 reovirus 3 infected; △——△, 87.92.6 (antiidiotypic hybrid). (Adapted from Ertl *et al.,* 1982.)

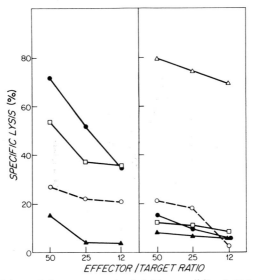

Fig. 12. Lysis of the antiidiotype-expressing hybridoma cell line is H-2 restricted. Tc cells derived from B10.D2 (H-2^d) but not B10.Br (H-2^k) mice effectively lyse the uninfected 87.92.6 (H-2^d) cell line in a 6-hr ^{51}Cr-release assay. O——O, P815 (H-2^d); ●——●, P815 reovirus infected; □——□, 87.92.6 (antiidiotypic hybrid); ▲——▲, L929 (H-2^k) uninfected; △——△, L929 reovirus infected. (Adapted from Ertl et al., 1982.)

antiidiotype-expressing 87.92.6 cells in conjunction with surface H-2 determinants. We conclude that the antireovirus 3 Tc must have an antigen-specific receptor capable of recognizing anti-Id3 antibodies on the hybridoma cell surface.

We cannot make a definite statement from these studies about the likelihood of there being one ("altered self hypothesis") or two receptors ("dual recognition hypothesis") on the Tc cell to explain H-2 restriction (Zinkernagel and Doherty, 1974). It seems unlikely that surface antiidiotypic immunoglobulin would combine with an H-2 antigen to form an "altered self" complex identical to the virus plus H-2 complex, however, which makes the two-receptor hypothesis more attractive. As the antiidiotypic cell line is a B cell, current studies are in progress to see if Tc-cell recognition of the antiidiotype is I or K/D region restricted. Lysis of the 87.92.6 cells could be effectively inhibited by free G5 immunoglobulin, as shown in Fig. 13. This inhibition is virus specific, as shown by failure of the G5 immunoglobulin to inhibit Sendai virus-specific Tc lysis of P815 Sendai virus-infected cells. This inhibition of Tc-mediated lysis is presumably caused by binding by the G5 immunoglobulin to surface anti-G5 determinants

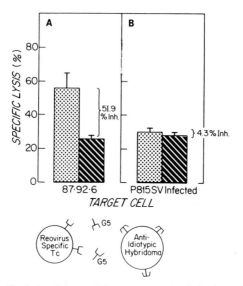

Fig. 13. Virus-specific lysis of the antiidiotype-expressing hybridoma line is inhibited by prior treatment of the antiidiotype with the G5 idiotypic hybridoma. (A), Reovirus 3-specific Tc; (B), Sendai virus-specific Tc. ⊠, NMS; ◨, GS. (Adapted from Ertl *et al.*, 1982.)

on the 87.92.6 cell. This finding implies that antiidiotype-recognizing Tc cells share antigen receptor idiotypes with B-cell hybridomas.

A limiting dilution analysis, summarized in Table III, indicates that lysis of reovirus-infected P815 cells (P815-3) and uninfected 87.92.6 cells is mediated by identical Tc-cell clones. Eighty per cent of the wells that lysed the 87.92.6 cell line also lysed reovirus 3-infected P815 (P815-3) cells. Of greater interest was the observation that 27% of the wells positive on P815-3 also lysed the antiidiotypic hybridoma, suggesting an idiotypically restricted Tc response to reovirus 3 infection. Further studies are in progress to examine these issues more closely with reovirus- and antiidiotype-specific Tc clones.

An analysis of Tc cells generated against reovirus variants provided further insights into the fine specificity of antiidiotype recognition. As previously mentioned, Spriggs and Fields (1982) showed that reovirus variants can be generated *in vitro* if wild-type virus is incubated with saturating amounts of neutralizing monoclonal anti-HA antibody. One such variant, the variant F virus, was utilized in these studies. This variant is no longer neutralized by the G5 monoclonal antibody. Previous studies (Finberg *et al.*, 1982) showed that this variant could both induce reovirus 3-specific Tc cells and be lysed by reovirus 3-specific

TABLE III

Lysis of P815.3 and 87.92.6 Cells Mediated by
Identical Tc-Cell Clones[a]

Target cell of positive well[b]	Percentage of population	Lysis[c]	
		P815.3	87.92.6
P815.3	27	+	+
	73	+	−
87.92.6	80	+	+
	20	−	+

[a] Adapted from Ertl et al. (1982).

[b] Limiting dilutions of responder cells were used in vitro to restimulate reovirus 3-sensitized BALB/c splenocytes. Seven days later, each well was tested for cytolytic activity on reovirus 3-infected P815 (P815-3) or uninfected 87.92.6 targets in a 6-h ^{51}Cr-release assay.

[c] Wells were considered positive if lysis was three standard deviations above spontaneous release.

Tc cells. As shown in Fig. 14, variant F-specific Tc cells effectively lysed reovirus 3-infected P815 cells but not the 87.92.6 cells, indicating a distinct specificity of these Tc cells. These findings suggest that the population of reovirus 3-induced Tc cells that lyse both reovirus

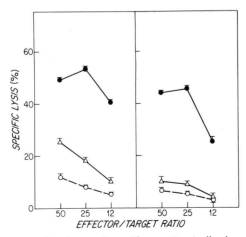

Fig. 14. Tc cells generated against reovirus with an antigenically altered HA do not lyse the monoclonal antiidiotype-expressing cell line. (A), Reovirus 3-specific Tc; (B) reovirus variant F-specific Tc. O--O, P815 uninfected; ●——●, P815 reovirus 3 infected; △——△, 87.92.6 (antiidiotypic hybrid). (Adapted from Ertl et al., 1982.)

3-infected targets and 87.92.6 recognize a G5 binding determinant, either the HA on wild-type virus or an anti-HA-binding determinant on the monoclonal antiidiotype. The variant virus presumably no longer expresses the G5-binding surface determinant and can therefore no longer induce a subset of Tc cells which recognize this determinant.

Taken together, these studies indicate that reovirus 3-specific Tc cells express structures on their cell surface that behave functionally like B-cell idiotypes and may share these idiotypes with a B-cell hybridoma (G5) reactive against the same antigenic determinants. It is possible to hypothesize from these findings that T-cell idiotypes may resemble B-cell idiotypes and indeed may utilize V-region genes to generate these structures. Furthermore, the demonstration of recognition of antiidiotypes by Tc cells suggests that recognition of antiidiotypic clones by Tc cells, and vice versa, could occur during the course of a normal immune response. Naturally occurring antiidiotypic clones theoretically could interact with idiotypes on Tc cells and lead to down-regulation of the Tc-cell response. Alternatively, Tc cells could lyse and eliminate auto-antiidiotypes during the immune response to viral infection. Having shown that idiotype-like receptors can occur on nonimmune cells (e.g., neurons), it is possible to speculate that immune cells and cell products could either lyse or alter the function of nonimmune cells bearing naturally occurring idiotypes or antiidiotypic structures. Such an occurrence has a precedent in the observation that antibodies to antiinsulin antibody can mimic the effect of insulin on nonimmune cells bearing the insulin receptor (Obberghen *et al.*, 1979). Auto-antiidiotypes generated in the course of an immune response to virus or other antigens could theoretically bind to idiotypes on CNS neurons and lead to the alteration of neurological function that occasionally follows viral infection or another immune challenge. Excitation of neurons by such an interaction could lead to spontaneous seizure generation; inhibition of cell function could potentially cause depression of neurological function, resulting in alterations in mental status (e.g., stupor, coma), motor performance (e.g., paralysis), or other pathophysiological ramifications.

V. Summary

These studies have shown that reovirus HA-recognizing structures, as defined by both xenogenic and monoclonal antiidiotypic antibodies, are shared by immunoglobulin- and reovirus-immune T cells as well as by nonimmune lymphoid and neuronal cells. One interpretation of these observations is that the apparent shared recognition of the antiidiotypes by the G5 monoclonal and other reovirus-binding cells is caused by antigen mimicry. In this case, it could be postulated that the antiidiotypes have a structural conformation sufficiently similar to that of the reovirus sigma 1 protein to permit binding to the reovirus receptor. It seems improbable that the antigen-combining site of both the xenogenic antiidiotype and the isologous monoclonal antiidiotype could sufficiently resemble the virus attachment protein to parallel so closely virus-binding behavior. As noted in Section III,A, two antireovirus 3 HA monoclonals, the G5 and A2 hybridomas, behaved differently in a competition-binding RIA with the rabbit anti-anti-3. These two monoclonals have both been shown to neutralize reovirus 3, and each competes with the other for binding to the reovirus 3 HA. If the rabbit antiidiotypic antisera were simply mimicking the conformation of the reovirus HA protein, one would have predicted that the A2 hybridomas would have successfully inhibited the binding of the absorbed mouse anti-reovirus 3 HA antisera to the rabbit anti-anti-3 antisera. We feel that the results of the studies are much more in keeping with a true idiotype–antiidiotype interaction and that the antiidiotype defines an idiotypic determinant on the HA-binding receptor on both cells and immunoglobulin.

The finding that the reovirus recognition structure is shared by immune and nonimmune cells does not imply that the reovirus receptor is necessarily identical on these populations. It is, of course, unlikely that the serologically defined reovirus recognition structure on neuronal and lymphoid cells is primarily a viral recognition receptor. We can postulate that the reovirus attachment protein binds to a cell surface structure necessary for an as yet undefined fundamental cell function. Nevertheless, the observation suggests that receptors of immune cells and somatic cells (e.g., neurons) may share structural similarities. In addition, our findings clearly show that the Tc cells share determinants that behave functionally as do the idiotypes of B cells with similar antigen specificity. These findings may suggest that these heterogeneous cell populations use a related family of genes to encode for these similar cell surface structures. At present, this notion is purely hypothetical. Confirmation will require either receptor amino acid sequencing or nucleic acid analysis of the relevant genomic fractions of these cell populations.

Acknowledgments

We would like to thank Jeffrey Drebin and Dr. Bernard N. Fields for reviewing this chapter and Ms. Sarah Curwood for the preparation of the manuscript. This work was supported by the National Institutes of Health (Grant NS 16998-02). Dr. Noseworthy is the recipient of a Centennial Fellowship of the Medical Research Council of Canada.

References

Babiss, L. E., Luftig, R. F., Weatherbee, J. A., Weihing, R., Ray, U. R., and Fields, B. N. (1979). Reovirus serotypes 1 and 3 differ in their *in vitro* association with microtubules. *J. Virol.* **30**, 863–874.

Binz, H., and Wigzell, H. (1975). Shared idiotypic determinants on B and T lymphocytes reactive against the same antigenic determinants. I. Demonstration of similar or identical idiotypes on IgG molecules and T-cell receptors with specificity for the same alloantigens. *J. Exp. Med.* **142**, 197–211.

Burstin, S. J., Spriggs, D. R., and Fields, B. N. (1982). Evidence for functional domains on the reovirus type 3 hemagglutinin. *Virology* **117**, 146–155.

Eichman, K., Ben-Neriah, Y., Hetzelberger, D., Polke, C., Givol, D., and Lonai, P. (1980). Correlated expression of V_H framework and V_H idiotypic determinants on T helper cells and on functionally undefined T cells binding group A streptococcal carbohydrate. *Eur. J. Immunol.* **10**, 105–112.

English, D., and Anderson, B. R. (1974). Single-step separation of red blood cells, granulocytes and mononuclear leukocytes on discontinuous density gradients of Ficoll-Hypaque. *J. Immunol. Methods* **5**, 249–252.

Ertl, H. C. J., Greene, M. I., Noseworthy, J. H., Fields, B. N., Nepom, J. T., Spriggs, D. R., and Finberg, R. W. (1982). Identification of idiotypic receptors on reovirus specific cytolytic T cells. *Proc. Natl. Acad. Sci. U.S.A.* **79**, 7479–7483.

Finberg, R. N., Weiner, H. L., Fields, B. N., Benacerraf, B., and Burakoff, S. J. (1979). Generation of cytolytic T lymphocytes after reovirus infection: Role of the S1 gene. *Proc. Natl. Acad. Sci. U.S.A.* **76**, 442–446.

Finberg, R. N., Spriggs, D. R., and Fields, B. N. (1982). Host immune response to reovirus: CTL's recognize the neutralization domain of the viral hemagglutinin. *J. Immunol.* **129**, 2235–2238.

Gomatos, P. J., and Tamm, I. (1962). Reactive sites of reovirus type 3 and their interaction with receptor substances. *Virology* **17**, 455–461.

Greene, M. I., and Weiner, H. L. (1980). Delayed hypersensitivity in mice infected with reovirus. Induction of tolerance and suppressor T cells to viral specific gene products. *J. Immunol.* **125**, 283–287.

Hetzelberger, D., and Eichman K. (1978). Recognition of idiotypes in lymphocyte reactions. I. Idiotypic selectivity in the cooperation between T and B lymphocytes. *Eur. J. Immunol.* **8**, 846–852.

Kees, U. R. (1981). Idiotypes on major histocompatibility complex-restricted virus-immune cytotoxic T lymphocytes. *J. Exp. Med.* **153**, 1562–1573.

Kim, S., Davis, M., Sinn, E., Patten, P., and Hood, L. (1981). Antibody diversity: Somatic hypermutation of rearranged V_H genes. *Cell* **27**, 573–581.

Kohler, F., and Milstein, C. (1975). Continuous cultures of fused cells secreting antibody of predefined specificity. *Nature (London)* **256**, 495–497.

Krammer, P. H., Rehberger, R., and Eichman, K. (1980). Antigen-receptors on major histocompatibility complex restricted T lymphocytes. I. Preparation and characterization of syngeneic antisera against trinitrophenyl-activated T cell blasts and demonstration of their speciality for idiotypes on cytolytic T lymphocytes. *J. Exp. Med.* **151**, 1166–1182.

Mendes, N. F., Tolnai, M. E. A., Silveira, N. P. A., Gilbertson, R. B., and Metzgar, R. S. (1973). Technical aspects of the rosette tests used to detect human complement receptor (B) and sheep erythrocyte-binding (T) lymphocytes. *J. Immunol.* **11**, 860–867.

Nepom, J. T., Weiner, H. L., Dichter, M. A., Tardieu, M., Spriggs, D. R., Gramm, C. F., Powers, M. L., Fields, B. N., and Greene, M. I. (1982a). Identification of a hemagglutinin-specific idiotype associated with reovirus recognition shared by lymphoid and neural cells. *J. Exp. Med.* **155**, 155–167.

Nepom, J. T., Tardieu, M., Epstein, R. L., Noseworthy, J. H., Weiner, H. L., Gentsch, J., Fields, B. N., and Greene, M. I. (1982b). Virus-binding receptors: Similarities to immune receptors as determined by anti-idiotypic antibodies. *Surv. Immunol. Res.* **1**, 255–261.

Noseworthy, J. H., Fields, B. N., Dichter, M. A., Sobotka, S., Pizer, E., Perry, L. L., Nepom, J. T., and Greene, M. I. (1983). Cell receptors for the mammalian Reovirus I. Syngeneic monoclonal anti-idiotypic antibody identifies a cell surface receptor for Reovirus. *J. Immunol.* **131**, 2533–2538.

Obberghen, V. E., Spooner, P. M., Kohn, C. R., Chernick, S. S., Garrison, M. M., Karlson, F. A., and Gruneld, C. (197). Insulin-receptor antibodies mimic a late insulin effect. *Nature (London)* **280**, 500–502.

Oi, V. T., Jones, P. P., Goding, J. W., Herzenberg, L. A., and Herzenberg, L. A. (1978). Properties of monoclonal antibodies to mouse Ig allotypes, H-2, and Ia antigens. *Curr. Top. Microbiol. Immunol.* **81**, 115.

Onodera, T., Toniolo, A., Roy, U. R., Jenson, A. B., Knazek, R. A., and Notkins, A. L. (1981). Virus-induced diabetes mellitus. XX. Polyendocrinopathy and autoimmunity. *J. Exp. Med.* **153**, 1457–1473.

Ozato, K., Mayer, N., and Sachs, D. H. (1980). Hybridoma cell lines secreting monoclonal antibodies to mouse H-2 and Ia antigens. *J. Immunol.* **124**, 533–540.

Sharpe, A. H., and Fields, B. N. (1981). Reovirus inhibition of cellular DNA synthesis: The role of the S1 gene. *J. Virol.* **38**, 389–392.

Sharpe, A. H., and Fields, B. N. (1982). Pathogenesis of reovirus infection. *In* "Comprehensive Virology" (H. Fraenkel-Conrat and R. R. Wagner, eds.). Plenum, New York.

Sherman, L. A., Burakoff, S. J., and Benacerraf, B. (1978). The induction of cytolytic T lymphocytes with specificity for p-azobenzenearsonate coupled syngeneic cells. *J. Immunol.* **121**, 1432–1436.

Spriggs, D. R., and Fields, B. N. (1982). Attenuated reovirus type 3 strains generated by selection of hemagglutinin antigenic variants. *Nature (London)* **297**, 68–70.

Takatsuki, A., and Tamura, G. (1971). Tunicamycin, a new antibiotic. III. Reversal of the antiviral activity of tunicamycin by aminosugars and other derivatives. *J. Antibiot.* **24**, 232.

Takatsuki, A., Kohno, K., and Tamura, G. (1975). Inhibition of biosynthesis of polyisoprenol sugars in chick embryo microsomes by tunicamycin. *Agric. Biol. Chem.* **39**, 2089–2091.

Weiner, H. L., Drayna, D., Averill, D. R., and Fields, B. N. (1977). Molecular basis of
reovirus virulence: The role of the S1 gene. *Proc. Natl. Acad. Sci. U.S.A.* **74,** 5744–
5748.

Weiner, H. L., Ault, K. A., and Fields, B. N. (1980a). Interaction of reovirus with cell
surface receptors. I. Murine and human lymphocytes have a receptor for the hemagglutinin of reovirus type 3. *J. Immunol.* **124,** 2143–2148.

Weiner, H. L., Greene, M. I., and Fields, B. N. (1980b). Delayed hypersensitivity in
mice infected with reovirus. I. Identification of host and viral gene products responsible for the immune response. *J. Immunol.* **125,** 278–282.

Weiner, H. L., Powers, M. L., and Fields, B. N. (1980c). Absolute linkage of virulence
with central nervous system cell tropism of reovirus to hemagglutinin. *J. Infect.
Dis.* **141,** 609–616.

Zinkernagel, R. M., and Doherty, P. C. (1974). Immunological surveillance against
altered self components by sensitized T lymphocytes in lymphocytic chorio-
meningitis. *Nature (London)* **251,** 547.

Chapter 17

Idiotypy in Autoimmune Central Nervous System Demyelinating Disease: Experimental Allergic Encephalomyelitis and Multiple Sclerosis

Robert B. Fritz

Department of Microbiology/Immunology
Emory University School of Medicine
Atlanta, Georgia

I. Introduction

In contrast to traditional views, autoimmunity may be considered the normal state in an immunocompetent individual. The network of idiotype–antiidiotype interactions postulated by Jerne (1974) is based upon the concept that an animal has the capacity to respond to antigenic determinants (idiotopes) on its own immune receptors and that a network of interacting immune responses acts to regulate the entire immune system. Thus, when an individual responds immunologically to an exogenous antigen, responses are generated against endogenous antigenic determinants (idiotopes) located on the receptor molecules of the immune system as well as to the exogenous epitopes. These antiidiotypic (anti-Id) responses act to regulate the immune system in a positive or negative manner. The anti-Id response itself is regulated by further receptor–antireceptor interactions. One set of receptor determinants (anti-Id) forms an internal image of the stimulating exogenous antigenic determinants within the context of the responding individual's own immune system. Thus, in this view, every immune response would have an autoimmune component. In the normal state, autoimmune reactions would be without pathological consequences. Only when the system becomes unbalanced in a manner causing pathological damage will clinical autoimmune disease be observed.

The mechanisms that lead to induction of spontaneous autoimmune disease in humans or in experimental animals are not well understood. A major obstacle in elucidation of the etiology of autoimmunity is that the antigens involved in the initiation of these responses are, in most cases, poorly characterized. Thus, one is unable to test the validity of Jerne's hypothesis vis-à-vis the autoimmune response. In order to do this, it would be necessary to localize the epitopes responsible for the deleterious components of the autoimmune response and to separate these from epitopes that induce nonpathological responses. If this were possible, relevant questions could be formulated about the regulation by the anti-Id network and the role of the internal image in autoimmunity.

An experimental model in which the antigen involved in the autoimmune response has been well characterized is experimental allergic encephalomyelitis (EAE), a T-cell-mediated demyelinating autoimmune disease of the central nervous system (CNS), which is readily induced in a number of animal species by the injection of highly purified myelin basic protein (MBP). In the Lewis (Le) rat model, it has been shown that a 19-amino-acid peptide (residues 68–88) contains the major encephalitogenic determinant (Chou et al., 1977; Martenson et al., 1977). Immunization with this peptide in complete Freund's adjuvant (CFA) leads to disease in 100% of the animals within 10–12 days (Kibler et al., 1977). In addition to EAE, immunized animals produce significant levels of antibody against the peptide (Fritz et al., 1979).

The application of these findings to studies of the role of the idiotypic network in autoimmune disease seem to be very appropriate. If it were possible to use anti-Id antibodies to down-regulate an ongoing pathological immune response by inhibition of T-helper activity, stimulation of T-suppressor activity, or elimination of effector T cells, specific control of autoimmunity might be achieved. For these reasons, a series of experiments was initiated to assess the role of the idiotype network in EAE.

The general approach was to immunize Le rats with the 19-amino-acid encephalitogenic fragment of guinea pig MBP, to characterize the humoral and cellular responses to this antigen, to purify and characterize antiencephalitogenic peptide antibodies, and to use these purified antibodies to immunize rabbits for the production of anti-Id antibodies. We then determined the idiotypic specificities of the rabbit antibodies and used these to attempt to modify EAE in the Le rat.

The rationale for our experiments was based on the finding that idiotopes on immunoglobulin V regions are serologically cross-reactive with an idiotope or idiotopes on T lymphocytes (Binz and Wigzell, 1975; Cozenza et al., 1977; Eichman, 1978). This finding raises the possibility of idiotypic intervention in the ongoing immune response. Indeed, it has been demonstrated that immune responses may be suppressed or enhanced by the administration of the appropriate anti-Id antibodies (Cozenza and Kohler, 1972; Hart et al., 1972; Eichman et al., 1978). Further, it has been possible to induce idiotype-bearing antigen-binding and non-antigen-binding immunoglobulin molecules by administration of anti-Id antibodies (Bluestone et al., 1981). The latter finding supports the concept of the internal image component of the immune response.

II. Experimental Studies

A. GUINEA PIG MYELIN BASIC PROTEIN AND ITS PEPTIDES

Myelin basic protein (MBP), which may be readily purified from CNS tissue of a number of different vertebrate species, is a molecule of approximately 170 amino acids having a molecular weight of approximately 18,000. Following its extraction from myelin, the protein retains little native conformation (Liebes et al., 1975). This is advantageous because antibodies prepared against the intact protein react well, for the most part, with peptides derived enzymatically from the protein.

MBP from the human, the cow, and the rat have been completely sequenced, whereas the sequence is known only for the encephalitogenic regions of guinea pig MBP (Dunkley and Carnegie, 1974; Shapira et al., 1971). The strategy for preparation of the enzymatic peptides derived from guinea pig MBP and the biological activity of each of these peptides are shown in Fig. 1. The major encephalitogenic activity of this protein for the Le rat lies between residues 68 and 88 (Chou et al., 1977). Immunization of Le rats with this peptide in CFA

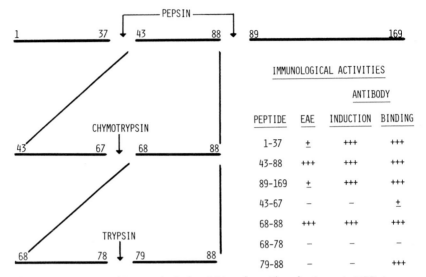

Fig. 1. Preparation and immunological activities of peptides of guinea pig MBP. Immunological activities: +++, high; ++, moderate; +, low; −, none.

leads to the induction of EAE, circulating antibody, and sensitized lymph node cells which can be assayed for the *in vitro* correlates of T-cell immunity. Significant cell-mediated immunity and antibody are induced against the nonencephalitogenic fragments 1–37 and 89–169 (Martenson *et al.*, 1975). Thus, the encephalitogenic epitope may be readily separated from other epitopes which do not induce pathological damage. The immunological activity of fragments of peptide 68–88 is shown in Fig. 1. Although neither fragment has immunogenic activity, peptide 79–88 acts as a hapten as it will react with preformed antibody to peptide 68–88 (Fritz *et al.*, 1979).

B. DEFINITION OF T-CELL AND B-CELL DETERMINANTS ON ENCEPHALITOGENIC PEPTIDE 68–88

For our studies, it was critical to determine whether T cells and B cells recognized the same or different epitopes on encephalitogenic peptides. This question was answered in two ways. The first was to compare immunological activities of guinea pig peptide 68–88 and the corresponding peptides from the Le rat and the cow. The amino acid sequence of all three peptides is known (Table I). Thus, the effect of known amino acid interchanges on the immunological activi-

TABLE I

Comparison of Peptide Sequence, Encephalitogenic Activity, and
Antibody-Binding Activity of Bovine, Guinea Pig, and Rat Peptides
68–88

	Peptide sequence[a]	EAE[b]	Ab binding[c]
Bovine	70 80 GSLPQKAQGHRPQDENPVVHF	±	+++
Guinea Pig	————S—( )–S————	+++	+++
Rat	————S—( )–T————	+	+++

[a] One-letter amino acid code. — indicates identity with bovine sequence, ( ) indicates deletion.

[b] Encephalitogenic activity. ±, low; +++, high.

[c] Binding to homologous or cross-reacting performed antibody.

ties of these peptides may be assessed readily. Table I is a summation of the results of these experiments. Residue 79 was critical for T-cell activity because an interchange of threonine for serine at this position markedly reduced the encephalitogenic activity of this molecule (Kibler *et al.*, 1977). The difference in encephalitogenic activity was even greater when the guinea pig peptide was compared with the bovine peptide. However, the residue at position 79 made little difference in the reactivity of these peptides with antibody induced by any one of them. By these criteria, then, the epitopes responsible for B-cell and T-cell activity were distinct.

An alternative approach to this problem was to cleave selectively amino acids from either the amino-terminal or the carboxy-terminal region of peptide 68–88 (Martenson *et al.*, 1977; Chou *et al.*, 1979). The smaller peptides were then compared for immunological activity with the parent peptide. The results of these experiments are shown in Table II. It is noteworthy that removal of the three hydrophobic carboxy-terminal amino acids by carboxypeptidase was sufficient to abrogate completely the reactivity of the peptide with its homologous antibody. T-cell activity of this peptide remained unchanged, however. The smallest fragment that retained full T-cell activity was peptide 71–85. The conclusion that may be drawn from these studies is that the T-cell epitope is centered on residue 79 and includes critical residues between 71 and 85, whereas the B-cell epitope includes residues 80–88. The latter conclusion was verified by competitive inhibition radioimmunoassay (RIA) using fragments of peptide 68–88

TABLE II

Encephalitogenic Activity of Fragments of Guinea
Pig Peptide 68–88

Peptide	EAE activity[a]	Ab binding[b]
68–88	+++	+++
68–85	+++	−
68–84	+	−
72–88	++	++

[a] EAE activity: +++, high; ++, moderate; +, low.
[b] Binding of peptides to antipeptide 68–88 antibody.

(Fritz *et al.*, 1977, 1979). Thus, although the epitopes are distinct, they occupy overlapping positions on the peptide.

C. INDUCTION OF ANTI-ANTIENCEPHALITOGENIC PEPTIDE ANTIBODIES

Because it was found in the above experiments that the epitopes were distinct for B and T lymphocytes reactive with the encephalitogenic peptide, it seemed likely that the receptors on these two cell types would also be distinct, and that the probability of their containing common or cross-reactive idiotopes would be small. However, the finding of cross-reactive idiotopes on B and T cells by several laboratories encouraged us to proceed with the production of anti-Id antibodies by immunization of rabbits with antiencephalitogenic peptides prepared from individual Le rats. Two questions prompted these studies. The first was whether antiencephalitogenic peptide antibodies from different rats contained common or cross-reactive idiotopes; the second was whether the administration of anti-Id antibodies to Le rats would modify the clinical course of EAE in any manner.

With respect to the first question, previous studies had shown that a significant degree of binding heterogeneity was found in antiencephalitogenic peptide antisera from different rats (Fritz *et al.*, 1977, 1979). In spite of this, all antisera recognized epitopes contained within the region 80–88 on the peptide. Thus, it was of interest to determine the degree of idiotypic heterogeneity displayed by these antisera.

Accordingly, pools of immune ascitic fluid from several individual rats were prepared, and antibodies were purified from them by affinity chromatography on peptide 43–88-Sepharose 4B. Because it was possible that affinity chromatography might select a subpopulation of

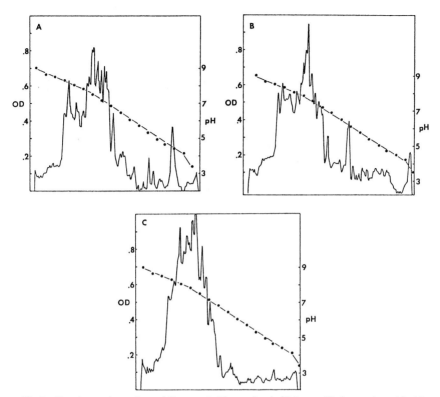

Fig. 2. Densitometric tracings of Coomassie Blue-stained affinity-purified rat antipeptide 68–88 antibodies after IEF. (A) and (B) represent two different purified antibodies; (C) is a tracing of DEAE-purified normal Le rat immunoglobulin. (Reprinted with permission from *Mol. Immunol.* **19;** Fritz *et al.* 1982, copyright Pergamon Press, Ltd.)

antibodies from the original heterogeneous population, the purified antibodies were characterized with respect to class, subclass, and specificity. Within the limits of experimental error, the populations of antibodies that were prepared from the affinity column had the same characteristics as did the antibodies in the unfractionated antisera (Fritz *et al.*, 1982). These and other experiments showed that the antibodies produced by rats immunized with peptide 68–88 were quite heterogeneous with respect to immunoglobulin class or subclass. The predominant classes of antibodies found in these antisera were either IgG_1 or IgG_2 and IgE. These antibodies were then further characterized by isoelectric focusing (IEF) (Fig. 2). In accordance with previous findings concerning specificity and class, charge heterogeneity of the purified antibodies was significant. Indeed, the purified antibodies were more heterogeneous than were control preparations of DEAE-purified normal Le rat immunoglobulin. The conclusion drawn from these studies was that although the rats were immunized with a small peptide containing one or at most a very small number of epitopes, the antibody response was heterogeneous with respect to class, charge, and specificity.

In order to determine whether anti-Id antibody raised by immunization with a single Le rat antipeptide antibody would cross-react with other antipeptide antibodies, purified antiencephalitogenic peptide antibodies from several different individual Le rats were used as immunogens to raise anti-Id antisera in rabbits (Fritz and Desjardins, 1982). Table III shows the specificity of the rat antipeptide antibodies used for production of the anti-Id antibodies. The resultant rabbit antisera were exhaustively absorbed with pooled, normal Le rat immunoglobulins coupled to Sepharose 4B until no reactivity against normal Le rat immunoglobulin was observed. Anti-Id antibody was assessed by the interference of the putative anti-Id with the ability of the antipeptide antibody to bind its radioiodinated ligand. The standard assay was a competitive inhibition-type RIA in which anti-Id antisera were assessed for their ability to inhibit the binding of a known amount of ^{125}I-labeled peptide by the antipeptide antisera. These assays were done in antigen excess because inhibition by anti-

TABLE III

Specificity of Rat Antipeptide Antibodies Used for
Production of Rabbit Antiidiotypic Antibodies[a]

Rat antiserum	Reactivity with peptide			Rabbit-Id number
	68–88	79–88	68–85	
378-3	+++[b]	+++	0	1
378-4	+++	++	+	2
12	+++	++	0	3
20	+++	+++	0	4
21	+++	+++	0	5
2078-1	±	±	+++	6

[a] Reprinted by permission from Fritz and Desjardins (1982), copyright American Association of Immunologists.

[b] +++, >90% inhibition of homologous reaction by the relevant peptide at a 10-fold molar excess; ++, 50–90% inhibition at a 10-fold molar excess; +, 20–50% inhibition at a 10-fold molar excess; ±, 1–10% inhibition at a 100-fold molar excess; 0, no inhibition at a 100-fold molar excess.

Id antibody was most pronounced when there was a minimum number of free antigen-binding sites available. Thus, all antipeptide antisera were diluted to the point at which they bound approximately 10% of the radiolabeled peptide in the absence of anti-Id antibody. Anti-Id antisera assayed in this manner were found to inhibit the binding of radiolabeled peptide to the homologous antipeptide antibodies by greater than 95%. These anti-Id antisera were then tested against a panel of Le rat antipeptide antibodies (Table IV). Interestingly, each anti-Id antiserum displayed a unique pattern of reactivity against the panel. Anti-Id antiserum 1 reacted predominantly with the antibodies used as immunogen and only weakly with other members of the panel. Comparison of the reactivities of anti-Id antisera 2 and 3 was interesting in that each serum cross-reacted with certain rat antisera, and yet each also recognized idiotopes that the others did not. These results did not show a correlation of fine specificity and idiotype. For example, anti-Id 1 and 2, which were raised by immunogens of different specificities, did not show any clear grouping when tested against the panel. These results showed that each antiserum recognized both

TABLE IV

Cross-Reactivity of Rabbit Antiidiotypic Antisera
with Rat Antipeptide 68–88 Antisera[a]

Rat antiserum	Inhibition of ^{125}I-Peptide 43–88 binding by rabbit anti-Id (%)				
	1	2	3	4	5
378-0	6[b]	50	6	90	88
378-1	4	17	36	90	92
378-3	91	23	42	93	89
3266A1	15	29	5	52	31
3277A2	8	20	8	36	37
3077B0	21	17	0	21	60
378-2	6	55	14	70	62
378-4	9	95	16	20	24
3277A0	11	8	21	3	25
3277A3	0	0	17	80	NT[c]
3277B3	0	40	45	84	54
3077B1	0	3	41	42	52

[a] Reprinted by permission from Fritz and Desjardins (1982), copyright American Association of Immunologists.
[b] CPM bound in the absence of anti-Id was 5000–6000. The negative control was approximately 200–400.
[c] Not tested.

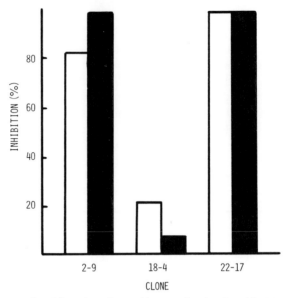

Fig. 3. Reactivity of antiidiotypic antisera with monoclonal antipeptide 68–88 antibodies as measured by inhibition of binding of monoclonal antibody to peptide 68–88. □, anti-Id-1; ■, anti-Id-2.

common and unique idiotopes. It is not possible to estimate from these data how many idiotopes were associated with these antibodies, nor is it possible to determine whether the heterogeneity was caused by multiple idiotopes on a single molecule or the presence of a large number of different molecules, each carrying a small number of idiotopes. It is clear, however, that a significant degree of idiotypic cross-reactivity was found among these antipeptide antisera.

It was then of interest to determine whether these antisera would cross-react with monoclonal antiencephalitogenic peptide antibodies. The results of such an experiment are shown in Fig. 3. Two of the three monoclonal antiencephalitogenic peptide antibodies carried idiotopes that were recognized by the anti-Id antisera tested. These results imply that the idiotopes recognized by the anti-Id antisera were common to many of the individual antibodies.

The antiidiotypic antisera were then tested for interstrain cross-reactivity by inhibition of antiencephalitogenic peptide antibody from Fisher rats (Table V). The data in this table indicate the presence of interstrain cross-reactive idiotopes on the peptide antibodies of Fisher rats. Again, the pattern of reactivity shown in this table indicates the presence of multiple cross-reactive idiotopes.

TABLE V

Inhibition of ^{125}I-Peptide 43–88 Binding to F344
Rat Antipeptide 68–88 Antibodies by Rabbit
Anti-Id Antisera[a]

Rat antiserum	Inhibition by rabbit anti-Id (%)			
	1	2	4	5
1	24	10	15	13
2	23	25	33	38
3	0	40	22	32
4	0	11	13	6
5	19	31	19	27

[a] Reprinted by permission from Fritz and Desjardins
(1982), copyright American Association of Immunologists.

Several of the anti-Id antisera were then tested to see whether they would have effect on EAE *in vivo*. Rats were injected intraperitoneally (ip) with 0.2 ml of absorbed antiidiotype or prebleed serum daily for 4 days. At the end of this time, they were challenged with peptide 68–88 in a regimen designed to induce EAE. The results of these experiments are shown in Table VI. In three separate experiments, animals treated with antiidiotype 1 had a longer incubation period and less severe symptoms of EAE than did the control animals treated

TABLE VI

EAE in Rats Treated with Rabbit Anti-Id[a]

Experiment number	Treatment	N[b]	Onset[c]	Average clinical grade
1	Prebleed	3/3	8.8	4.1 ± 0.6
	Anti-Id-1	3/3	10.0	1.7 ± 1.3
2	Prebleed	4/4	9.0	4.3 ± 0.9
	Anti-Id-1	4/4	10.8	3.4 ± 0.8
	Anti-Id-2	4/4	9.5	5.5 ± 0.4
3	Prebleed	4/4	9.0	3.8 ± 0.5
	Anti-Id-1	4/4	11.0	2.9 ± 1.6
	Anti-Id-2	4/4	9.3	5.0 ± 1.4

[a] Reprinted by permission from Fritz and Desjardins (1982), copyright
American Association of Immunologists.
[b] Number of animals with symptoms/number in experiment.
[c] Average day of onset of EAE.

TABLE VII

In Vitro Proliferative Response of Lymph Node Cells of
Anti-Id-Treated Peptide 68–88-Challenged Le Rats[a]

	SI[b,c]		
		Anti-Id	
Stimulant	Control	1	2
PHA	233 ± 44	403 ± 19	254 ± 82
Peptide 68–88	3.7 ± 1.4	1.3 ± 0.4	1.7 ± 0.5
GPBP	4.8 ± 1.0	1.2 ± 0.5	2.8 ± 0.4

[a] Reprinted by permission from Fritz and Desjardins (1982), copyright American Association of Immunologists.
[b] Stimulation Index, CPM experimental CPM control.
[c] Cells taken 10 days after challenge.

with preimmune serum. In contrast, treatment with antiidiotype 2 resulted in more severe signs of EAE compared to control animals. None of the other anti-Id antibodies tested were found to have any significant effect *in vivo*.

In light of the findings *in vivo* of the anti-Id treatment, it was of interest to test the *in vitro* proliferative response of lymphocytes from treated animals cultured in the presence of guinea pig MBP or peptide 68–88. The results of these experiments are shown in Table VII. Lymph node cell (LNC) from peptide 68–88-sensitized animals treated with preimmune serum gave stimulation indices of 3.7 and 4.8 for peptide 68–88 and guinea pig MBP, respectively. LNC from anti-Id 1-treated sensitized animals had corresponding values of 1.3 and 1.2, which are below the level of a significant response of 1.5. These data are in keeping with reduced clinical EAE in anti-Id 1-treated animals. LNC from anti-Id 2-treated sensitized animals gave stimulation indices of 1.7 and 2.8 for guinea pig MBP and peptide 68–88, slightly above the level of significance but less than control values.

III. Discussion

Experimental allergic encephalomyelitis (EAE) is an appealing model with which to carry out studies on the relationship of the idiotype network and autoimmunity. The primary structure of the inducing antigen is known for MBP from several species; therefore, the effect of amino acid interchanges on the immune response and the idiotypic network may be easily studied. The epitopes responsible for induction of the immune process leading to demyelinating disease have been characterized for the guinea pig, rabbit, Le rat, and several inbred strains of mice (Eylar *et al.*, 1970; Shapira *et al.*, 1971; Martenson *et al.*, 1977; Chou *et al.*, 1977; Pettinelli *et al.*, 1982; Fritz *et al.*, 1983). In the Le rat and in mice, immunization of susceptible animals with peptides carrying these epitopes induces EAE, serum antibody, and the sensitization of lymphocytes that are responsive to antigen *in vitro*. Thus, the methodology is available for studies of idiotypic regulation of this response.

It is apparent from the data presented that antibodies to peptide 68–88 carry cross-reactive idiotopes. However, the observed degree of cross-reactivity was dependent upon the anti-Id serum used in the assay. Certain of the anti-Id antisera were highly cross-reactive, whereas others were much less so.

Each anti-Id serum displayed a different pattern of reactivity with the panel of antipeptide antibodies, which implied the presence of multiple idiotopes. The total number of reactive idiotopes is not known. It is noteworthy that systems with a predominant cross-reactive idiotype, such as the antiazophenylarsonate (ARS) system in A/J mice, are in reality made up of a family of related idiotypes, both public and private (Lamoyi *et al.*, 1980). Similarly, correlation of fine specificity with idiotype was not absolute in the ARS system (Kresina *et al.*, 1982).

The question of idiotypic cross-reactivity on B and T lymphocytes in the MBP system was not completely resolved by our studies. From the data presented, it is apparent that certain of the anti-Id antisera do affect T-cell function, but the mechanism is not known at the present time. The effects could be caused by either qualitative or quantitative differences in the antibodies injected.

The results were surprising because the more cross-reactive anti-Id antibodies (4 and 5) had no visible effect on EAE, whereas anti-Id 1 and 2, which were less cross-reactive, affected the response in either a positive or a negative manner. This might possibly be caused by a reaction with idiotypes on different subpopulations of regulatory T cells.

Ben Nun *et al.* (1981a) approached the question of control of EAE in a different, but related, manner. They developed antigen-specific lines of rat T lymphoblasts which are capable of transferring EAE to naive syngeneic recipients. Rats pretreated with irradiated or mitomycin C lymphoblasts were resistant to challenge with MBP in CFA

(Ben-Nun *et al.*, 1981b). Protection was caused, presumably, by immunity directed against the MBP receptor on the lymphoblasts. Significantly, the recipients were protected from EAE induced by injection of MBP, but were not protected if MBP-sensitized lymphoblasts were passively transferred into the recipients (Ben-Nun and Cohen, 1981). These data imply that protection is active during the induction phase of EAE but not during the effector phase.

IV. Relevance of These Studies to Human CNS Demyelinating Disease

For purposes of brevity, this discussion will be limited to multiple sclerosis, although it may be relevant to other central nervous system (CNS) demyelinating diseases as well. Multiple sclerosis (MS) is a disease of unknown etiology. However, there is good reason to believe that immunological mechanisms play an important role in the pathogenesis of this disease. A characteristic feature of MS is the presence of oligoclonal immunoglobulins in the cerebrospinal fluid (CSF). There is evidence that these immunoglobulins are locally synthesized within the CNS (Sandberg-Wollheim, 1977). It is speculated that these immunoglobulins are synthesized in response to specific neuroantigens. This speculation is yet unproven in spite of many attempts to show specificity of the oligoclonal immunoglobulins for CNS antigens. The failure to find a predominant specificity for these oligoclonal antibodies does not preclude a role for them in the disease process, however.

Because oligoclonal immunoglobulin bands are present in the CSF of about 90% of MS patients and are predominantly IgG_1, it is entirely possible that they are representative of a specific immune response. Using this rationale, several laboratories have prepared anti-Id antibodies using CSF oligoclonal immunoglobulins as antigen (Nagelkerken *et al.*, 1980; Ebers, 1982). When anti-Id antibodies were used to screen panels of MS CSF, in only one instance was evidence of cross-reactivity obtained, and that was a weak reaction in 1 of 14 patients (Baird *et al.*, 1980). Thus, consistent with the inability to show antigen specificity for oligoclonal immunoglobulins, cross-reactive idiotopes have been found only very rarely. In the face of these findings, one is left to ask whether idiotype studies of human CSF or of experimental model systems are of any value for understanding of or therapy for MS.

Perhaps the most relevant aspect of the studies of experimental demyelinating CNS disease is that they allow a model to be designed for human CNS disease. In EAE, it is clear that MBP is the inciting antigen; in MS the inciting agent is not MBP, but it may be viral in nature. In both EAE and MS, the mechanisms which lead to pathological damage have yet to be defined; however, the following observations and speculations may be relevant.

When effector cells from an MBP-sensitized donor are transferred into a syngeneic naive recipient animal, clinical and histological EAE follow within a few days. An important question is, how do the sensitized cells damage the CNS, particularly when MBP is not exposed on the myelin surface (Poduslo and Braun, 1975; Wood et al., 1977)? The answer is unknown, but it may be speculated that IA^+ vascular endothelial cells, which are capable of antigen presentation in vitro (Hirschberg et al., 1980), present MBP or fragments of MBP to the effector cells, which then set up a local delayed-type hypersensitivity reaction at the site of antigen presentation. This, in turn, leads to damage of the blood–brain barrier, which results in infiltration of B and T lymphocytes, macrophages, and other cells.

One could then ask whether a similar process could be induced by the presence of non-CNS antigens in an animal sensitized to these antigens. In one key study (Wisniewski and Bloom, 1975), it was shown that injection of purified protein derivative (PPD) into the CNS of mycobacteria-sensitized guinea pigs led to (DTH) lesions in the CNS. Presumably, a similar situation could occur in an individual with a vigorous immune response to viral antigen in the peripheral system and viral antigen in the CNS. Localized DTH reactions could occur, infiltration of plasma cells and other cells would occur at the site of the lesion, and release of antiviral (or other) antibodies would occur in the CNS. If several diverse agents could initiate this process, it is likely that specificity to neuroantigens would not be observed, and idiotypic cross-reactivity of CSF immunoglobulins would be highly unlikely.

However, if B and T cells in the deleterious response carried common idiotypes in this situation, it might be possible to down-regulate the response with idiotypic intervention. The animal models then become highly relevant because one can deal with a system in which the antigen is well defined and the disease can be induced at will. Thus, the effect of idiotypic manipulations can be readily assessed. Of course, to be successful for human disease, manipulation must be possible after the disease process has already begun. We have recently developed a mouse model of chronic relapsing EAE and have begun using this model in our idiotypic studies because the clinical picture is similar to that of MS.

Ackowledgments

The author thanks Mrs. Claire Guest for assistance in preparation of the manuscript. These studies were supported by USPHS Research Grants NS 10721 and NS 11418.

References

Baird, L. G., Tachovsky, T. G., Sandberg-Wollheim, M., Koprowski, H., and Nisonoff, A. (1980). *J. Immunol.* **124**, 2324.
Ben-Nun, A., and Cohen, I. R. (1981). *Eur. J. Immunol.* **11**, 949.
Ben-Nun, A., Wekerle, H., and Cohen, I. R. (1981a). *Eur. J. Immunol.* **11**, 195.
Ben-Nun, A., Wekerle, H., and Cohen, I. R. (1981b). *Nature (London)* **292**, 60.
Binz, H., and Wigzell, H. (1975). *J. Exp. Med.* **142**, 197.
Bluestone, J. A., Epstein, S. L., Ozato, K., Sharrow, S. O., and Sachs, D. H. (1981). *J. Exp. Med.* **154**, 1305.
Chou, C.-H. J., Chou, F. C.-H., Kowalski, T. J., Shapira, R., and Kibler, R. F. (1977). *J. Neurochem.* **28**, 115.
Chou, C.-H. J., Fritz, R. B., Chou, F. C.-H., and Kibler, R. F. (1979). *J. Immunol.* **123**, 1540.
Cozenza, H., and Köhler, H. (1972). *Proc. Natl. Acad. Sci. U.S.A.* **69**, 2701.
Cozenza, H., Julius, M. H., and Augustin, H. H. (1977). *Immunol. Rev.* **34**, 3.
Dunkley, P. R., and Carnegie, P. R. (1974). *Biochem. J.* **141**, 243.
Ebers, G. C. (1982). *Scand. J. Immunol.* **16**, 151.
Eichman, K. (1978). *Adv. Immunol.* **26**, 195.
Eichman, K., Falk, I., and Rajewsky, K. (1978). *Eur. J. Immunol.* **8**, 853.
Eylar, E. H., Caccam, J., Jackson, J. J., Westall, F. C., and Robinson, A. B. (1970). *Science* **168**, 1220.
Fritz, R. B., and Desjardins, A. E. (1982). *J. Immunol.* **128**, 247.
Fritz, R. B., Chou, C.-H. J., Randolph, D. H., Desjardins, A. E., and Kibler, R. F. (1977). *J. Immunol.* **121**, 1865.
Fritz, R. B., Chou, F. C.-H., Chou, C.-H. J., and Kibler, R. F. (1979). *J. Immunol.* **123**, 1544.
Fritz, R. B., Desjardins, A. E., and Shapira, R. (1982). *Mol. Immunol.* **19**, 665.
Fritz, R. B., Chou, C.-H. J., and McFarlin, D. E. (1983). *J. Immunol.* **130**, 191.
Hart, D. A., Wang, A. L., Paulak, L. L., and Nisonoff, A. (1972). *J. Exp. Med.* **135**, 1283.
Hirschberg, H., Bergh, O. J., and Thorsby, E. (1980). *J. Exp. Med.* **152**, 249s.
Jerne, N. K. (1974). *Ann. Immunol. (Paris)* **125C**, 373.
Kibler, R. F., Fritz, R. B., Chou, F. C.-H., Chou, C.-H. J., Peacocke, N. Y., Brown, N. M., and McFarlin, D. E. (1977). *J. Exp. Med.* **146**, 1323.
Kresina, T. F., Rosen, S. M., and Nisonoff, A. (1982). *Mol. Immunol.* **19**, 1433.
Lamoyi, E., Estress, P., Capra, J. D., and Nisonoff, A. (1980). *J. Immunol.* **124**, 2834.
Liebes, L. F., Zand, R., and Phillips, W. D. (1975). *Biochim. Biophys. Acta* **405**, 27.

Martenson, R. E., Levine, S., and Sowinski, R. (1975). *J. Immunol.* **114**, 592.

Martenson, R. E., Nomura, K., Levine, S., and Sowinski, R. (1977). *J. Immunol.* **118**, 1280.

Nagelkerken, L. M., Aalberse, R. C., Van Walbeek, H. K., and Out, T. A. (1980). *J. Immunol.* **125**, 384.

Pettinelli, C. B., Fritz, R. B., Chou, C.-H. J., and McFarlin, D. E. (1982). *J. Immunol.* **129**, 1209.

Poduslo, J. F., and Braun, P. E. (1975). *J. Biol. Chem.* **250**, 1099.

Sandberg-Wollheim, N. (1977). *Scand. J. Immunol.* **3**, 717.

Shapira, R., McKneally, S. S., Chou, F., and Kibler, R. F. (1971). *J. Biol. Chem.* **246**, 4630.

Wisniewski, H. M., and Bloom, B. R. (1975). *J. Exp. Med.* **141**, 346.

Wood, D. D., Epand, R. M., and Moscarello, M. A. (1977). *Biochim. Biophys. Acta* **467**, 120.

Chapter 18

Idiotypes in Myasthenia Gravis

Donard S. Dwyer

Max Planck Gesellschaft
Klinische Forschungsgruppe für Multiple Sklerose
Würzburg, Federal Republic of Germany

and

Ronald J. Bradley[1], Shin J. Oh[2], and John F. Kearney[3]

The Cellular Immunobiology Unit of the Tumor Institute
Departments of Microbiology[3], Psychiatry[1], and Neurology[2]
The Comprehensive Cancer Center
University of Alabama at Birmingham
Birmingham, Alabama

I. Introduction

The maintenance of self-tolerance through immunoregulatory events is of central importance to the notion of idiotypic networks. As envisioned by Jerne (1974), every exogenous antigen encountered by the immune system has an internal counterpart represented by certain V-region antigenic determinants on immunoglobulins known as idiotopes. Further, he proposed that regulation of an immune response might occur via a network of interacting idiotype–antiidiotype antibodies. Recently, there has been an accumulation of evidence that supports these ideas (Eichmann, 1978; Bona, 1981). In the broadest sense, the idiotype–antiidiotype interaction can be considered an autoimmune response because idiotopes are themselves components of self. Thus, the question can be asked, how is tolerance maintained to other self determinants because this tolerance is obviously breached in the case of idiotopes? There are numerous examples of autoimmune diseases involving a variety of self antigens; therefore, self tolerance is not absolute. Idiotypic interactions and autoimmunity can then be considered separate manifestations of the same problem. Myasthenia gravis (MG) offers a unique opportunity to analyze the immunoregulation of a disease state in which these two aspects of functional immunity can be studied simultaneously. In this chapter, we will first describe some experimental findings relevant to MG and then discuss recent data concerning idiotypic analysis of this autoimmune disease.

II. Autoantibodies Against the Acetylcholine Receptor (AChR)

A. SPONTANEOUS OCCURRENCE IN HUMANS WITH MYASTHENIA GRAVIS (MG)

MG is a human neuromuscular disease characterized by weakness and fatigability of skeletal muscle (Lindstrom and Dau, 1980). The impairment of synaptic transmission at the muscle endplate is caused by an autoimmune response against the AChR. Autoantibodies against this receptor can be detected in the serum of 80–90% of the MG patients tested (Lindstrom, 1977). Generally, however, there is not an exact correlation between antibody titer and disease severity (Lindstrom et al., 1976), although average titers do increase with disease severity (Bradley et al., 1979; Tindall, 1981). Passive transfer of human MG antibodies into mice produces symptoms of muscle weakness characteristic of MG (Toyka et al., 1975). In addition, MG patients undergoing plasmapheresis show a decrease in anti-AChR titers and a concomitant improvement in their clinical picture (Pinching et al., 1976; Dau et al., 1977). Although these studies do not address the precise mechanisms involved in the causation of MG, they demonstrate the crucial role played by autoantibodies in this disease.

B. AUTOANTIBODIES FOLLOWING IMMUNIZATION OF ANIMALS WITH AChR

Early attempts to produce antisera against purified AChR provided the first direct link between anti-AChR antibodies and MG. Patrick and Lindstrom (1973) immunized rabbits with AChR purified from the electric organs of *Torpedo californica* and observed that the animals became weak. Others confirmed these findings (Lennon *et al.*, 1975; Sanders *et al.*, 1977), and the basis for an animal model of MG, known as experimental myasthenia gravis (EMG), was established. Elegant studies by Berman and Patrick (1980a,b) were aimed at identifying genetic factors that affect the induction of EMG. In particular, they were searching for contributions by the mouse major histocompatibility locus (*H-2*), as well as genes encoded by the immunoglobulin heavy chain locus *Igh-C*. Mice of various inbred strains, as well as congenic mice, were immunized with AChR and then examined for deficits in muscle strength. Certain H-2 haplotypes appeared to be associated with increased susceptibility to EMG. In general, mice with H-2^b were high responders, whereas those with H-2^d and H-2^k were low responders. In addition, Berman and Patrick found that *Igh-C* genes influenced the development of EMG. Further studies with congenic mouse strains indicated that the immunoglobulin genes that influence susceptibility mapped to the V_H region. Anti-AChR antibody titers were similar for all strains of mice tested. Taken together, these data imply that anti-AChR antibodies of a particular specificity are critical for the induction of muscle weakness in mice. Another interpretation of the *Igh-C* mapping experiments would be that all mice mount a humoral response against AChR; however, certain idiotypes encoded by V_H genes are more easily regulated via anti-idiotypic antibodies or T cells whose specificity is also inherited or germline and is encoded by or linked to the same V_H locus. Therefore, mice inherit the ability to regulate an immune response via idiotype. These possibilities will be discussed in more detail later.

Other investigators have examined the regulation of lymphocyte responsiveness to AChR by *H-2* genes (Christadoss *et al.*, 1979). Lymph node cells from mice primed with AChR were tested for thymidine uptake after *in vitro* stimulation with AChR under specific experimental conditions. It was concluded that control of the lymphocyte-proliferative response to AChR *in vitro* maps to the I-A subregion of the mouse *H-2* gene complex. Thus, the studies mentioned here indicate that the immune response to AChR and the development of

EMG are regulated by genes encoded by mouse *H-2* and *Igh-C* regions.

III. Experimental MG: Production of Monoclonal Antibodies (mAbs) and T-Cell Lines Specific for AChR

A more precise analysis of the anti-AChR response in animals is now possible because of the availability of mAbs against AChR, as well as the propagation of T-cell lines that recognize the receptor protein. Various groups have produced mAbs against electric fish AChR (Gomez *et al.*, 1979; Moshly-Rosen *et al.*, 1979), and mAbs that cross-react with muscle AChR have been used to induce EMG in rats (Lennon and Lambert, 1980; Richman *et al.*, 1980; Tzartos and Lindstrom, 1980). We previously reported the production of EMG in mice using a BALB/c γ_I, κ mAb (ACR-24) which was raised against AChR purified from electroplax of *Narcine braziliensis* (Dwyer *et al.*, 1981). In order to quantify the deficits in muscle strength, mice were inoculated with the ACR-24 hybridoma as a source of anti-AChR antibodies. When tumor growth became visible, muscle function was tested via repetitive nerve stimulation. Results of electrophysiological testing of a mouse showing only mild physical symptoms of weakness and a control animal carrying an irrelevant hybridoma are shown in Fig. 1. Overall, we found decrements of the fifth response compared to the first, greater than 25% for about 30% of the mice tested. It may be that regulatory elements account for the failure to produce obvious weakness in all individual mice.

The contribution of T lymphocytes to immunoregulation in MG has largely been a neglected area of research. However, recent developments which permit continuous T-cell propagation promise to shed new light on regulatory pathways. Wekerle and co-workers (1981) successfully propagated rat T-cell lines that react with *Torpedo*, eel, and muscle AChR. Generally, the T-cell lines react most strongly with the type of AChR used during immunization; however, cross-reactivity against AChR from other sources has also been observed (Schalke *et al.*, 1982). These T lymphocytes have the surface phenotype of inducer cells, as judged by staining with mAb reagents. When the T cells were administered to rats which were then challenged with AChR, there was an enhancement of anti-AChR titers and the development of weakness (Hohlfeld *et al.*, 1981). It will be interesting to determine whether both T- and B-cell responses to AChR can be

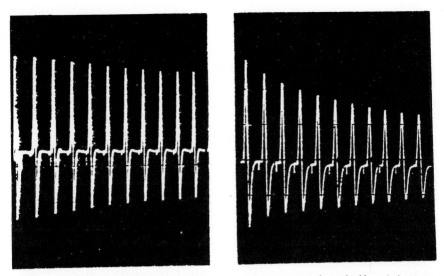

Fig. 1. Compound action potentials of mouse gastrocnemius muscle evoked by sciatic nerve stimulation at 100 Hz. Control mouse potentials are shown on the left; these are from a mouse bearing an irrelevant mouse hybridoma. Measurements from a mouse bearing the ACR-24 hybridoma producing mAb against AChR are shown on the right. The mouse with control hybridoma has a decrement of the fifth response compared to the first response of 11%. For the experimental ACR-24-bearing mouse, the decrement is 32%.

regulated by common elements, namely, antiidiotype antibodies, thus providing a unifying scheme for immunotherapy of the human disease.

IV. Idiotypic Analysis in MG

A. PRODUCTION OF ANTIIDIOTYPE ANTIBODIES IN ANIMAL MODELS

Building on the experimental foundations already described, various laboratories have now begun to produce antiidiotype antibodies that react with anti-AChR immunoglobulins. These antiidiotype reagents have been produced to analyze the idiotypic profile exhibited by antireceptor antibodies. In 1978, Schwartz *et al.* reported the production of antiidiotype antibodies by immunizing mice with "educated" spleen cells obtained from a second set of mice that had been challenged with AChR. These antiidiotype antibodies cross-reacted with anti-AChR antibodies from other mouse strains and other species, including rabbits and monkeys. However, because the antiidiotypic antiserum was not absorbed against normal mouse IgG, the results must be interpreted with caution. In addition, this group (Fuchs et al., 1981) isolated anti-AChR antibodies from the serum of two immunized rabbits and then injected these antireceptor antibodies back into the same animals to produce auto-antiidotypes (although the presence of antiidiotype was not demonstrated). The animals were then reimmunized with AChR, and the antiidiotypes reportedly protected rabbits against the development of EMG. However, other groups (Lennon and Lambert, 1981) have not had success with this type of strategy.

Lennon and Lambert (1981) described their work characterizing the idiotypes of five mAbs raised against Torpedo AChR, four of which also bound to muscle receptor. Antiidiotypic antisera were prepared by immunizing rats with the five purified anti-AChR mAbs. One of the mAbs elicited an immune response directed against individual idiotypes only. The other four mAbs shared an idiotypic determinant; however, three of these also had identical light chains, as determined by isoelectric focusing. Using these antiidiotype reagents, it was then possible to look for similar idiotypes among anti-AChR antibodies in the serum of rats immunized with receptor. The cross-reactive idiotype was detected in the serum of 6 of the 15 rats that were tested. Next, animals were immunized with a mAb bearing the cross-reactive idiotype to elicit an antiidiotype response. These rats were then challenged with AChR to determine whether the induced antiidiotype antibodies conferred protection against the subsequent development of EMG. However, they observed no protective influence in animals producing demonstrable antiidiotype antibodies.

Recent provocative findings in the AChR system illustrate the potential of idiotypic interactions in MG. Wassermann et al. (1982) immunized rabbits with Bis Q, a rigid synthetic AChR agonist, to induce antibody production. The anti-Bis Q antibodies were purified with a Bis Q affinity column and were found to resemble closely the AChR, as judged by pharmacologic properties. These purified antibodies were then injected into a second set of rabbits to elicit an antiidiotype response. Some of the antiidiotype antibodies that were produced by the rabbits bound to AChR from muscle tissue. This type of finding was reported previously with other ligand–receptor systems (Sege and Peterson, 1978). Thus, the anti-Bis Q antibodies resemble AChR, and antibodies made against them mimic anti-AChR antibodies seen in MG. In fact, two of three rabbits showed some symptoms of MG during the peak of their antiidiotype response. The authors mention the possibility that such a cascade of idiotype–antiidiotype interactions could inadvertently lead to an autoimmune response.

B. IDIOTYPIC ANALYSIS OF ANTI-AChR ANTIBODIES AND NATURALLY OCCURRING ANTIIDIOTYPE ANTIBODIES IN MG

The research on idiotype expression in EMG has been complemented by efforts aimed at idiotypic analysis of antibodies in humans suffering from MG. Lefvert (1981) has purified anti-AChR antibodies from MG sera and then challenged rabbits with the purified antibodies. Thus far, two antiidiotypic antisera have been described that react specifically with the antireceptor antibodies. These rabbit antisera were then used to examine various MG sera for antibodies sharing idiotypes with the original immunizing antibodies. One of the antisera reacted with antibodies from 2 of 49 MG patients, whereas the other recognized a common idiotype in 16 of the 49 sera tested. These findings indicated that as many as 30% of MG patients may have serum anti-AChR antibodies that share certain idiotypes.

Research in our laboratory has recently led to the discovery of naturally occurring antiidiotype antibodies in MG serum (Dwyer *et al.*, 1983a). This finding is the topic of the remainder of this chapter. During the development of an enzyme-linked immunoabsorbent assay (ELISA) for measuring anti-AChR antibodies (Dwyer *et al.*, 1983b), we detected antiidiotype antibodies in MG serum. In the ELISA, a mAb (ACR-24) that reacts with muscle AChR was coated onto microtiter plates, followed by the addition of a detergent extract of muscle tissue containing AChR. AChR was bound to the plate via the mAb; from this point on, the assay resembled a conventional ELISA. With this assay, it was possible to measure anti-AChR antibodies in the serum of 80% of MG patients. In addition, it was observed that certain MG sera reacted with ACR-24 in the absence of AChR, a condition that was used to assess background binding. Further studies showed that these particular sera did not react with other BALB/c antibodies, ruling out antiimmunoglobulin isotype activity as a cause of this binding.

In order to determine more precisely whether this binding activity resulted from antiidiotype antibodies, several sera that reacted most strongly with ACR-24 were selected for purification of the anti-ACR-24 immunoglobulin. The sera, denoted SId, DId, and VId, were obtained from patients who had anti-AChR titers of 0.05, 0.08, and 0.1 n*M*, respectively. The purification and binding properties of the antiidiotype antibodies from sera have been described elsewhere (Dwyer *et al.*, 1983a). To summarize, it was found that the purified antiidiotypes bound only to ACR-24 and not to other BALB/c or A/J $\gamma1,\kappa$ antibodies or to BALB/c antibodies of other isotypes. In addition, the binding of these purified serum antibodies to ACR-24 was inhibited by AChR, which is consistent with the behavior of binding site-related antiidiotype antibodies. It was further demonstrated by several distinct methods that the purified antiidiotypes did not contain AChR–anti-AChR complexes. We therefore concluded that the purified human antibodies were indeed recognizing idiotypic determinants expressed by the murine monoclonal antibody ACR-24.

Complementary studies aimed at isolating human mAbs against AChR by somatic cell hybridization with the human myeloma line, GK-5, led to the production of a human line that secretes antiidiotype antibodies with properties similar to those of antibodies purified from MG sera. For these experiments, peripheral blood lymphocytes (PBLs) were isolated from blood drawn from MG patients. The PBL were cultured for 48 h with pokeweed mitogen and then fused with GK-5, a variant of GM1500 $GTGAL_2$ (Croce *et al.*, 1980) which does not synthesize the parental γ_2 heavy chains (Kearney, 1983). The resultant hybrids (13 of 48 wells) were tested for binding of AChR and ACR-24 with the ELISA. One hybridoma, denoted SR11, produced antibody that showed specific binding to ACR-24 and was cloned for use in further studies. Because all of the purified antiidiotype antibodies, including SR11, had κ light chains, the heavy chain isotypes were determined in order to assess the heterogeneity of these antibodies. These results are shown in Fig. 2. Monoclonal anti-IgG subclass reagents were used for these assays. As expected, SR11 expressed only μ heavy chains; however, the purified serum antiidiotype antibodies displayed a variety of isotype profiles. Each of the independently isolated antiidiotype antibodies contained a different dominant isotype; generally, for each, more than one heavy chain isotype was detected. These results imply that the serum antiidiotypes are heterogeneous at least with respect to heavy chain isotype. It remains to be tested whether the immunoglobulins of the different isotypes are clonally related.

Next, it was important to explore the possibility that an idiotypic counterpart for ACR-24 exists in MG sera. For these experiments, we examined numerous serum samples from two patients who had shown antiidiotypic activity during the course of their disease. From a series

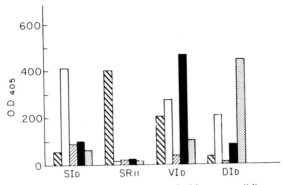

Fig. 2. Heavy chain isotype distribution of the purified human antiidiotype antibodies. For these assays, microtiter plates were coated with ACR-24 (5 μg/ml), followed by the addition of the various purified antiidiotype antibodies or the human monoclonal antiidiotype antibody (SR-11). Next, monoclonal antihuman immunoglobulin reagents which had been labeled with alkaline phosphatase were introduced into the wells. Substrate was added, and the reaction values were determined with an ELISA multiscan (Flow Laboratories) after 30 min. ◩, IgM; □, IgG1; ▨, IgG2; ■, IgG3; ▦, IgG4.

of these samples, two (166,432) were chosen because they had high anti-AChR titers (890.0 and 21.8 nM, respectively) but low levels of antiidiotype (O.D.$_{405}$: 0.071 and 0.030). With these MG sera, it was hoped that two important questions might be answered: (1) Do MG sera contain an idiotypic counterpart to ACR-24 (i.e., can MG serum antibodies compete with ACR-24 for binding by antiidiotype)? (2) Can the purified antiidiotype antibodies prevent binding of some MG anti-AChR antibodies from binding to receptor?

To answer the first question, the ELISA was used to determine whether MG serum antibodies could compete with ACR-24 for binding by antiidiotype. From Table I, it is clear that with increasing amounts of serum there is increased inhibition of antiidiotype binding to ACR-24. This finding demonstrates that there is indeed an idiotypic counterpart to ACR-24 among the serum antibodies from certain MG patients. For the second question, we evaluated the purified antiidiotypes for their ability to inhibit binding of serum antibodies to AChR. An immunoprecipitation assay (Dwyer *et al.*, 1979) was used for this evaluation. For this assay, AChR ^{125}I-labeled α-bungarotoxin complexes were incubated with MG sera either in the absence or the presence of increasing concentrations of antiidiotype, and AChR–antibody complexes were then precipitated by adding a second antibody. In this case, as shown by the data at the bottom of Table I, the

TABLE I

Evidence for ACR-24 Idiotype in MG Serum

Serum antibody	Dilution[a]	% inhibition (ELISA)	
		SId	DId
166	1 : 10	76	83
	1 : 80	62	55
	1 : 640	40	28
432	1 : 10	85	77
	1 : 80	59	27
	1 : 640	34	6

Antiidiotype antibody	Dilution[b]	% inhibition (IMP)	
		166	432
SId	1 : 1	37	46
	1 : 3	15	36
	1 : 15	6	17
DId	1 : 1	41	49
	1 : 3	16	31
	1 : 15	3	5

[a] Serum was diluted in borate-buffered saline containing 1.0% BSA, 0.1% NaN_3, and 0.05% Tween 20.
[b] The starting solution of antiidiotype contained 40 $\mu g/ml$ of purified antibody protein.

purified antiidiotype antibodies prevented the binding of some MG antibodies to human AChR.

These findings have two important implications. First, they provide evidence that certain MG patients have idiotypic counterparts to ACR-24 among their serum antibodies directed against muscle AChR. Thus, the naturally occurring antiidiotype antibodies may arise in response to idiotypic determinants on autologous anti-AChR antibodies and only fortuitously bind to the murine monclonal, ACR-24. Second, the antiidiotype antibodies can inhibit the binding of some MG antibodies to muscle AChR. If this is true *in vivo* as well, then the antiidiotype antibodies may have a beneficial effect by decreasing the number of anti-AChR antibodies that are capable of binding to the receptor or have suppressive effects on the T and B cells involved in the production of these antibodies.

TABLE II

Relationship of Anti-AChR and Antiidiotype Serum Antibody Titers to the
Diagnostic Classification of MG Patients Compared with Normal Sera

Diagnostic classification	Anti-AChR titer (nM)	Number positive	Antiidiotype	Number positive
I	2.99 (4.82)	8/9	0.115 (114)	2/9
IIO	0.05 —	0/1	0.052 —	0/1
IIA	28.45 (119.6)	22/28	0.176 (0.165)	13/28
IIB	1.02 (1.70)	6/7	0.164 (0.148)	3/7
IIC	86.9 (55.6)	4/4	0.113 (0.125)	1/4
Control	0.03 (0.01)	0/24	0.047 (0.025)	0/24

[a] The percentage of MG patients with anti-AChR or anti-Id antibody, respectively.

Inhibition by antiidiotypes could explain, in part, why there is not a perfect correlation between anti-AChR titers and disease severity. In patients with high levels of antiidiotype antibodies, the ability to detect anti-AChR antibodies will be reduced because antiidiotype binding can interfere with the assay used for measurement. Thus, the measured titer of anti-AChR antibodies may not accurately reflect the quantity of circulating autoantibodies. Naturally, the same limitation is encountered when measuring serum antiidiotypes. In this instance, high levels of anti-AChR antibodies would bind available serum antiidiotype and would preclude their measurement in the ELISA. Some support for this idea appears in Table II.

Sera from MG patients or normal controls were examined for anti-AChR antibodies with the immunoprecipitation assay and for antiidiotype antibodies with the ELISA. The patients were classified according to their clinical diagnosis: I, ocular MG; IIO, previously generalized MG now in complete remission; IIA, mild, generalized MG; IIB, moderate generalized MG; and finally IIC, severe generalized MG. Several points can be made from an analysis of these data. First, consistent with previous reports, there is not a very good correlation between disease severity and anti-AChR antibody titer. Second, about 38% of the 49 MG patients tested had measurable serum antiidiotype antibodies. A value was considered positive if it was three standard deviations above the mean for the controls or greater than 0.125 O.D. units. Finally, there appears to be a nonrandom distribution of antiidiotype antibodies in relation to the different diagnostic classifications. Occular MG patients have low levels of both anti-AChR antibodies and antiidiotype; only two of nine patients were positive. Interestingly, patients with the highest anti-AChR titers (IIC) also tended to have low levels of antiidiotype. As mentioned above, this finding could be caused by complexing of anti-AChR antibodies with antiidiotype antibodies, thus preventing their measurement in the ELISA. The highest levels of antiidiotype, as well as the largest number of positive patients, were found with the mild (IIA) and moderate (IIB) forms of MG. With the exception of the ocular MG group, lower levels of antiidiotype antibodies are associated with more severe symptoms. It is tempting to speculate that antiidiotype antibodies are suppressing the autoimmune response; however, there is little direct evidence to support this notion.

Interpretation of the observed distribution of antiidiotype antibodies is further complicated by the type of treatment that the patient receives. This is illustrated in Fig. 3. MG patients were grouped according to whether they had received prednisone or a thymectomy prior to the time the serum sample was obtained. The third group consisted of MG patients who were receiving either anticholinesterase drugs or no medication when the blood was drawn for testing. Clearly, the patients without alteration in immune function as a result of immunosuppressive drugs or thymectomy had the highest levels of antiidiotype antibody. In addition, 50% of the MG patients in this group

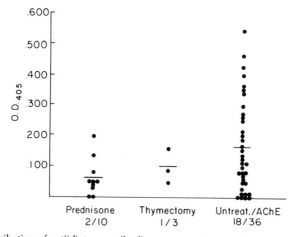

Fig. 3. Distribution of antiidiotype antibodies among patients undergoing various therapies for MG. Patients were categorized according to whether they (A) were receiving prednisone, (B) had already had a thymectomy, or (C) were receiving anticholinesterase medication or were untreated at the time the serum sample was obtained. Individual measurements of the ELISA are shown to indicate the range of values seen in a given category. The bar represents the mean value for the group.

were positive for antiidiotype, whereas less than one-third of the patients in the other groups were positive. These data suggest that immunosuppression or thymectomy reduces the level of serum antiidiotypic antibodies in patients with MG. Because both of these therapies affect the T-cell compartment, it appears that T cells are instrumental in the production of these particular antiidiotypes. The T-cell involvement could occur as a result of specific help, which is provided to the B cells synthesizing antiidiotype. Alternatively, idiotypic structures on relevant T cells could deliver a stimulatory signal to B cells bearing antiidiotype on their surface. Certainly, there could be other explanations for these findings. Nevertheless, it is interesting that prednisone therapy or thymectomy are associated with low levels of antiidiotype.

The data in Fig. 3 describe the static measurement of antiidiotype antibodies. Serum samples obtained serially from 10 MG patients who had been followed over a long period of time were then examined for anti-AChR antibodies and antiidiotype to obtain a clearer picture of the dynamics of the interaction between these two antibodies. In Fig. 4, a time course profile is shown for a representative patient who was treated for more than 4 years in the Neurology Clinic in Birmingham.

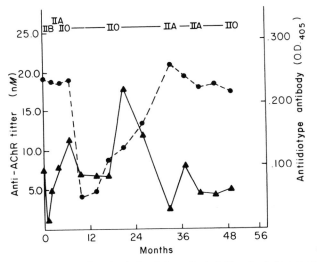

Fig. 4. Longitudinal study of antibody levels in a single MG patient. Serum samples were collected intermittently over a period of more than 4 years. The samples were assayed for anti-AChR antibodies (●---●) with the immunoprecipitation assay and for antiidiotype antibodies (▲——▲) with the ELISA. The clinical status is represented at the top by IIA, IIO, etc. (see text). AChE and Pred. refer to anticholinesterase drugs and prednisone, respectively, which were initiated at the first time point and continued throughout treatment.

It is obvious from these data that both anti-AChR titer and anti-idiotype can vary markedly during the course of MG. At the time the first serum sample was taken, the patient was placed on anticholines-terase medication and prednisone. The patient's condition began to improve and remained stable for 2.5 years. At that point, there was an exacerbation of symptoms which persisted for 1 year until the patient again showed improvement. Some of these clinical features were ac-companied by changes in antibody levels. For instance, there was a marked drop in antiidiotype antibody when the patient was placed on prednisone; however, antiidiotype levels recovered 4 months later. As the patient entered the first remission phase, anti-AChR titers fell dramatically, whereas antiidiotypic antibodies began to increase. During the exacerbation period, there was a concurrent sharp increase in anti-AChR antibodies and a decrease in antiidiotype levels. These findings provide further support for the interpretations given above. Specifically, prednisone appears to depress antiidiotype levels, and excess anti-AChR immunoglobulin can absorb or block antiidiotype antibody in serum (see Fig. 4, the 33-month time point).

Based on the data from the 10 MG patients examined, some general-izations can be made. First, over the course of MG in a single patient, anti-AChR and antiidiotype antibodies showed numerous fluctua-tions. Thus, with the exception of prolonged remission periods, anti-body levels were not very stable from one serum sample to the next. Second, the entry of a patient into remission was nearly always accom-panied by a decrease in the anti-AChR antibody titer. There was no consistent effect on antiidiotype with remission, although if the pa-tient remained symptom free for a long period of time, antiidiotype antibody levels usually fell to near control values. From the serial profile data, two broad patterns of fluctuation could be identified. The most common pattern could be characterized by an inverse relation-ship between antiidiotype levels and anti-AChR antibodies. Thus, high anti-AChR levels were associated with low levels of antiidiotype antibodies; conversely, as antiidiotype levels increased, anti-AChR levels were often falling. On occasion, the rise and fall of antibody levels appeared to be slightly out of phase. In two of the patients, anti-AChR and antiidiotype antibodies rose simultaneously throughout most of the period examined. Naturally, many of the patients showed both of these patterns sometime during the course of their disease. Finally, as mentioned previously, immunosuppressive drugs and thy-mectomy appear to influence antiidiotype antibody.

In order to investigate this last issue in a more systematic fashion, the following analysis was performed. The 10 patient profiles (as in

Fig. 4) were examined for situations in which immunosuppressive drug therapy was initiated, a thymectomy was performed, or the anti-AChR antibody titer increased by more than 25% (because this has been associated with a decrease in antiidiotype). The change in antiidiotype antibodies following one of these events was evaluated and then plotted as the percentage decrease from the serum sample taken just prior to the situation of interest. These data are shown in Fig. 5. The introduction of prednisone therapy or a thymectomy was always followed by a decrease in antiidiotype antibodies, sometimes by more than 80%. A 25% or more increase in anti-AChR antibody was often followed by a decrease in antiidiotype; however, the decreases were generally smaller, and in two instances the levels of antiidiotype antibodies actually increased. Finally, a fourth group was added to show decreases in antiidiotype antibody which are not associated with any of the above situations and which was therefore termed "spontaneous decrease." Again, the spontaneous decreases are typically smaller than those associated with the initiation of immunosuppressive drugs. Thus, these data complement those discussed in earlier sections. From Fig. 3, it is clear that a patient who has received either prednisone or a thymectomy sometime in the past is likely to have low levels of antiidiotype antibody. Figure 5 shows that, in association with pred-

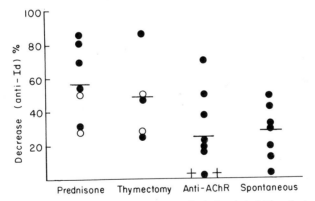

Fig. 5. Effect of various factors on antiidiotype antibody levels in MG patients. Ten patient profiles, as in Fig. 4, were examined for factors that affected antiidiotype levels. If patients received prednisone or a thymectomy, the first serum sample obtained after these treatments was compared with the sample taken at the time the treatment was initiated. The results are expressed as the percentage decrease between the pre- and posttreatment samples. Similarly, when the anti-AChR titer increased by more than 25%, the change in antiidiotype level was measured for the same time period. The term "spontaneous" refers to decreases which occurred in the absence of any identifiable factor. The + symbols denote patients who showed an increase in antiidiotype antibody. Their values are not plotted on this graph.

nisone or thymectomy, there is a decrease in antiidiotype levels. Thus, these two treatments appear to have not only immediate but also long-term effects on antiidiotype antibodies. Their influence on anti-AChR antibodies has already been well documented (Bradley *et al.*, 1979; Sanders *et al.*, 1979).

V. Summary

We previously reported the discovery of naturally occurring antiidiotype antibodies in MG; additional characterization of these antibodies was described here. These human antiidiotypes bind not only to the mouse monoclonal antibody, ACR-24, but also to an idiotypic counterpart which can be found in the serum of certain MG patients. The antiidiotype antibodies are heterogeneous with respect to heavy chain isotype and are found most frequently in the serum of patients with mild to moderate symptoms of MG. Immunosuppressive drugs or thymectomy are typically associated with a decrease in antiidiotype, although a causal relationship has not been established. Finally, the common finding that in a given patient there is an inverse relationship between anti-AChR antibodies and antiidiotype levels suggests that the antiidiotype antibodies are somehow involved in the regulation of MG.

A physiologic role for these antiidiotype antibodies would have important implications for the study and treatment of MG. Most significantly, it would imply that immune regulation through idiotypic networks can and does occur in MG. Therefore, it may be possible to identify dominant or regulatory idiotypes on anti-AChR antibodies derived from MG patients which allow suppression of the aberrant autoimmune response. If progress is made toward this goal, one can imagine the possibility of specific immunotherapy involving antiidiotype antibodies. Because we have already developed a human monoclonal antiidiotype antibody, the technological aspects will probably not be the limiting factor for immunotherapy.

Before therapeutic strategies involving antiidiotype become a reality, we must have a better understanding of how these networks operate in animal models of MG. With other antigen systems, it has been reported that antiidiotype antibodies can either enhance or suppress a given immune response (Eichmann, 1975). Kelsoe *et al.* (1981) were able to enhance or suppress the level of idiotype-bearing antibodies by varying the dose of the antiidiotype antibody which the animals received. In light of these findings, it is critical to control the direction of the immune response before applying antiidiotypic therapy to MG patients.

At present, there are few data available from animal models of MG regarding idiotypic regulation. Nevertheless, some clues may exist. The genetic mapping studies of Berman and Patrick (1980b) showed that not only H-2 genes but also genes mapping to the immunoglobulin V_H region are important for the development of EMG. This could imply that antibodies of certain restricted specificities can cause EMG in these mice. Another possibility is that the apparent V_H locus linkage of EMG susceptibility may be related to idiotype–antiidiotype regulation. One set of linked V_H genes could specify important idiotypes which are the target of idiotypic regulation. Alternatively, there may be another independent set that encodes antiidiotypic structures which are crucial for the prevention of autoimmunity. Thus, animals displaying high susceptibility to the development of EMG may fail to express an essential target regulatory idiotype among their anti-AChR antibodies, or they may simply fail to develop the appropriate antiidiotype antibodies to regulate properly the autoimmune response. It is interesting that the murine ACR-24 idiotype has a counterpart among human anti-AChR antibodies. This may indicate that a similar spectrum of V_H structures reactive with AChR molecules is conserved between species and causes MG in humans.

Acknowledgments

The authors wish to thank Drs. H. Kubagawa and M. Cooper for helpful advice and criticism and Mrs. Ann Brookshire for preparation of the manuscript. This work was supported by U.S.P.H.S. grants CA 16673, CA 13148, and AI 14782. D. Dwyer is the recipient of a Muscular Dystrophy Association Award, and J. F. Kearney is the recipient of research career development award AI 00338.

References

Bona, C. A. (1981). "Idiotypes and Lymphocytes." Academic Press, New York.

Berman, P. W., and Patrick, J. (1980a). *J. Exp. Med.* **151**, 204–223.

Berman, P. W., and Patrick, J. (1980b). *J. Exp. Med.* **152**, 507–520.

Bradley, R. J., Dwyer, D. S., Morley, B., Robinson, G., Kemp, G. E., and Oh, S. J. (1979). *Prog. Brain Res.* **49**, 441–448.

Christadoss, P., Lennon, V. A., and David, C. (1979). *J. Immunol.* **123**, 2540–2543.

Croce, C. M., Linnenbach, A., Hall, W., Steplewski, Z., and Koprowski, H. (1980). *Nature (London)* **288**, 488–491.

Dau, P. C., Lindstrom, J. M., Cassel, C. K., Denys, E. H., Shew, E., and Spitler, L. (1977). *N. Engl. J. Med.* **297**, 1134–1140.

Dwyer, D. S., Bradley, R. J., Oh, S. J., and Kemp, G. E. (1979). *Clin. Exp. Immunol.* **37,** 488–491.

Dwyer, D. S., Kearney, J. F., Bradley, R. J., Kemp, G. E., and Oh, S. J. (1981). *Ann. N.Y. Acad. Sci.* **377,** 143–157.

Dwyer, D. S., Bradley, R. J., Urquhart, C. K., and Kearney, J. F. (1983a). *Nature (London)* **301,** 611–614.

Dwyer, D. S., Bradley, R. J., Urquhart, C. K., and Kearney, J. F. (1983b). *J. Immunol. Methods* **57,** 111–119.

Eichmann, K. (1975). *Eur. J. Immunol.* **5,** 511–516.

Eichmann, K. (1978). *Adv. Immunol.* **26,** 195–254.

Fuchs, S., Bartfeld, D., Moshly-Rosen, D., Souriyon, M., and Feingold, C. (1981). *Ann. N.Y. Acad. Sci.* **377,** 110–124.

Gomez, C., Richman, D., Berman, P., Burres, S., Arnason, B., and Fitch, F. (1979). *Biochem. Biophys. Res. Commun.* **88,** 575–582.

Hohlfeld, R., Kalies, I., Heinz, F., Kalden, J., and Wekerle, H. (1981). *J. Immunol.* **126,** 1355–1359.

Jerne, N. K. (1974). *Ann. Immunol. (Paris)* **125C,** 373–389.

Kerney, J. F. (1983). In preparation.

Kelsoe, G., Reth, M., and Rajewsky, K. (1981). *Eur. J. Immunol.* **11,** 418–423.

Lefvert, A. K. (1981). *Ann. N.Y. Acad. Sci.* **377,** 125–142.

Lennon, V. A., and Lambert, E. H. (1980). *Nature (London)* **285,** 238–240.

Lennon, V. A., and Lambert, E. H. (1981). *Ann. N.Y. Acad. Sci.* **377,** 77–96.

Lennon, V. A., Lindstrom, J. M., and Seybold, M. E. (1975). *J. Exp. Med.* **141,** 1365–1372.

Lindstrom, J. (1977). *J. Clin. Immunol. Immunopathol.* **7,** 36–43.

Lindstrom, J. M., and Dau, P. (1980). *Annu. Rev. Pharm. Toxicol.* **20,** 337–362.

Lindstrom, J. M., Seybold, M. E., Whittingham, S., and Duane, D. (1976). *Neurology* **26,** 1054–1059.

Moshly-Rosen, D., Fuchs, S., and Eshhar, Z. (1979). *FEBS Lett.* **106,** 389–392.

Patrick, J., and Lindstrom, J. (1973). *Science* **180,** 871–872.

Pinching, A. J., Peters, D. K., and Newsom-Davis, J. (1976). *Lancet* **2,** 1373–1376.

Richman, D., Gomez, C., Berman, P., Burres, S., Fitch, F., and Arnason, B. (1980). *Nature (London)* **286,** 738–739.

Sanders, D. B., Johns, T. R., Eldefrawi, M. E., and Cobb, E. E. (1977). *Arch. Neurol. (Chicago)* **34,** 75–81.

Sanders, D. B., Howard, J. F., Johns, T. R., and Campa, J. F. (1979). *In* "Plasmapheresis and the Immunobiology of Myasthenia Gravis" (P. Dau, ed.), pp. 289–306. Houghton Mifflin, Boston, Massachusetts.

Schalke, B. C., Ben-Nun, A., Kalies, I., Cohen, I., Kalden, and Wekerle, H. (1982). *Immunobiology* **162,** 414.

Schwartz, M., Novick, D., Givol, D., and Fuchs, S. (1978). *Nature (London)* **273,** 543–545.

Sege, K., and Peterson, P. A. (1978). *Proc. Natl. Acad. Sci. U.S.A.* **75,** 2443–2447.

Tindall, R. S. (1981). *Ann. N.Y. Acad. Sci.* **377,** 316–331.

Toyka, K. V., Drachman, D. B., Pestronk, A., and Kao, I. (1975). *Science* **190,** 397–399.

Tzartos, S. J., and Lindstrom, J. M. (1980). *Proc. Natl. Acad. Sci. U.S.A.* **77,** 755–759.

Wassermann, N. H., Penn, A. S., Freimuth, P. I., Treptow, N., Wentzel, S., Cleveland, W. L., and Erlanger, B. F. (1982). *Proc. Natl. Acad. Sci. U.S.A.* **79,** 4810–4814.

Wekerle, H., Hohfeld, R., Ketelsen, U., Kalden, J., and Kalies, I. (1981). *Ann. N.Y. Acad. Sci.* **377,** 455–476.

Chapter 19

Antiidiotypic Antibodies as Immunological Internal Images of Hormones

A. D. Strosberg

Laboratory of Molecular Immunology
Institut Jacques Monod (Institut de Recherche en Biologie Moléculaire)
Centre National de la Recherche Scientifique and University Paris VII
Paris, France

I. Introduction

The comparison of different proteins that bind the same ligand has been the focus of many studies. Analyses of different antibodies that bind given haptens have revealed similarities between the sequences and the predicted tridimensional structures of the combining sites. For example, in one study guinea pig antibodies directed against an acidic hapten, arsonate, were found to contain several lysyl or arginyl basic residues in the first and second hypervariable regions of the heavy chain; antibodies directed against a basic hapten, trimethylammonium, contained acidic side chains such as those of glutamyl and aspartyl residues in corresponding parts of the protein (Koo and Cebra, 1974).

In other studies, antibodies have also been compared by immunological methods. For this purpose, antiidiotypic antibodies were raised against the variable regions of antiarsonate (Capra *et al.*, 1982; Margolies, 1983; Nisonoff, 1983) or antiphosphorylcholine antibodies (Clevinger *et al.*, 1983; Schilling *et al.*, 1980). The antiidiotypes reacted with antiphosphorylcholine antibodies, whether induced or spontaneously appearing as myeloma proteins, again demonstrating that structural similarities exist among different proteins which bind the same ligand.

It was therefore logical to investigate whether this conservation held true even among acceptor or receptor proteins synthesized by different cells and of different genetic origin. This immunological approach was used by Sege and Peterson (1978) to analyze the possible similarities between antiinsulin receptor antibodies and antiidiotypic antibodies directed against the antihormone immunoglobulins. Their early results, obtained in rabbits, were confirmed in mice by Shechter *et al.* (1982). We will discuss these and other similar studies at length later in the chapter.

Although the underlying premise in the insulin study, as in others, is that proteins (antibodies or receptors) that bind the same ligands share common properties of the ligand-binding site, an alternative hypothesis has emerged as a direct consequence of the elegant network concept proposed by Jerne (1974). According to this theory, in the interaction between the antiidiotype and the idiotype, it would be the idiotype (the antihormone antibody) that acts as the antibody and the antiidiotype that acts as the ligand, literally behaving as the "internal image" of the hormone.

It is not easy to visualize how antiidiotypic antibodies might actually mimic the structure of a small ligand. Such molecular mimicry may be imagined if the ligand is a polypeptide hormone composed of the same amino acid building blocks as the antihormone antibody. When the ligand is a synthetic compound, the imitation must depend on tridimensional similarity. A survey by Niall and Tregear (1979) suggests that structurally unrelated molecules may indeed resemble each other closely in spatial configuration.

II. Similarities in Binding Properties of Receptors and Antibodies

Similarities in binding properties of receptors and antibodies have been described in several studies. Marasco and Becker (1982) showed that antibodies against the chemotactic peptide formylmethionyl leucylphenylalanine raised in several animals from two different species are extremely similar in binding specificity to the neutrophil surface receptor for chemotactic formyl peptides. Hoebeke *et al.* (1979) described antibodies raised against the β-adrenergic catecholamine antagonist L-alprenolol which were able to bind a number of other antagonists with binding constants in the same order of potency as the β-adrenergic receptor itself. Thus, L-propranolol was best recognized both by the antibodies and the receptor, although affinities for other ligands, including agonists such as isoproterenol or epinephrine, were much lower.

Wassermann *et al.* (1982) used a derivative of Bis Q (*Trans*-3,3'-bis[α-(trimethylammonio)methyl]azobenzene bromide), a potent agonist of the acetylcholine receptor, to raise rabbit antibodies that mimicked the binding characteristics of the acetylcholine receptor with respect to the order of binding of decamethonium (an agonist) over hexamethonium (an antagonist).

A number of studies have documented binding properties of insulins of a variety of origins for inhibitory antiinsulin antibodies, on the one hand, and insulin receptors, on the other. Again, extensive similarities were found. In addition, the elucidation of the polypeptide chain organization of the insulin receptor has apparently revealed structural similarities with immunoglobulins: Two pairs of two different chains are linked to each other by disulfide bonds.

The structural resemblance between different proteins that bind the same ligands may have a conceptual basis as is schematically represented in Fig. 1. The part of the receptor responsible for recognizing (for instance) the various polypeptide hormones corresponds to the antibody variable region. Transmission of the signal of recognition

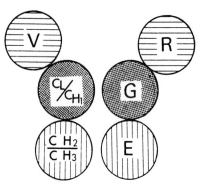

Fig. 1. Conceptual homologies between the antibody molecule and the hormone receptor. Both types of multifunctional structures comprise a recognition moiety (R or V) capable of binding specifically either the antigen or the hormone, a component responsible for signal transmission (C or G), and an effector part (CH$_2$, CH$_3$, or E) responsible for the biological response induced by antigen binding (such as complement fixation or interaction with Fc receptors) or by hormone binding (adenylate cyclase activation, opening of ion channels or phosphorylation). R, receptor; G, GTP binding regulatory protein; E, effector (cyclase); V, variable antigen binding parts; C$_L$, light chain constant region; CH$_1$, CH$_2$, CH$_3$, heavy chain constant domains.

occurs through the antibody C$_L$, CH$_1$ and hinge domains or through the GTP-binding regulatory protein (in other receptor systems through phosphorylating catalytic units). Finally, the triggering of the biological signal is caused by the immunoglobulin Fc part, to which may correspond the adenylate or guanylate cyclase components.

III. Interaction of Antiidiotypic Antibodies with Receptors

We will first review recent data describing the interaction of anti-idiotypic antibodies with various hormone receptors (Table I). These results will be discussed individually, and common observations will be compared at the end of the chapter.

A. ANTIIDIOTYPIC ANTIBODIES RAISED AGAINST ANTIBODIES TO RETINOL-BINDING PROTEIN (RBP) INTERACT WITH THE RBP RECEPTOR

Antibodies against RBP were prepared in rats, and antiidiotypic antibodies against these were raised in rabbits and made specific by

TABLE I

Antiidiotypic Antibodies Which Recognize Receptors

Immunogen	Receptor	Antibody-Induced Signal	Cell	References
Insulin	Insulin receptor	Oxidation and uptake of glucose Inhibition lipolysis	Adipocyte	Sege and Peterson (1978) Shechter et al. (1982)
Retinol	RBP	Retinol uptake	Intestinal epithelial cell	Sege and Peterson (1978)
Catecholamine	β-adrenergic receptor	Adenylate cyclase activation or inhibition	Nucleated erythrocyte	Schreiber et al. (1980) Homcy et al. (1982)
Thyrotropin	Thyrotropin receptor	Adenylate cyclase activation Increased I transport Follicle formation	Thyroid cell	Farid et al. (1982)
Chemotactic peptide	Chemotactic peptide receptor		Neutrophil cell	Marasco and Becker (1982)
Nicotinic agonist Bis Q	Nicotinic acetylcholine receptor			Wasserman et al. (1982)

removal of antiisotypic antibodies or by affinity chromatography on an Ig–agarose gel. Possible anti-RPB antibodies were removed from the antiidiotypic sera by absorption on a RBP–agarose gel (Sege and Peterson, 1978). The specificity of the antiidiotypic antibodies for anti-RPB antibodies was demonstrated in both binding and immunoprecipitation experiments. RBP completely inhibited the interaction between the anti-RBP Fab fragments and the antiidiotypic antibodies in a concentration-dependent manner.

Intestine epithelial cells have cell-surface receptors for RBP, and IgG from antiidiotypic antiserum bound significantly better to these cells than did the control IgG from the preimmune serum. The "specific" binding was inhibited by the anti-RBP antibodies. It was not reported whether RBP also inhibited this binding, or conversely, whether RBP binding to the receptors was inhibited by the antiidiotypic antibodies. However, the antibodies did impede RBP-mediated [^{3}H]retinol uptake of intestine epithelial cells.

B. ANTIIDIOTYPIC ANTIBODY AGAINST INSULIN ANTIBODIES INTERACTS WITH THE MEMBRANE-BOUND INSULIN RECEPTORS

Specific rat antibodies against bovine insulin were isolated by affinity chromatography on an insulin-containing Sepharose gel and injected into two rabbits (Sege and Peterson, 1978). The IgG fractions from the antiidiotypic antisera were isolated on a Sepharose column containing *Staphylococcus aureus* protein A, and antibodies directed against common determinants of rat IgG (isotypes) were removed by absorption on an immunoadsorbent containing rat IgG. Prior to use, the antiidiotypic IgG fractions were passed over the insulin gel to remove antiinsulin antibodies and then over a gel filtration column to eliminate free insulin.

Antiidiotypic antibody activity was demonstrated using radioiodinated monovalent rat antiinsulin Fab fragments. Free Fab fragments were separated from bound Fab fragments on Sephadex G200. In immunoprecipitation experiments, insulin was found to inhibit completely the binding of Fab fragments to the antiidiotypes.

Competition experiments were performed between insulin and the antiidiotypic antibodies for binding to insulin receptors on rat epididymal fat cells. The presence of the antibodies caused almost complete inhibition of insulin binding to the receptors.

The IgG fractions of antiiidiotypic antisera from two different rabbits increased α-aminoisobutyric acid uptake by young rat thymocytes to the same extent (50%) as did insulin, although the amounts of protein required for stimulation differed by several magnitudes.

Shechter *et al.* (1982) immunized mice with insulin and found that they spontaneously developed both antiinsulin and antiinsulin receptor antibodies. The antireceptor antibodies displaced labeled insulin from its specific binding sites on fat cells. In addition, the antireceptor antibodies mimicked the biological effects of insulin in stimulating the oxidation of glucose and its incorporation into lipids and in inhibiting lipolysis. It was possible to block the binding of the antibodies to insulin receptor by antiinsulin antibodies, some of which were shown to actually bind to the antireceptor antibodies, suggesting an idiotype–antiidiotype interaction. According to the authors, the immunization against the hormone may be sufficient to activate an idiotype–antiidiotype network, of which some components may act as the immunological internal image of the hormone and behave as antireceptor antibodies.

A number of questions were raised by this study. The foremost concerns how both idiotypes and antiidiotypes can coexist and function in the same serum without neutralizing each other. In our own studies using a catecholamine hormone antagonist as the immunizing agent, such a neutralization indeed masked part of the response (Lü *et al.*, 1983; Couraud *et al.*, 1983). In the case of the insulin study, several competing antibodies could coexist, and the resulting response may represent only the summation of a number of positive and negative interactions.

Another question, partially answered in the report of Shechter *et al.* (1982), concerns the possibility that the insulin-like activity may actually be attributed to two different kinds of antibodies: (1) the "internal image" antiidiotypic antibodies whose structure of the variable region would "mimic" insulin and (2) the antiinsulin antibodies complexed with insulin, which would bind the receptor because of the insulin component of the complex. Because mild trypsinization of fat cells, a treatment which greatly decreases the response to insulin, did not affect the response to the insulin-like antibody, the authors concluded that insulin and insulin-like antibodies interact with different sites on the receptor. This finding, however, appears to be contradictory in view of the competition between insulin and the antibodies for binding to the receptor: How can the interaction with different parts of the receptor result in such a mutual inhibition? How does the mild trypsinization observed here relate to similar observations with the insulin-like effects of concanavalin A? If the effects of insulin-like antibodies and concanavalin A on fat cells are both unaffected by mild trypsinization, whereas the action of insulin is not, does it not follow that only the hormone combines with the receptor itself, although the antibodies and the lectin interact with adjacent proteins or glycoproteins? Clearly, these points need further clarification.

C. ANTIIDIOTYPIC ANTIBODIES THAT MIMIC THE BIOLOGICAL ACTIVITY OF THYROTROPIN

Rabbits immunized with rat antihuman thyroid-stimulating hormone (TSH or thyrotropin) produce immunoglobulins which do not bind the hormone but inhibit the binding of bovine thyrotropin to the porcine thyroid receptor in a dose-dependent manner up to 50% of the total binding (Farid *et al.*, 1982). Direct interaction of the antiidiotypic antibodies to porcine thyroid cell membranes was saturable and could be inhibited as much as 64% at 160 mU/ml by increasing concentrations of the free bovine hormone. In the presence of Gpp(NH)p, a nondegradable synthetic analog of GTP, the antiidiotypic antibodies increased thyroid membrane adenylate cyclase activity by 40% over the enzymatic activity induced by nonspecific immunoglobulin. The rate of incorporation of $Na^{131}I$ into cultured thyrocytes was also increased in a dose-dependent manner by the antiidiotypic antibodies, which induced the organization of these cells into follicles between 5 and 7 days of culture.

D. ANTIIDIOTYPIC ANTIBODIES THAT REACT WITH THE FORMYL PEPTIDE CHEMOATTRACTANT RECEPTOR OF NEUTROPHIL CELLS

In a study by Marasco and Becker (1982), antiidiotypic antibodies against rabbit antibodies to the chemoattractant peptide formyl Met-Leu-Phe were raised in mice, guinea pigs, and goats. The goat antibodies bound to rabbit polymorphonuclear leukocytes and the corresponding $F(ab')_2$ fragments partially inhibited the binding of the formyl Met-Leu-Phe peptide to the same cells. Both the antipolymorphonuclear leukocyte receptor and the antiidiotype activities were lost after passage over an affinity gel containing antibody against the formyl Met-Leu-Phe peptide.

In this study, the authors investigated the possibility that the antipeptide antibodies display ligand-recognition sites similar to those of the peptide receptor. Antibodies to these common structures (idiotopes on the antibodies) would cross-react with both the receptor and the antihormone antibodies. Conservation of the idiotypic determinants was shown on nearly all rabbit and rat antiformyl Met-Leu-Phe antibodies examined by the ability of antibodies produced in rabbits immunized with the chemoattractant conjugated to either goat IgG or keyhole limpet hemocyanin to bind $F(ab')_2$ goat antiidiotype. The same was true for the capacity displayed by various rat antiformyl Met-Leu-Phe to block the binding of rabbit antibodies of the same specificity to goat antiidiotype adsorbed to *Staphylococcus aureus*. It should, however, be stressed that the similarity in binding capacity does not in itself suggest that the proteins will cross-react. The data presented by Marasco and Becker (1982) are also compatible with the existence, among the antiidiotypic antibodies, of a very minor subpopulation which constitutes the immunological internal image of the chemoattractant peptide.

The authors could not demonstrate that the antiidiotypic antibodies mimicked the biological activity of this peptide. However, this was explained by the fact that the preimmune control IgG preparations themselves induced locomotion, and in the presence or absence of cytochalasin B, granule enzyme release. These "nonspecific" effects thus could mask a hypothetical specific effect by the antiidiotypic internal image.

E. INDUCTION OF EXPERIMENTAL MYASTHENIA GRAVIS BY ANTIIDIOTYPIC ANTIBODIES

Immunization of rabbits with antibodies directed against Bis Q, a potent analog of acetylcholine (Wassermann *et al.*, 1982), yielded antisera which recognized rat, torpedo, or eel acetylcholine receptor in complement fixation and enzyme immunoassay. The binding was inhibited by the free ligand Bis Q. Two of the three rabbits showed signs of muscle weakness similar to that seen after immunization with the purified receptor. One of the rabbits was injected intramuscularly with neostigmine and showed temporary improvement. Another showed posttetanic exhaustion of hind limb muscles after stimulation of the sciatic nerve at 30 Hz. The third rabbit, despite a significant titer of antiidiotypic antibodies, demonstrated no signs of muscle weakness.

Interestingly, the response to anti-Bis Q was transient in one animal, both with respect to antireceptor titer and to symptoms of experimental myasthenia gravis. Maximal titer and muscle weakness occurred after the first boost and remained high until the second boost, after which the titer dropped three- to fourfold and signs of weakness disappeared. Subsequent boosting apparently caused tolerance: The antireceptor titer dropped to the range found in nonimmunized animals.

F. ANTI-β-ADRENERGIC LIGAND ANTIIDIOTYPIC
   ANTIBODIES BIND THE β-ADRENERGIC RECEPTOR
   AND STIMULATE ADENYLATE CYCLASE

Antibodies were raised in rabbits against alprenolol, a potent antagonist of the β-adrenergic catecholamine hormones (Hoebeke et al., 1979). These antibodies were shown to bind other antagonists and even agonists. The common determinant on these ligands appeared to be the ethanolamine side chain.

Antiidiotypic antibodies were raised against the immunoglobulin fractions of the rabbits immunized with alprenolol. The antiidiotypic nature of these new antibodies was demonstrated by their ability to inhibit the binding of radiolabeled alprenolol to their specific antibodies in a dose-dependent manner. It was possible to isolate the antiidiotypes on an idiotype-containing affinity column (Schreiber et al., 1980; Couraud et al., 1983).

The antiidiotypic antibodies also inhibited the binding of alprenolol to the membrane-bound β-adrenergic receptor, again in a dose-dependent manner, but the inhibition was not competitive with the ligand binding, suggesting that antibody and catecholamine agonists or antagonists bind at different sites on the receptor, just as two different antigens may bind to the same antibody at the same combining site.

Direct binding of the antiidiotypic antibodies to the β-adrenergic receptors of various types of cells was demonstrated using a number of methods. Immunofluorescent antirabbit antibodies revealed fluorescence on cells covered with the antiidiotypes, such as avian erythrocytes, P815 mastocytoma, or S49 lymphoma cells, all of which have β-receptors. Human or rabbit erythrocytes or S49 mutant cells either devoid of or greatly deficient in receptors displayed only background fluorescence (Strosberg et al., 1982). The binding of the antiidiotypes to the β-receptors was quantitated by using radiolabeled antirabbit antibodies. A semiquantitative assay based on hemagglutination of receptor-bearing erythrocytes was also used.

Binding of the antiidiotypic antibodies also resulted in activation (Schreiber et al., 1980) or inhibition (Homcy et al., 1982) of basal or catecholamine-sensitive adenylate cyclase. The synergistic effect between the hormone and the antibodies again confirmed that binding to the β-receptor, although producing similar results, was not necessarily competitive and thus did not always occur at exactly the same site. Interestingly, no synergistic effect on adenylate cyclase activation was observed between the antibodies and guanyl trinucleotides such as GTP or its synthetic analog Gpp(NH)p.

The synthesis of anti-β-receptor antibodies in response to immunization by anticatecholamine hormone antibodies was found to be transient and occurred in sharp peaks, differing in number and intensity from rabbit to rabbit. Similar observations were made in mice. When hormone-binding ability was measured in the sera of the animals immunized with antihormone antibodies, peaks of catecholamine-binding activity alternated with peaks of receptor-binding activity. These successive responses may reflect different stages in the network of idiotype–antiidiotype interactions proposed by Jerne (1974) (Fig. 2). According to this model, Ab1 (the idiotype) would induce the production of Ab2 (antiidiotype), which in turn would stimulate the synthesis of Ab3 (anti-antiidiotype). Each of these pairs of antigen-antibodies would interact by mutual complementarity, resulting in partial or complete neutralization. Subsets of the Ab2 and Ab3 antibodies may sufficiently resemble the original antigen against which either Ab1 or Ab2 is directed. This molecular mimicry of hormones and receptors

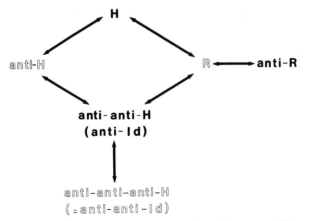

Fig. 2. A network of immunological interactions involving a hormone and its specific receptor and antibodies. The symmetrical positions of the antihormone antibodies (anti-H) and the receptor (R) around the hormone (H) are mirrored by those of the anti-R and the anti-anti-H antibodies around R. The network of interactions is extended by the emergence of anti-anti-anti-H antibodies which are antiidiotypic (anti-Id) toward the anti-anti-H immunoglobulins.

by immunological internal images would result in specific interactions which can be accurately measured in our system, in which radiolabeled ligands and sensitive enzymatic assays are available.

The neutralization of Ab1 by Ab2 and of Ab2 by Ab3 could indeed be demonstrated after separating the various antibody subpopulations on the appropriate affinity columns: alprenol–agarose for Ab1 or Ab3 and idiotype (Ab1)–agarose for Ab2. The purified Ab2 fraction contained no catecholamine-binding antibodies, whereas the purified Ab3 had little or no β-adrenergic-binding activity. As expected, quantitation showed that not all antiidiotypic antibodies bind receptor and that antihormone antibodies constitute only a subset of the anti-antiidiotype antibodies (Couraud et al., 1983).

The study of the antiidiotypic response against antihormone antibodies revealed two phenomena not commonly observed in previous experimental analyses: the spontaneous appearance of auto-antiidiotypic antibodies (Shechter et al., 1982) and the rapid disappearance of antiidiotype antibodies apparently through neutralization by an auto-anti-antiidiotypic antibody (Couraud et al., 1983; Wassermann et al., 1982). One may indeed wonder why these autologous antibodies have not been observed in the more conventional studies of idiotypic responses. In these studies, the synthesis of antiidiotypes is induced through immunization with antibodies from other animals, and even from other species, and this synthesis is stable over long periods without reported variations. However, because these antiidiotypic antibodies do not bind to autologous receptors for hormones, they are unable to trigger any hormone- or neurotransmitter-mediated physiological responses, in contrast to the antibodies against the insulin, acetylcholine, or catecholamine antibodies. Possibly it is the potential detrimental effect that stimulates an autologous immune reaction against the antiligand antibodies and leads to their rapid removal from the circulation.

IV. Antiidiotypic Antireceptor Antibodies and Autoimmune Diseases

Several pathological developments in man have been related to the action of autoantibodies binding to receptors on the surface of normal cells of the individual. In myasthenia gravis patients, the serum contains antibodies which bind, and in some instances block, the nicotinic acetylcholine receptor at the neuromuscular junction (Fuchs et al., 1980). Patients suffering from Graves' disease have antibodies that stimulate the thyroid gland by activating receptors for the thyrotropin causing aberrant hypersecretion of thyroid hormones and apparent hyperthyroidism (Drachman, 1978). A very rare form of insulin-resistant diabetes is apparently caused by the presence in the patient's serum of antiinsulin receptor antibodies (Kahn et al., 1981). Finally, Venter et al. (1980) have reported the presence of anti-β-adrenergic receptors in patients with allergic asthma and rhinitis.

It is probable that the very rare pathological developments result from the synthesis of antireceptor antibodies that mimic the hormone or its antagonists by binding to the receptor at the same site as the natural ligand. Unaffected individuals may make antireceptor antibodies which bind to the receptor but do not compete with the hormone, and thus do not trigger the biological response.

One may indeed wonder whether the antireceptor antibodies that mimic the hormone may have arisen against antihormone antibodies rather than against receptor. Patients treated with exogenous insulin may develop antiinsulin antibodies, and responses to other hormones and their synthetic analogs used for therapeutic purposes are just as likely to occur. The possibility that autoidiotypic antibodies to auto-antihormone antibodies arise spontaneously has been verified effectively in mice by Shechter et al. (1982).

The only documented instance in which an experimental induction of antiidiotypic antibodies actually led to pathological developments was described by Wassermann et al. (1982). In this study, the same symptoms of experimental myasthenia gravis usually seen after injection of purified acetylcholine receptor were induced by antiidiotypic antibodies which bind to the acetylcholine receptor. The partially paralyzed rabbit could be cured instantaneously by injection of neostigmine, an inhibitor of acetylcholinesterase, commonly used in the treatment of myasthenia gravis patients.

Other situations have been described in which auto-antiidiotypic responses may intervene in pathological processes. In one example in B-cell tumor-bearing mice, antiidiotypic antibodies were observed to bind to the surface immunoglobulin of the proliferating B lymphocytes and intervene in their lysis by activated complement. In an analogy to these experimental situations, several teams of cancerologists have initiated the treatment of patients with B-cell tumors using antibodies raised against the monoclonal immunoglobulin produced by the tumor.

Antireceptor antibodies may display both stimulatory and inhibitory activity toward receptor-linked effector systems. Thus, Graves' hyperthyroidism is explained by the presence of long-acting thyroid-stimulating (LATS) antibodies, whereas thyrotoxicosis may be caused by antibodies that block TSH receptors (Orgiazzi *et al.*, 1976). The apparent decrease of acetylcholine receptors in myasthenia gravis is attributed to the antibody-induced removal of the receptors. Anti-idiotypic antibodies, which behave as directed against hormone or neurotransmitter receptors, display the same duality of effects. For instance, anticatecholamine antiidiotypic antibodies may be found that either stimulate or inhibit adenylate cyclase.

Because of these observations, it is surprising that single effects may be observed using conventional polyclonal and thus multispecific antiidiotypic antibodies. Mutual compensation would be likely to cancel opposite effects. In this respect, monoclonal antiidiotypic antibodies yield results that are much more easily interpreted. However, because the transient character of the expression of antireceptor antiidiotypic antibodies has been described by several groups, the timing and selection of monoclonal antibodies become critical.

V. The Nature of the Interaction between the Antiidiotypic Antibody and the Receptor

A schematic representation (Fig. 3) may account for the observations: The hormone (H) binds at the site (S) to the receptor, which in the bound or activated state (R^+) will trigger the effector (C). This same

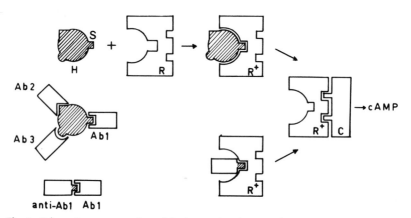

Fig. 3. Schematic representation of the interactions between hormone (H), receptor (R and R^+), cyclase (C), and antibodies (Ab1, Ab2, and Ab3). The antigenic site S is recognized by both the receptor and antibody Ab1.

S site, which is likely to protrude into the solvent because it is recognized by a membrane-bound receptor, therefore possesses the properties of the potential antigenic and immunogenic determinants. When antibodies are raised against the hormone, some (Ab1) are directed against the S site. Antiidiotypic antibodies induced against the Ab1 antibodies might indeed have the same configuration of the S site and therefore bind to the hormone receptor, triggering the hormone-specific effector function.

This simplified scheme does not explain all the facts. Not all antibodies that bind to the receptor trigger the effector function; some may actually inhibit the hormone action, as would an antagonist. The antibody is not expected to bind to the receptor in exactly the same way as the hormone. The antibody-combining site is larger than the small ligand, and many more interactions probably will occur between the amino acid residues of the immunoglobulin and those of the receptor. The kinetics of the interactions need not be the same, either: A small ligand is likely to dissociate faster than an antibody. Binding constants of antibodies may cover a wide range of values, whereas that of the hormone is unique.

The nature of the interaction between the antiidiotypic antibody and the receptor has been difficult to analyze without the use of monoclonal antiidiotypic antibodies. However, reports have now been published in which monoclonal antireceptor antibodies raised against purified receptor are described. Although the antireceptor antibodies may react with any antigenic determinant of the receptor, it is probable that an antiidiotypic antibody would bind only to the hormone recognition site. Such antibodies are expected to inhibit hormone binding. The few antireceptor antibodies that are inhibitory have been described for the acetylcholine system by Moshly-Rosen *et al.* (1979) and by Lindström *et al.* (1976), and for the epidermal growth factor by Schreiber *et al.* (1980).

VI. Potential Applications of Antiidiotypic Antibodies in Basic Research

The finding by different groups of investigators that antireceptor antibodies can be raised by immunization with antihormone antibodies should be very useful in practical applications. These antireceptor antibodies can be obtained without prior purification of the receptor; they can in fact be used for this purpose. Because the antiidiotypic antibodies probably will react with the hormone-binding site of the receptor, the specificity of these antibodies should not be restricted to any species as long as the binding site is conserved. Results in the β-adrenergic system indicate that rabbit anticatecholamine antiidiotypic antibodies bind to β-adrenergic receptors from human HeLa cells, murine lymphoma S49, or mastocytoma P815 cells, and turkey and duck erythrocytes.

Large-scale isolation of the receptor can be carried out using the antiidiotypic antibodies. However, for this purpose, monoclonal rather than polyclonal reagents should be used. The polyclonal response is both diverse (agonistic, antagonistic effects) and transient (rapid disappearance of the antireceptor antibody, possibly because of the synthesis of an anti-anti-antibody). The monoclonal antibody, which corresponds to an "immortalized" clone selected from among the many clones producing the antiidiotypic antibodies, is both stable and available in large quantities.

VII. Medical Applications of Antiidiotypic Antibodies

The antiidiotypic antihormone receptor antibodies may arise spontaneously in a number of autoimmune diseases, as we have discussed, and may be detrimental to the health of the patient. However, situations may exist in which the antiidiotypes may actually be useful. Examples include situations in which these antibodies could replace an unavailable hormone or one that is degraded before reaching the receptor, or in which a deficient receptor cannot interact with the hormone but could possibly still be recognized by the antibody.

Antiidiotypic antibodies able to recognize membrane-bound receptors may eventually be considered useful tools in the treatment of disease. Levy and his collaborators (Miller et al., 1982) have initiated a series of in vivo studies by injecting mouse monoclonal antiidiotypic antibodies into leukemic patients. In this case, the receptor was the idiotype, that is, the immunoglobulin expressed on the surface of the B cells of the patients with a B-cell leukemia. By binding to this receptor, the antibody triggered the disappearance of the leukemic cells, probably by activation of complement. Along the same line of thought, Ertl et al. (1982) raised an antiidiotypic antibody against an antibody specific for the hemagglutinin of reovirus. The monoclonal antiidiotypic antibody detected the hemagglutinin receptor on somatic cells. Cytolytic T lymphocytes specific for cells infected with reovirus type 3 lysed the hybridoma cells expressing the antihemag-glutinin receptor antiidiotypic antibody.

Another use of antiidiotypic antibodies utilizes their ability to mimic the structure of drugs. Antagonist-like antiidiotypic antibodies could potentially replace synthetic antagonists with detrimental secondary effects or could be invaluable in systems for which antagonists have not yet been isolated or prepared. Antibodies binding to β-adrenergic receptor have already been shown to block the binding of catecholamine agonists or antagonists (Schreiber *et al.*, 1980; Couraud *et al.*, 1983). Fab fragments derived from antidigoxin antibodies were recently given to patients with an accidental overdose of this drug for the purpose of detoxification. In this case, no immunological reaction to the antibody fragments was observed. Likewise, Fab or even Fv fragments of antiidiotypic antibodies may be used to stimulate or block receptors in a specific way. Alternatively, these Fv molecules may be used as models for the synthesis of new therapeutic compounds.

VIII. Prospects

The concept emerging from the data reviewed here is that antireceptor antibodies may be obtained, either spontaneously or by experimental design, without immunization with receptor. This may have far-reaching consequences both in diagnostic and therapeutic terms and in fundamental applications.

A. DIAGNOSTIC

In a number of diseases, some of which are discussed here, it has been suspected that autoantibodies against receptors actually intervene in pathological development. It is usually assumed that these antibodies arise through accidental exposure of receptor or cross-reactive molecules to the immune system. The experimentally obtained antiidiotypic antibodies that bind to receptors, however, suggests that an alternative explanation for such an exposure may exist: The antireceptor antibodies could originally arise against antihormone antibodies directed against circulating hormone or ingested analogs. In view of this possibility, it would certainly be worthwhile to look for antiidiotypic reactivity in diseases characterized by antireceptor antibodies.

B. THERAPEUTIC

The use of antiidiotypic antibodies as therapeutic aids has hitherto been based on the interactions between idiotypes on B leukemia cells and antiidiotypic antibodies raised in mice and was used to search for and destroy the target cells (Miller *et al.*, 1982). In a similar manner, antireceptor activity of antiidiotypic antibodies could, however, be used in a number of situations.

Antagonist-like antiidiotypic antibodies may prove to be invaluable in blocking receptors for which synthetic "inhibitors" either are not available or display detrimental side effects. The antibodies could be used directly, preferably as Fv fragments, or to serve as models for synthesis of new hypervariable region-like peptides. Similarly, agonist-like antibodies might be used when the hormone is unavailable or unable to interact with a deficient receptor which could still be recognized by the antibody.

C. FUNDAMENTAL APPLICATIONS

The ability to raise antireceptor antibodies without prior purification of the receptor itself should be of considerable help in systems in which the lack of appropriate isolation methods has often precluded progress in the understanding of receptor physiology. The site-directed specificity of the antiidiotypic antibodies increases their usefulness, because inhibitory antireceptor antibodies are usually the most difficult to obtain even in systems in which receptor molecules are relatively easy to purify in sufficient quantities to allow immunization.

Many of the studies described in this chapter are recent and still in process, and the full implications of the data are yet to be explored. However, the importance of antireceptor antiidiotypic antibodies has already been recognized, and their future should include new and exciting findings in the fields of immunoendocrinology and neuroimmunology.

Acknowledgments

Original research reviewed in this chapter was supported by grants from the Centre National de la Recherche Scientifique (79.7.054), the Délégation Général à la Recherche Scientifique et Technique (79.7.0780), Fonds de la Recherche Médicale Française, and the Association pour le Développement de la Recherche sur le Cancer.

References

Capra, J. D., Slaughter, C., Milner, E. C. B., Estess, P., and Tucker, P. W. (1982). *Immunol. Today* 3, 332–339.

Clevinger, B., Thomas, J., Davie, J., Schilling, J., Bond, M., Hood, L., and Kearney, J. (1983). *Nature (London)* (in press).

Couraud, P.-O., Lü, B.-Z., and Strosberg, A. D. (1983). *J. Exp. Med.* 157, 1369–1378.

Drachman, D. B. (1978). *N. Eng. J. Med.* 298, 136–142.

Ertl, H. C. J., Greene, M. I., Noseworthy, J. H., Fields, B. N., Nepom, J. T., Spriggs, D. R., and Finberg, R. W. (1982). *Proc. Natl. Acad. Sci. U.S.A.* 79, 7479–7483.

Farid, N. R., Pepper, B., Urbina-Briones, R., and Islam, N. R. (1982). *J. Cell. Biochem.* 19, 305.

Fuchs, S., Schmidt-Hopfeld, H., Tridenta, G., and Terrab-Hazdai, R. (1980). *Nature (London)* 287, 162–164.

Hoebeke, J., Vray, B., Foriers, A., and Strosberg, A. D. (1979). *Protides Biol. Fluids* 27, 443–446.

Homcy, C. J., Rockson, S. G., and Haber, E. (1982). *J. Clin. Invest.* 69, 1147–1154.

Jerne, N. K. (1974). *Ann. Immunol. (Paris)* 125C, 373–389.

Kahn, C. R., Baird, K. L., Flier, J. S., Grunfeld, C., Harmon, J. T., Harrison, L. C., Karlsson, F. A., Kasuga, M., King, G. L., Lang, U. C., Poskalny, J. M., and Van Obberghen, E. (1981). *Recent Prog. Horm. Res.* 37, 477–538.

Koo, P. H., and Cebra, J. J. (1974). *Biochemistry* 13, 184–195.

Lindstrom, J., Lennon, V. A., Seybold, M. E., and Wittingham, S. (1976). *Ann. N.Y. Acad. Sci.* 174, 283.

Lü, B.-Z., Couraud, P.-O., Schmutz, A., and Strosberg, A. D. (1983). *Ann. N.Y. Acad Sci.* (in press).

Marasco, W. A., and Becker, E. L. (1982). *J. Immunol.* 128, 963–968.

Margolies, M. (1983). *Ann. N.Y. Acad. Sci.* (in press).

Miller, R. A., Maloney, D. G., and Levy, R. A. (1982). *N. Engl. J. Med.* 307, 687.

Moshly-Rosen, D., Fuchs, S., and Eshhar, Z. (1979). *FEBS Lett.* 106, 389–392.

Niall, H. D., and Tregear, G. W. (1979). *N. Engl. J. Med.* 301, 940–941.

Nisonoff, A. (1983). *Ann. N.Y. Acad. Sci.* (in press).

Orgiazzi, J., Williams, D. L., Chopra, I. J., and Solomon, D. H. (1976). *J. Clin. Endocrinol. Metab.* 42, 341–348.

Schilling, J., Clevinger, B., Davie, J. M., and Hood, L. (1980). *Nature (London)* 283, 35–40.

Schreiber, A. B., Couraud, P. O., Andre, C., Vray, B., and Strosberg, A. D. (1980). *Proc. Natl. Acad. Sci. U.S.A.* 77, 7385–7389.

Sege, K., and Peterson, P. A. (1978). *Proc. Natl. Acad. Sci. U.S.A.* 75, 2443–2447.

Shechter, Y., Maron, R., Elias, D., and Cohen, E. R. (1982). *Science* 216, 542–545.

Strosberg, A. D., Couraud, P. O., Durier-Trautmann, O., and Delavier-Klutchco, C. (1982). *Trends Pharmacol. Sci.* 3, 272–285.

Venter, C., Fraser, C. M., and Harrison, L. C. (1980). *Science* 207, 1361–1363.

Wassermann, N. H., Penn, A. S., Freimuth, P. I., Treptow, N., Wentzel, S., Cleveland, W. L., and Erlanger, B. F. (1982). *Proc. Natl. Acad. Sci. U.S.A.* 79, 4810–4817.

Chapter 20

Immunization to Insulin Generates Antiidiotypes That Behave as Antibodies to the Insulin Hormone Receptor and Cause Diabetes Mellitus

Irun R. Cohen,[1] Dana Elias,[1,2] Ruth Maron,[1] and Yoram Shechter[2]

Department of Cell Biology[1] and Hormone Research[2]
The Weizmann Institute of Science
Rehovot, Israel

I. Hormone Receptor Antibody: The Immune System Image of a Hormone

The binding of insulin to its receptor at the surface of a target cell triggers specific biochemical responses that influence glucose homeostasis (Czech, 1977). However, similar biochemical responses may be triggered by the binding to target cells of other ligands, such as lectins or insulin receptor antibodies (Czech, 1980). Insulin is superior to other ligands in that it functions as a regulatory element in an endocrinological network that activates the information inherent in the insulin receptor in accord with the metabolic needs of the body. Insulin receptor antibody, in contrast, is merely an interloper; its activation of the insulin receptor is unconnected to glucose homeostasis. This chapter will discuss insulin receptor antibodies that arise spontaneously as antiidiotypes to specific insulin autoantibodies and thus function as elements in an immunological network (Jerne, 1974). These antiidiotypic antibodies seem to regulate the expression of the idiotypic antibodies. However, in their role as receptor antibodies, the antiidiotypes have a pernicious effect on insulin receptors and on glucose homeostasis. Thus, an internal image of insulin generated by an idiotype–antiidiotype network of autoantibodies profoundly influences the flow of information in the endocrinological network.

II. The Insulin Molecule: Structure–Function Relationships

To bind to the insulin-combining site of the insulin receptor, an antiidiotypic antibody must mimic the conformation of that portion of insulin that also binds to the receptor (Nisonoff and Lamoyi, 1981). This can be appreciated by considering the tertiary structure of the insulin molecule. Insulin (MW about 5600) is formed by two disulfide-linked polypeptide chains of 21 and 30 amino acids, the A and B chains, respectively (Ryle *et al.*, 1955). The chains are folded in such a way that the molecule has the shape of a flat, triangular wedge (Blundell *et al.*, 1972; Ranghino *et al.*, 1981; Talmon *et al.*, 1983). Figure 1 shows a schematic diagram of the face of the insulin molecule. Insulin has been highly conserved in evolution, and most mammalian species have identical amino acid sequences throughout 85% or more of the molecule (Dayhoff, 1972). Moreover, the substitutions that have appeared have tended to accumulate in one part of the molecule. For example, mouse insulins differ from those of pig, beef, sheep, horse, or man at as many as six positions: A4, A8–10, B3, or B30. These residues are not in the primary sequence but nevertheless are folded to form the contiguous patch pictured at the top of the molecule in Fig. 1. The conserved portions of the insulin molecule contain that part that seems to fit the hormone receptor, the receptor site (Fig. 1). Other parts of the conserved portion of insulin would appear to be external to the receptor site. The function of these external sites is not clear, but it is probable that they contribute to the conformation of the receptor site.

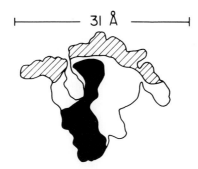

Fig. 1. The insulin molecule. A schematic view of the structure of insulin derived from Talmon *et al.* (1983), Ranghino *et al.* (1981), and De Meyts *et al.* (1978), showing the areas with variable or conserved amino acid residues. The variable patch on ungulate insulins probably contains foreign antigens for mouse T cells, whereas the conserved areas include the receptor and external sites with self-epitopes seen by mouse B cells. ⊘, Variable residues/foreign antigens: conserved residues/self-antigens; ●, receptor site; ○, external site.

The insulins of guinea pigs and related species seem to represent an evolutionary deviation from the mainstream of mammalian insulins. Mouse or rat insulins differ from pig insulin by three substitutions, but guinea pig insulin differs from pig insulin by 18 of its 51 amino acids (Blundell *et al.*, 1972). These substitutions occur in the areas conserved in other species, as well as in the variable patch, so that guinea pig insulin is structurally different from the other mammalian insulins (Blundell *et al.*, 1972; Neville *et al.*, 1973). Functionally, guinea pig insulin is only about 10% as efficient as ungulate insulins in activating the insulin receptors of rat adipocytes (Blundell *et al.*, 1972). Presumably, guinea pig insulin is an adequate ligand for the insulin receptor of guinea pigs.

From an immunological point of view, a mouse immunized to beef or pig insulins would be confronted with foreign antigens associated with the variable patch together with self-antigens associated with the conserved region shared by mouse insulin (Fig. 1). Moreover, some self-antigens would be formed by the receptor-binding site of the molecule and others by epitopes external to the receptor site. A guinea pig, in contrast to a mouse, would see foreign antigenic determinants throughout the ungulate insulin molecule. This difference may be important because, as we shall see below, mice and guinea pigs seem to respond differently to immunization with ungulate insulins.

Another functional relationship between insulin structure and the immune response is exemplified by a division of labor between T and

B lymphocytes. The T lymphocytes of mice seem to pay careful attention to the foreign variable patch of ungulate insulins and, under *H-2* gene control, can discriminate between single amino acid substitutions in this area (Cohen and Talmon, 1980). In contrast, the bulk of the antibodies made by a mouse in response to one insulin are totally cross-reactive with other insulins, including its own (Keck, 1975). Thus, helper T lymphocytes scrutinize the variable portion of insulin with its foreign antigens and induce B lymphocytes to make autoantibodies to the conserved self-antigenic portion.

III. Four Questions

On the basis of the fact that mice can be induced to produce insulin autoantibodies, we asked four questions:

1. On immunization to ungulate insulins, do mice make insulin antibodies to the receptor site on the molecule?
2. Do such idiotypic antibodies spontaneously induce antiidiotypes with a conformation similar to that of the receptor-site epitope?
3. Would such antiidiotypic antibodies bind to insulin receptors and act as insulin-receptor autoantibodies?
4. Do such spontaneous antiidiotypic (receptor) antibodies function to affect glucose homeostasis as well as to regulate expression of idiotypic antibodies?

In essence, we wished to learn whether a specific idiotype–antiidiotype network is generated by immunization to insulin and whether the products of this immunological network could short-circuit an endocrinological network.

IV. Experimental Approach

To study these questions, we immunized mice of responsive *H-2* genotypes (Keck, 1975) to beef or pig insulins emulsified in adjuvant, followed by a secondary booster inoculation 21 days later (Shechter *et al.*, 1982). Individual mice were bled at intervals to investigate their serum for antibodies.

Insulin antibodies were detected using a solid-state radioimmunoassay (Eshhar *et al.*, 1979). Receptor antibodies were measured by induction of insulin-like effects in rat adipocytes and by displacement of insulin from its receptors (Sege and Peterson, 1978). The insulin-like effects included augmented glucose transport (Czech, 1977), antilipolysis (Fain *et al.*, 1966), and lipogenesis (Moody *et al.*, 1974), which we used as our routine measure of insulin-like activity. Specific idiotypes and antiidiotypes were defined by their mutual binding and neutralization. For example, insulin receptor antibodies were identified as antiidiotypes because their lipogenic effects on adipocytes were inhibitable by affinity-purified insulin antibodies (idiotypes). Likewise, specific idiotypic insulin antibodies were characterized by their ability to interact with the receptor (antiidiotypic) antibodies. Glucose homeostasis was assayed by serial glucose tolerance tests and measurement of blood glucose after periods of fasting. The state of the glucose receptors on the adipocytes of the mice was studied by specific binding of labeled insulin *in vitro* (Cuatrecasas, 1971, 1973) and by the magnitude of the lipogenic response of the adipocytes to stimulation with insulin. A summary of the results of these studies and the conclusions they support form the substance of this chapter. The experiments are detailed in two published articles (Shechter *et al.*, 1982) and in two others that have been accepted for publication (Shechter *et al.*, 1984; Elias *et al.*, 1984).

V. Insulin Receptor Antibodies Generated as Specific Antiidiotypes

Figure 2A illustrates the kinetics of unspecific insulin antibody detected in the sera of mice after a primary immunization with beef insulin and a secondary boost 21 days later. Figure 1B shows, in relative titers, the kinetics of two kinds of activities found in these sera: insulin receptor (antiidiotypic) antibodies and specific idiotypic insulin antibodies. The insulin-like receptor antibodies were of the IgG_2 class (Shechter *et al.*, 1984). We could find no evidence of insulin itself in complex with these IgG_2 receptor antibodies, and the receptor antibodies were distinct from the insulin antibodies. It is noteworthy that the bulk of the insulin antibodies in these sera belonged to the IgG_1 class and thus differed in isotype from the IgG_2 antiidiotypic receptor antibodies. The receptor antibodies were identified as antiidiotypes because they specifically bound to guinea pig insulin antibodies (Shechter *et al.*, 1982) and because their insulin-like effects were inhibited by affinity-purified mouse insulin antibodies, idiotypes (Elias *et al.*, 1984). Antiidiotypic receptor antibodies

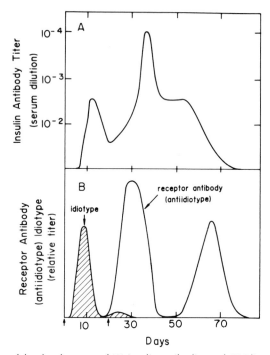

Fig. 2. Kinetics of the development of (A) insulin antibodies and (B) idiotypes and antiidiotypic receptor antibodies. Mice of the (C3H/eB × C57BL/6)F₁ hybrid strain were immunized by
two injections (arrows) (each into a different hind footpad) of beef insulin (25 μg) emulsified in
complete Freund's adjuvant. Insulin antibodies were measured by a solid-phase radioimmunoassay (Eshhar et al., 1979), antiidiotypic receptor antibodies by lipogenesis in adipocytes,
and idiotypes by the ability of affinity-purified insulin antibodies to inhibit the lipogenic activity
of the receptor antibodies (Shechter et al., 1982). The curves are constructed from the results of
two different experiments involving 20 individual mice.

were also found to appear in mice that had not been boosted by a
second immunization to insulin (Shechter et al., 1984).

Figure 2B also shows that the specific idiotypes that interacted with
the antiidiotypic receptor antibodies were confined to the primary
phase of the antibody response. Specific idiotypes were hardly detectable in the much higher secondary peak of insulin antibodies. In
contrast to the specific idiotypes, all the antiidiotypic receptor antibodies were found in two peaks that appeared after the booster immunization, and none were detectable in the primary response. Thus,
primary immunization to insulin generated relatively low titers of
insulin antibodies that included the specific idiotype. This idiotype-
positive primary response appeared to prime the mice for production

of antiidiotypes which emerged with the kinetics of a secondary response immediately upon booster immunization to insulin. Network theory (Jerne, 1974; Hart *et al.*, 1972) would suggest that the antiidiotypes suppressed the specific idiotypes which primed them. The cyclical expression of the antiidiotypic antibodies could be explained by an undetected second cycle of idiotypic antibodies or by more distant elements in the network such as anti-antiidiotypes (Paul and Bona, 1982).

Network theory would also explain the insulin receptor binding of the antiidiotypes as a fortuitous consequence of their mimicry of the conformation of the receptor site of insulin (Sege and Peterson, 1978; Nisonoff and Lamoyi, 1981; Strosberg *et al.*, 1981). Considering the structure–function relationships of the insulin molecule (Fig. 1), we suggest that the specific idiotypes probably recognized an epitope at the receptor site of insulin. Experimental support for this conjecture was obtained by immunizing mice with insulin molecules chemically modified so as to abolish their interaction with the hormone receptor. We found that the mice responded by producing high titers of antibodies to unmodified insulin. Thus the modified insulins preserved sufficient native structure to cross-react immunologically with unmodified insulin. Nevertheless, the mice produced no antiidiotypic receptor antibodies (Shechter *et al.*, 1984). It is reasonable to conclude that the chemical modification abolished both the hormone receptor site of the molecule and the critical epitope for the specific idiotype-antiidiotype network.

The antiidiotypic antibodies, being complementary to the idiotypes, could be imagined to have shapes similar to that of the receptor site of the hormone. Antibodies that look like the receptor site of insulin should be able to bind to the insulin receptors of target cells and thus behave as receptor antibodies. Although this interpretation of our results seems obvious and best fits the bias of this volume, we shall be much more confident when we succeed in isolating hybridomas and studying monoclonal antibodies (Kull *et al.*, 1982) with these specificities.

VI. Selectivity of the Immunological Network

One may wonder at the specificity of the immunological network, which suppresses the primary idiotypic insulin antibodies but not the nonidiotypic insulin antibodies that comprised the augmented secondary response (Fig. 1). It may be claimed that the insulin-like effects of the specific antiidiotypes provided an especially sensitive assay that favored detection of this particular idiotype–antiidiotype interaction, and that suppression of other idiotypes by more silent antiidotypic antibodies may have gone unnoticed. Nevertheless, a comparison of the responses of mice and guinea pigs to ungulate insulins suggests that activation of network control may be selective.

We have found that guinea pigs highly immunized to ungulate insulins have relatively high titers of specific idiotype but no detectable antiidiotypic antibodies (Shechter *et al.*, 1982). That is, guinea pig insulin antibodies bound the antiidiotypic (receptor) antibodies present in the sera of insulin-boosted mice, whereas the guinea pig sera themselves were negative for receptor antibodies. Hence, the late secondary immune response of guinea pigs to ungulate insulin was in contrast to that of mice, the latter manifesting insulin-like antiidiotypic antibodies but no specific idiotypes. This paradox may be explained if we consider the structures of ungulate, mouse, and guinea pig insulins (see Section II). It is apparent that the receptor site of ungulate insulin may be more of a self-epitope for mice than it is for guinea pigs. Therefore, the development of regulatory antiidiotypic antibodies in mice could be associated with the identity of the specific idiotypes as autoantibodies to the receptor site of mouse insulin. In contrast, the same idiotypes in guinea pigs are not autoantibodies (Neville *et al.*, 1973) because the receptor site of ungulate insulin is not a self-epitope for guinea pigs (Table I). Thus, guinea pigs may be less prone to suppress the specific idiotype than are mice. This argument implies that the idiotype–antiidiotype network may be more attuned to regulating autoantibodies (mice) than foreign antibodies (guinea pigs) directed against the same epitope (the ungulate insulin receptor site). How the antiidiotypic network might make such a distinction is a question for investigation. However, it is conceivable that the network is primed to deal with autoidiotypes as a result of immu-

TABLE I

Development of Regulatory Antiidiotype (Receptor Antibody) Is Correlated with Autoimmunity to a Self-Epitope

Host	Ungulate insulin receptor site epitope	Idiotype	Production of regulatory antiidiotype (receptor antibody)
Mouse	Self	Autoantibody	Yes
Guinea pig	Foreign	Not autoantibody	No

nological experience with the self-epitopes that constitute the individual. It should also be noted that idiotypes that specifically recognize the receptor site of insulin must mimic to some extent the combining site of the insulin receptor. Such a resemblance might also favor a specific antiidiotypic response primed by the individual's own insulin receptor. Thus, the presence in relatively high concentration of insulin and insulin receptor in the individual may serve as "internal-internal images" of the idiotypes of the specific antiidiotypic and idiotypic antibodies and prime the network for expression of these antibodies upon immunization with ungulate insulins.

VII. Effect of Antiidiotypic (Receptor) Antibodies on Glucose Homeostasis

Irrespective of one's concept of the machinations that drive the immunological network, it is clear that antiidiotypic antibodies with receptor activity can be generated by immunization to insulin. A practical question is whether these antibodies can enter and short-circuit the endocrinological network responsible for glucose homeostasis. To answer this question, we investigated individual mice with or without antiidiotypic receptor antibodies by provoking glucose imbalance through glucose loading or fasting (Elias et al., 1984).

Figure 3 shows the mean blood glucose concentrations of mice deprived of food for 8 h as a function of time after immunization to insulin. For comparison, the kinetics of insulin antibodies, specific idiotypes, and antiidiotypic receptor antibodies in these mice are shown in Fig. 2. It can be seen that the development of antiidiotypic receptor antibodies was associated with two distinct trends in the fasting glucose concentration. Hypoglycemia (about 20 mg% glucose) appeared around days 40–50. Prolongation of fasting to 18 h during this period led to the death of some mice, presumably because of severe hypoglycemia. The phase of hypoglycemia could be explained by uncontrolled activation of insulin receptors by the insulin-like antiidiotypic receptor antibodies, a state of functional "hyperinsulinemia."

Paradoxically, the phase of hypoglycemia was followed by a period of fasting hyperglycemia in which the blood glucose reached levels of about 115 mg%, almost twice that of normal mice. This phase of dysregulation could be explained by the development of resistance to the effects of insulin or insulin-like antibodies, a state of "hypoactivity" of insulin receptors.

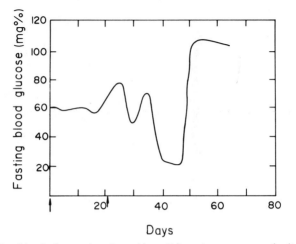

Fig. 3. Fasting blood glucose in mice with antiidiotypic receptor antibodies. Mice (see legend for Fig. 2) were deprived of food for 8 h, and the concentration of blood glucose was measured using a Beckman Glucose Analyzer II (glucose oxidase method).

The abnormal responses to fasting were accompanied by intolerance to glucose loading. Figure 4 shows the superimposed glucose tolerance curves of three kinds of mice: normals and those tested 36 or 58 days after immunization to insulin when they had high levels of idiotypic receptor antibodies (see Fig. 2). The immunized mice in

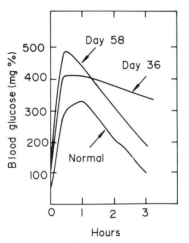

Fig. 4. Glucose tolerance curves. Normal control mice or mice that had been immunized to insulin (see legend for Fig. 2) 36 or 58 days earlier were injected intraperitoneally with glucose (5 gm/kg), and the blood glucose was measured at 0 and 20 min and at 1, 2, and 3 h.

either state showed abnormal responses characterized by high peak levels and prolonged elevation of blood glucose after a glucose load. Thus, mice with antiidiotypic receptor antibodies suffered from abnormal regulation of blood glucose, a kind of diabetes mellitus. At present, we cannot attribute the disease exclusively to the receptor antibodies because the mice also had insulin antibodies and probably other abnormalities. However, our impression from studying individual mice is that the degree of glucose dysregulation seemed to be associated with the magnitude of the antiidiotypic receptor antibodies rather than with the insulin antibodies. Hopefully, the role of each type of antibody can be clarified by using monoclonal antibodies. In any case, it is obvious that the products of the immunological network do short-circuit the endocrinological network and disturb homeostasis.

VIII. Down-Regulation and Desensitization of Insulin Receptors

The finding of a phase of fasting hyperglycemia (Fig. 3) suggested that the antiidiotypic receptor antibodies might influence the insulin receptors so as to produce resistance to insulin. Insulin resistance could be explained by at least two types of receptor abnormalities: down-regulation (Pollet and Levey, 1980) and desensitization (Marshall and Olefsky, 1980). Down-regulation denotes a decrease on target cells of the number of insulin receptors that can be measured by the binding of radiolabeled insulin. Desensitization refers to a decrease in the magnitude of the biochemical response triggered by the binding of insulin to the available receptors. It has been shown that binding of insulin to only about 2% of a cell's receptors is sufficient to trigger a maximal lipogenic response in normal adipocytes (Kono and Barham, 1971). Therefore, desensitization is detected by a decrease in the maximal lipogenic response that can be elicited by optimal concentrations of insulin.

Figure 5 shows that isolated adipocytes from mice with antiidiotypic receptor antibodies bound about 40% of the radiolabeled insulin bound by adipocytes from unimmunized mice. Note that the concentration of insulin producing 50% of maximal binding was unaffected in the mice with antiidiotypic receptor antibodies. This indicates that there was no decrease in affinity of binding of insulin to the available receptors. The degree of down-regulation of 60% was about half of

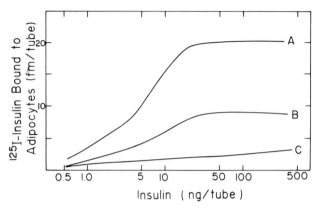

Fig. 5. Down-regulation of insulin receptors. Adipocytes were obtained from normal control mice, mice with antiidiotypic receptor antibodies, and obese mice with a genetic receptor defect (Kahn, 1980), and the amount of available insulin receptors was measured by the binding of radiolabeled insulin. (Cuatrecasas, 1971)

that found in genetically obese mice (*ob/ob*) that suffer from diabetes because of a receptor defect (Kahn, 1980).

Figure 6 shows that the receptors that were available in the adipocytes of mice with antiidiotypic receptor antibodies were partially desensitized. The adipocytes showed suboptimal lipogenesis at the plateau response when stimulated by high amounts of insulin. Thus, the presence of the antiidiotypic receptor antibodies was associated with both a decreased number of insulin receptors and a diminished sensitivity of the remaining insulin receptors to insulin. The mechanisms responsible for those receptor abnormalities are unknown. Exposure to insulin has been shown to increase the resistance of target cells to subsequent stimulation by a second contact with insulin (Gavin *et al.*, 1974). Thus, the antiidiotypic receptor antibodies may have affected the adipocytes of the mice by mechanisms similar to those inducible by insulin itself, whatever they may be. In general, the augmented resistance to insulin could be a function of receptor or postreceptor alteration of the target cells. In any case, the insulin resistance could be looked upon as a compensatory adaptation to the functional hyperinsulinemia mediated by the insulin-like receptor antibodies.

We have yet to catalog the other adaptations that must certainly occur in the endocrinological network, such as production of endogenous insulin, glucagon, and growth and other hormones.

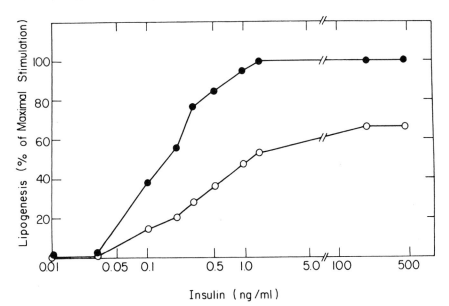

Fig. 6. Desensitization of insulin receptors. Adipocytes were obtained from normal mice (●) or from mice with antiidiotypic insulin receptor antibodies (○), and the degree of lipogenesis was measured as a function of the amount of added insulin. (Marshall and Olefsky, 1980)

IX. Receptor Antibodies in Human Patients

Receptor antibodies are considered to cause several human diseases, such as Graves disease, in which thyroid-stimulating hormone receptors are hyperactivated by receptor antibodies (Hall *et al.*, 1975); myasthenia gravis, in which the acetylcholine receptor is blocked (Fuchs, 1979); and severe insulin-resistant diabetes associated with acanthosis nigricans involving the insulin receptor (Flier *et al.*, 1976). Antibodies to β-adrenergic receptors are also suspected of being important in allergic diseases (Venter *et al.*, 1980), and it is probable that receptor antibodies will be discovered in additional diseases, particularly those of the endocrine and nervous systems, in which ligand–receptor interactions are important for normal function. Our observation that receptor antibodies may arise as antiidiotypic antibodies suggests that a similar mechanism could operate in certain patients. Thus, some receptor antibodies may turn out to be a secondary result of network regulation of primary autoimmunity to receptor ligands. For example, some patients suffering from Graves disease might have primary autoimmunity to the thyroid-stimulating hormone, with hyperthyroidism resulting from receptor antibodies that are antiidio-types.

An obvious question is the relationship between the antiidiotypic receptor antibodies in the mice and the receptor antibodies described in the rare patient with diabetes and acanthosis nigricans (Flier *et al.*, 1976). What we know about both conditions at this time leads us to believe that the antiidiotypic receptor antibodies in the immunized mice are not an experimental model of the receptor antibodies in diabetes associated with acanthosis nigricans. Acanthosis nigricans diabetics manifest an extreme resistance to treatment with insulin and some may have a primary defect of their insulin receptors that is independent of the presence of receptor antibodies (Podskalny and Kahn, 1982). In contrast, the hallmark of the diabetes in the mice was its clinical mildness. Given free access to food, the mice appeared to be well, if somewhat fatter than their control brethren. Their bio-chemical diabetes was demonstrable through provocation by fasting or glucose load, and receptor changes were relatively mild, although significant. This is certainly not the case with acanthosis nigricans patients whose diabetes is controllable only with the greatest diffi-culty.

Insulin antibodies are not uncommon in humans with easily man-ageable diabetes, and if such persons do make antiidiotypic receptor antibodies, they certainly do not have the clinical course characteris-tic of the ancanthosis nigricans patients. Therefore, we believe that the clinical condition for which the immunized mice are a model will turn out to be much more subtle and more widespread than the acan-thosis nigricans diabetes syndrome. Recently, we detected relatively benign IgM insulin receptor antibodies in children suffering from insulin-dependent diabetes mellitus (Maron *et al.* 1983). It remains to be seen whether these receptor autoantibodies are in fact antiidio-types.

X. Summary: Four Answers

The message of this chapter can be summarized by the answers to the four questions raised above (see Section II).

1. On immunization to ungulate insulins, mice produce spontane-ously insulin receptor antibodies that are also antiidiotypes.
2. These antibodies are functional and both regulate expression of the idiotypic antibodies and modify insulin receptors to affect glucose homeostasis.

3. Behavior of the antiidiotypes as receptor antibodies suggests that the combining sites of the antiidiotypes might mimic the structure of the receptor site of insulin.
4. A corollary to these conjectures is that the specific idiotypes are autoantibodies to the receptor site of mouse insulin.

References

Blundell, T., Dodson, G., Hodgkin, D., and Mercola, D. (1972). *Adv. Protein Chem.* **26**, 279–402.

Cohen, I. R., and Talmon, J. (1980). *Eur. J. Immunol.* **10**, 284–289.

Cuatrecasas, P. (1971). *Proc. Natl. Acad. Sci. U.S.A.* **68**, 1264–1268.

Cuatrecasas, P. (1973). *J. Biol. Chem.* **248**, 3528–3534.

Czech, M. P. (1977). *Annu. Rev. Biochem.* **47**, 359–384.

Czech, M. P. (1980). *Diabetes* **29**, 399–409.

Dayhoff, M. O., ed. (1972). "Atlas of Protein Sequence and Structure," pp. D186–D187. Nat. Biomed. Res. Found., Washington, D.C.

De Meyts, P., Van Obberghen, E., Roth, J., Wollmer, A., and Brandenburg, D. (1978). *Nature (London)* **273**, 504–509.

Elias, D., Maron, R., Cohen, I. R., and Shechter, Y. (1984). *J. Biol. Chem.* (in press).

Eshhar, Z., Strassmann, G., Waks, T., and Mozes, E. (1979). *Cell. Immunol.* **47**, 378–389.

Fain, J. N., Kovacev, V. P., and Scow, R. O. (1966). *Endocrinology* **78**, 773–778.

Flier, J. S., Kahn, C. R., Jarett, D. B., and Roth, J. (1976). *J. Clin. Invest.* **58**, 1442–1449.

Fuchs, S. (1979). *Curr. Top. Microbiol. Immunol.* **85**, 1–29.

Gavin, J. R., III, Roth, J., Neville, D. M., Jr., De Meyts, P., and Buell, D. N. (1974). *Proc. Natl. Acad. Sci. U.S.A.* **71**, 84–88.

Hall, R., Smith, B. R., and Mukhtar, E. D. (1975). *Clin. Endocrinol.* **4**, 213–230.

Hart, D. A., Wang, A., Pawlak, L. L., and Nisonoff, A. (1972). *J. Exp. Med.* **135**, 1293–1300.

Jerne, N. K. (1974). *Ann. Immunol. (Paris)* **125C**, 373–384.

Kahn, C. R. (1980). *Metab. Clin. Exp.* **29**, 455–466.

Keck, K. (1975). *Nature (London)* **254**, 78–79.

Kono, T., and Barham, F. W. (1971). *J. Biol. Chem.* **246**, 6210–6216.

Kull, F. C., Jr., Jacobs, S., Su, Y. F., and Cuatrecasas, P. (1982). *Biochem. Biophys. Res. Commun.* **106**, 1019–1026.

Maron, R., Elias, D., de Jongh, B. M., Bruining, G. J., van Rood, J. J., Shechter, Y., and Cohen, I. R. (1983). *Nature* **303**, 817–818.

Marshall, S., and Olefsky, J. M. (1980). *J. Clin. Invest.* **66**, 763–772.

Moody, A. J., Stan, M. A., Stan, M., and Gliemann, J. (1974). *Horm. Metab. Res.* **6**, 12–16.

Neville, R. W. J., Weir, B. J., and Lazarus, N. R. (1973). *Diabetes* **22**, 851–853.

Nisonoff, A., and Lamoyi, A. (1981). *Clin. Immunol. Immunopathol.* **21**, 397–406.

Paul, W. E., and Bona, C. (1982). *Immunol. Today* **3**, 230–234.

Podskalny, J. M., and Kahn, C. R. (1982). *J. Clin. Endocrinol. Metab.* **54**, 261–268.

Pollet, R. J., and Levey, G. S. (1980). *Ann. Intern. Med.* **92**, 663–680.

Ranghino, G., Talmon, J., Yonath, A., and Cohen, I. R. (1981). *In* "Structural Aspects of

Recognition and Assembly in Biological Macromolecules" (M. Balaban, J. L. Sussman, W. Traub, and A. Yonath, eds.), pp. 263–279. Balaban ISS, Philadelphia, Pennsylvania.

Ryle, A. P., Sanger, F., Smith, L. F., and Kitai, R. (1955). *Biochem. J.* **60**, 541–556.

Sege, K., and Peterson, P. A. (1978). *Proc. Natl. Acad. Sci. U.S.A.* **75**, 2443–2447.

Shechter, Y., Maron, R., Elias, D., and Cohen, I. R. (1982). *Science* **216**, 542–545.

Shechter, Y., Elias, D., Maron, R., and Cohen, I. R. (1984). *J. Biol. Chem.* (in press).

Strosberg, A. D., Couraud, P. O., and Schreiber, A. (1981). *Immunol. Today* **2**, 75–79.

Talmon, J., Ranghino, G., Yonath, A., and Cohen, I. R. (1983). *Immunogenetics* **18**, 79–89.

Venter, J. C., Fraser, C. M., and Harrison, L. C. (1980). *Science* **207**, 1361–1362.

Chapter 21

Induction of Protective Immunity Using Antiidiotypic Antibodies: Immunization against Experimental African Trypanosomiasis

David L. Sacks

Immunology and Cell Biology Section
Laboratory of Parasitic Diseases
National Institute of Allergy and Infectious Diseases
National Institutes of Health
Bethesda, Maryland

I. Introduction

Treatment with antiidiotypic (anti-Id) antibodies can, under certain experimental conditions, induce lymphocytes and antibodies of complementary specificity. Injection of anti-Id antibodies has been shown in several experimental systems to induce antigen-specific helper T cells (1–4) and to enhance the expression of the corresponding idiotype in subsequent antibody responses (5–9). More recently, administration of anti-Id has been reported to induce the production of antigen-binding idiotype-positive molecules in the absence of exposure to antigen (10–12). Collectively, these experiments provide clear evidence that idiotypic regulation of the immune system can occur and that antigen-independent mechanisms exist for the expansion of B- and T-cell clones bearing the appropriate idiotype. The application and extension of these findings to the induction of immunity to microbial agents are of obvious interest.

In these studies, we have attempted to immunize mice against African trypanosomiasis using antiidiotypic antibodies (13). Infection with African trypanosomes, the etiological agents of sleeping sickness, is characterized by a cycling parasitemia, with each cycle consisting of increasing parasitemia, host antibody production, parasite clearance, and the appearance of trypanosomes of different variable antigen types (VATs) (reviewed in Ref. 14). This antigenic variation apparently occurs spontaneously, with antibody playing a selective role in the elimination of major VATs. It is the ability of the parasite to produce antigenic variants of its surface glycoprotein coat which is responsible for the cycling parasitemia and the chronicity of the infection.

Experimental African trypanosomiasis was chosen as a model for anti-Id-induced antimicrobial immunity for two reasons: first, protective monoclonal antibodies bearing a defined idiotype can be raised against the variable surface antigens of these parasites; second, low concentrations of antibody directed against these antigens are sufficient to protect mice against challenge with parasites expressing the homologous VAT. In these studies, the regulatory activities of anti-Id antibodies *in vivo* were examined for their ability to influence the expression of the corresponding idiotype prior to and during the course of infection with *Trypanosoma rhodesiense* and, more importantly, for their ability to immunize mice against infection with these parasites. In addition, the genetic control of idiotype expression was examined, as well as the nature of the idiotype–antiidiotype interactions which might lead to immunity in these systems.

II. Immunization with Anti-Id Antibodies

In these studies, anti-Id antibodies were raised against three monoclonal antibodies, 7H11, 11D5, and B7B1, each of which has specificity for distinct epitopes on the VAT of a clone of *Trypanosoma rhodesiense*, WRATat-1.1. In addition, each of these monoclonal antibodies protects mice against challenge with WRATat-1.1, as determined by passive transfer and *in vitro* neutralization.

Anti-Id antibodies were raised by immunization of SJL/J mice with each of the three protein A-purified monoclonal antibodies. Antisera were absorbed against normal BALB/c IgG and MOPC 21-coupled Sepharose 4B to remove antiallotype and anti-MOPC 21 idiotype activities. The idiotypic specificities of the three antisera were confirmed in a competitive radioimmune assay (RIA). The binding of radiolabeled monoclonal antibodies by the homologous anti-Id was shown to be restricted in each case to Id by the failure of NMIg, MOPC 21, and the heterologous Ids to inhibit binding. Following previous studies (1,9) in which the subclass of anti-Id was found to influence its regulatory effect, IgG_1, shown to be capable of priming for idiotype expression, was purified from each of the three anti-Id antisera as well as from control, normal SJL sera. We chose to administer the three IgG_1 anti-Ids together in order to improve the chances of inducing immunity. Doses ranging from 250 ng to 4 μg of each anti-Id were administered ip in saline 3–4 weeks before challenge. Infection of BALB/c mice with 100 cloned WRATat-1.1 organisms results in fluctuating waves of blood parasitemia, of which 95–100% of the parasites in the first peak bear the original VAT (11). Trypanosomes in the subsequent peaks bear new VATs; therefore, any immunity induced by anti-Id administration will presumably affect only the first-wave parasitemia. The successful induction of a specific anti-VAT response would be expected to have three alternative effects on the infection: (a) complete protection, in which the infecting VAT is eliminated before new VATs are able to emerge and no blood parasitemia is ever observed, (b) reduced first-wave parasitemia, or (c) selection against parasites bearing the original VAT in favor of different VATs in the first wave, observed as VAT switching.

In fact, all three effects were observed. As shown in Table I, mice treated with normal SJL IgG_1 had typical primary parasitemias, except for an aberrant mouse in which the original VAT was not expressed. Within each of the three groups of mice treated with either 250 ng, 1 μg, or 4 μg of the three anti-Ids' were mice which had normal infections, no detectable blood parasitemia, reduced parasitemia, or

TABLE I

Outcome of Primary Parasitemia in BALB/c Mice Immunized with Antiidiotypic Antibodies

Treatment	Normal	Protected	Reduced	Switched	Altered infection/total
Normal SJL IgG_1	9	0	0	1	1/10
Anti-Id IgG					
250 ng	4	2	1	3	6/10
1 μg	5	3	1	1	5/10
4 μg	2	2	2	4	8/10

switched VAT. No obvious dose effect was observed. Considered together, of the 30 mice treated with anti-Id, 63% had altered infections, with complete protection (23%) and VAT switching (27%) being the dominant effects.

III. Idiotype Expression in Anti-Id-Treated Mice

Sera obtained pre- and postchallenge were analyzed in a competitive RIA (see the legend for Fig. 1) for the presence of each of the three idiotypes. In Fig. 1, mice were grouped according to the outcome of the initial parasitemia. Control mice that received normal SJL IgG$_1$ and had normal infection had either very low or undetectable levels of the 7H11 idiotype in their sera both 2 weeks before and 3 days after infection. The detection of low levels of the 7H11 idiotype in the majority of mice 2 weeks after infection suggests a shared idiotype which is normally expressed in response to the first-wave parasites that bear the WRATat-1.1 VAT. Anti-Id-treated mice which had normal infection all had low or undetectable levels of the 7H11 idiotype when examined 3 days after challenge. In contrast, high levels of the idiotype were found 3 days after challenge in all mice which displayed some degree of immunity. In these animals, in which the concentration of WRATat-1.1 VAT remained minimal, the levels of 7H11 idiotype generally declined after 2 weeks of infection. Thus, anti-Id administration appeared to affect 7H11 Id expression in the majority of treated mice, and the presence of the Id in high levels shortly after challenge was associated with immunity.

The 11D5 Id also appears to be a shared BALB/c idiotype expressed in the majority of mice in response to WRATat-1.1 infection. In addition, the majority of anti-11D5 Id-treated mice had detectable levels of 11D5 Id-bearing molecules in their sera prior to challenge. However, unlike the 7H11 Id experience, the levels of 11D5 Id in sera shortly after infection did not distinguish anti-Id-treated immune animals from either control infected or anti-Id-treated nonimmune animals.

Finally, the B7B1 idiotype also arose in the majority of BALB/c mice in response to infection; however, it did not appear to be readily inducible by anti-Id, as it was only rarely detected prior to infection and its levels after antigen exposure did not appear to be enhanced in the anti-Id-treated mice. Thus, the contribution of the 11D5 and B7B1 Ids to the immunity observed is not indicated by the experience of BALB/c mice treated simultaneously with the three anti-Ids. How-

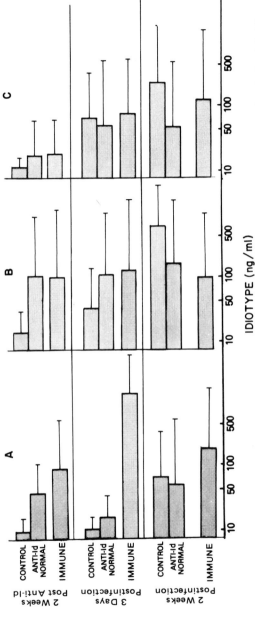

Fig. 1. Idiotype levels in BALB/c sera determined at intervals after anti-Id administration and infection with WRATat-1.1. Mice are grouped according to the outcome of primary parasitemia. Id concentrations in sera were determined in a solid-phase RIA in which the capacity of serum to inhibit the binding of ^{125}I-labeled Id to the homologous anti-Id was measured. Briefly, microwell plates were coated with affinity-purified anti-Id (50 μl, 20 μg/ml) for 18 h at 4°C, washed with PBS, and incubated for 1 h with 50% fetal calf serum in PBS, washed, and incubated for 3 h at 4°C with saline or sera, either undiluted or diluted 1 : 10 in saline. After washing, the homologous ^{125}I-labeled Id (chloramine T method) (50,000 cpm/50 μl) was added to each well and incubated for 3 h at 4°C. The plates were washed extensively, and individual wells were counted. The assay was standardized with known concentrations of purified Id as inhibitors. Bars represent arithmetic means ±1 standard deviation. (A) Expression of the 7H11 idiotype; (B) expression of the 11D5 idiotype; and (c) expression of the B7B1 idiotype.

TABLE II

Anti-Id Immunization of BALB/c Mice against
WRATat-1.1 Challenge

Experiment number	Anti-Id administered			
	NMIg	7H11	11D5	B7B1
1	0/10[a]	8/10	2/10	0/10
2A	0/9	6/9	0/8	0/8[b]
2B[c]	0/8	0/8	NT[d]	NT

[a] Number of mice without VAT-1.1 in primary parasitemia/number tested.
[b] 11D5 and B7B1 anti-Id's administered together.
[c] Challenge with 100 NIHTat-1 trypanosomes.
[d] Not tested.

ever, in order to address this point directly, BALB/c mice were immunized with each of the anti-Ids individually. In these experiments, mice were administered 20 μg of whole affinity-purified anti-Id and challenged 6–8 weeks later with 100 WRATat-1.1 trypanosomes. In experiment 1 in Table II, immunization with anti-7H11 Id alone resulted in exclusively VAT switching in 80% of the animals, whereas anti-11D5 Id immunization affected only 20% and anti-B7B1 Id none at all. In experiment 2A, similar results were obtained, except that no anti-11D5 Id-treated mice displayed immunity. Administration of anti-7H11 Id alone was therefore sufficient to immunize mice, and the effect was again associated with the more rapid and enhanced expression of the 7H11 idiotype after challenge (data not shown). Also included in experiment 2B were mice immunized with anti-7H11 Id but then challenged with a heterologous non-cross-reacting VAT-bearing *T. rhodesiense* clone, NIHTat-1. Of these, none displayed any immunity, including VAT switching, despite having detectable levels of the 7H11 idiotype before infection. Thus, the immunity induced by anti-7H11 Id was specific for the parasite bearing the VAT for which the 7H11 monoclonal antibody has specificity.

IV. Genetic Control of Idiotype Induction

In these experiments, other inbred mouse strains were injected with a pooled preparation containing 20 μg of each of the three anti-Ids. Mice were challenged 6–8 weeks later with parasite clone WRATat-1.1. As seen in Table III, only mice that bore the *a* heavy

TABLE III

Anti-Id Immunization of Various Mouse Strains
against WRATat-1.1 Challenge

Mouse strain[a]	Igh-C	H-2	Immune/total[b]
BALB/c	a	d	8/10
BALB/B	a	b	4/8
C57BL/10	b	b	0/10
A/J	e	a	0/10
C.B20	b	d	0–10

[a] All mice immunized with a pooled preparation of 20 μg
each of anti-7H11, -11D5, and -B7B1 Ids 6 weeks before
challenge with 100 WRATat-1.1.
[b] Immunity determined as the absence of VAT-1.1-bear-
ing parasites in primary parasitemia.

chain allotype demonstrated immunity, in each case VAT switching. Allotype congenic recombinant mice (CB20) had infections indistinguishable from those of nonimmunized BALB/c mice. Thus, the induction of immunity appeared to be linked to Ig-constant region genes.

Antisera made in these inbred mouse strains in response to infection or anti-Id treatment prior to infection were tested for expression of each Id to examine the genetic requirements for expression. Figures 2, 3, and 4 show the various idiotype levels of individual anti-Id-treated or -untreated mice 6 weeks after administration of anti-Id and just prior to infection, 4 days postinfection, and 12 days postinfection. The 7H11 idiotype was produced only by BALB/c and BALB.B mice in response to WRATat-1.1 infection (Fig. 2). In addition, only in these strains was the 7H11 idiotype induced by anti-Id. This idiotype was detectable in low levels on day 0 and once again in significantly increased levels on day 4. In all other mouse strains tested, including CB20, the 7H11 idiotype was only rarely expressed. The expression of the 11D5 idiotype in response to both infection and anti-Id immunization appears to be under similar genetic control (Fig. 3). It was induced only in mice bearing genes linked to Igh-C^a. The expression of the B7B1 idiotype did not appear to be allotype restricted insofar as this Id was present in response to infection in the majority of mice regardless of strain (Fig. 4). Administration of anti-B7B1 Id did not result in the induction of B7B1 Id-bearing molecules prior to antigen exposure in any mouse strain, nor did it result in the enhancement of B7B1 Id expression in the subsequent response to infection.

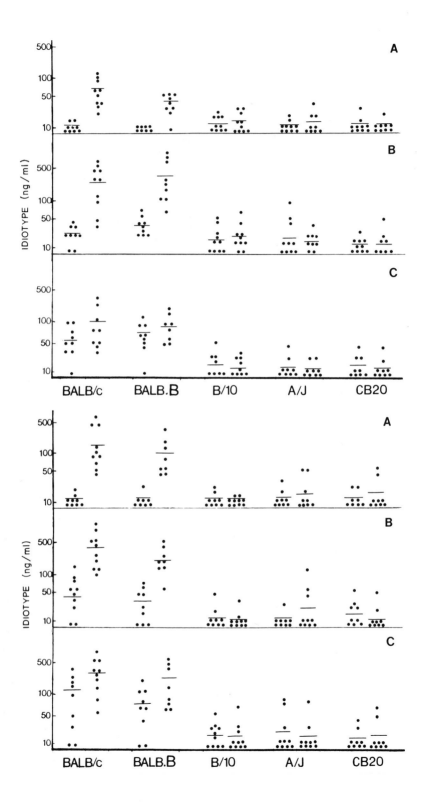

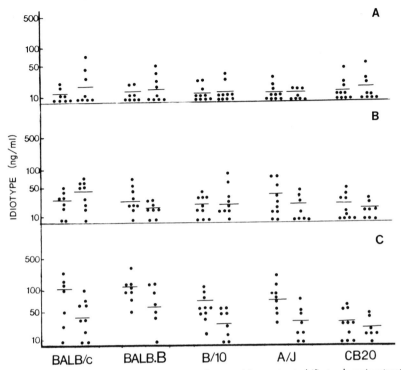

Figs. 2–4. Idiotype levels in various strains of mice, either untreated (first column) or treated (second column) with 20 μg each of anti-7H11, -11D5, and -B7B1 Ids 6 weeks prior to challenge with WRATat-1.1. Idiotype levels were determined as in Fig. 1. Lines represent arithmetic means. Fig. 2 (p. 408, top), 7H11; Fig. 3 (p. 408, bottom), 11DS; Fig. 4, B7B1. In all, (A) day 0, (B) day 4; (C) day 12.

In summary, then, the 7H11 and 11D5 Ids are strictly allotype linked, and Id-bearing molecules can be found in 80–100% of infected or anti–Id-immunized mice bearing the appropriate allotype. An influence of the H-2 haplotype was not apparent in the limited number of strains examined. These results are not unexpected, given that most classical idiotypic markers have been shown to be inherited together with the heavy chain locus (1,8–11,15). The simplest interpretation of the data would imply polymorphism of the structural genes encoding heavy chain idiotypic phenotypes. Alternatively, it has been argued that control by the Igh locus is indirect, through antiidiotypic gene products, and that normally silent clones can be revealed through idiotypic selection (16,17) (induction by anti-Id) or polyclonal activation (18). It should be emphasized that in these experiments the administration of anti-Id never induced immunity and only very rarely induced the expression of idiotype-bearing molecules in allotype-inappropriate mouse strains.

V. Specificity of Induced Idiotypes

The 7H11 and 11D5 Ids, although both allotype linked and readily inducible by anti-Id, differ in one crucial respect: Anti-Id-induced 7H11 expression is associated with immunity, whereas anti-Id-induced 11D5 expression is not. The basis for this difference cannot be attributed to an intrinsic difference in the antiparasite activities of the Id-bearing antibodies themselves. Titration of 7H11-neutralizing activity was no greater than that of 11D5. The difference, therefore, in the immunizing potential of the anti-Ids will undoubtedly be found in the specificity of the Id-bearing clones and molecules which they induce. Sera from all pooled anti-Id-treated mice of the appropriate allotype showed activity in RIA for both the 7H11 and 11D5 Ids which were detectable prior to infection. The material detected in these assays, designated Ab3, could, as previously discussed by Sachs *et al.* (8), include the following: (a) induced immunoglobulin molecules bearing shared idiotopes with 7H11 and 11D5, termed Id', and (b) antibody molecules bearing idiotopes unrelated to 7H11 and 11D5 produced as an immune response to V-region determinants on the allogenic anti-Ids, termed anti-anti-Id. It has been argued (19) that anti-anti-Id would not comprise more than a small fraction of these molecules because the injection of one low dose of anti-Id in saline is not a conventionally immunogenic protocol. In addition, it seems unlikely that the immune response to anti-Id would be allotype linked.

Thus, we believe that the majority of anti-Id-induced molecules are Id'. The question, then, is reduced to the specificity of Id'. The induction of Id-bearing, non-antigen-binding molecules by anti-Id has been reported in a number of systems (8,10–12). We are unable to demonstrate that any Id-bearing molecules that are induced prior to infection have any specificity for the parasite. Antibody was not detectable by RIA or immunofluorescence using as antigen either purified VAT or fixed trypanosomes. Still, these assays for antibody are far less sensitive than those for Id detection. Attempts to neutralize WRATat-1.1 infectivity by preincubation with either 7H11 or 11D5 Id' were unsuccessful. Finally, absorption of Id' with WRATat-1.1 did diminish the concentration of subsequently detectable Id, but to no greater degree than absorption with a heterologous clone, NIHTat-1. Thus, the specificities of both 7H11 and 11D5 Ids detected prior to infection remain unknown. It should be stressed that the levels of these idiotypes, which appear in response to either infection and/or anti-Id, are far lower than those reported in the more classical idiotype systems. The idiotypes analyzed here represent minor components of an extremely heterogeneous response to the surface glycoprotein coat of these parasites, in contrast to the dominant idiotypes which have been analyzed in response to organic haptens and carbohydrates. Thus, although the parasite system presents certain disadvantages in terms of analysis, the fact that manipulation of one or two minor clones can indeed enhance immunity becomes all the more encouraging for idiotype manipulations in other microbial (parasite) systems for which response heterogeneity is apt to be the rule.

A. ENHANCEMENT OF IDIOTYPE EXPRESSION AFTER INFECTION

In most systems for which the administration of anti-Id has been shown to enhance the expression of Id-bearing antibody, the effect has been generally seen in a subsequent response to antigen (5,6,8,9,16). In this regard, the expression of the 7H11 Id in anti-Id-treated mice was significantly increased shortly after infection, strongly suggesting that the majority of Id-bearing molecules detected at this time were parasite specific. The association of immunity with the more rapid and enhanced expression of the 7H11 Id within 3 days after challenge suggests that the immunity may not simply have been mediated by preexisting antibody, for which it is difficult to provide evidence, but may have resulted from the early activation by antigen of increased numbers of 7H11 Id-bearing antigen-specific clones, established as a consequence of anti-7H11 Id immunization. Enhancement of 11D5 Id expression measurable after infection was not apparent in mice pretreated with anti-11D5 Id. Thus, it is possible that the induction of idiotypic memory by anti-11D5 Id compared to anti-7H11 Id included very few Id-positive clones that had specificity for VAT-1.1. Why might this be so? One possibility is that 7H11-bearing VAT-1.1-specific clones have a larger precursor frequency than 11D5. We consider this unlikely because during a normal response to WRATat-1.1 infections, the 11D5 Id appears earlier and in higher concentration than the 7H11-Id.

B. INHIBITION OF ANTIGEN BINDING
BY ANTIIDIOTYPES

Alternatively, a difference in the nature of the anti-Ids themselves might explain their different biological activities. What is the nature of the idiotopes reactive with the respective anti-Ids? The following experiment was designed to determine the relative concentrations of combining site-specific anti-Id antibodies in the respective populations of anti-7H11 Id and anti-11D5 Id. Serial dilutions of each anti-Id were preincubated with an equivalent concentration of radiolabeled Id. The material was then reacted with plates coated with VAT-1.1 antigen. Figure 5 shows that 15 μg of anti-7H11 Id was sufficient to inhibit 50% of the binding of 7H11 to antigen. In contrast, more than

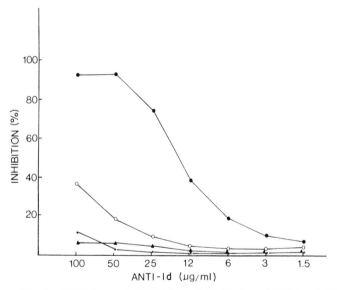

Fig. 5. Ability of anti-7H11 or anti-11D5 Id to inhibit binding of 7H11 and 11D5 Ids to purified VAT-1.1. Antigen plates were prepared by incubating microwell plates with 50 μl of purified VAT-1.1 (500 μg/ml) overnight at 4°C. Plates were washed with PBS, incubated for 1 h with 50% fetal calf serum in PBS, and washed again. Affinity-purified anti-Ids were serially diluted in PBS and incubated with an equivalent volume (100 μl) of ^{125}I-labeled 7H11 or 11D5 (100,000 cpm) for 3 h at 4°C. The reaction mixtures were then added (50 μl) to the antigen plates and incubated for an additional 3 h at 4°C before washing and counting. Data are plotted as the percentage of inhibition of control binding of ^{125}I-labeled Ids preincubated with saline. Preincubation mixtures were as follows: [125]I-7H11 plus anti-7H11 Id, ●; [125]I-11D5 plus anti-11D5 Id, ○, [125]I-7H11 plus anti-11D5 Id, ▲; [125]I-11D5 plus anti-7H11 Id, *.

100 μg of anti-11D5 Id was required to inhibit 50% of 11D5 binding. The inhibitory effect of anti-7H11 Id was apparent only when preincubated with the homologous Id, and the binding of 7H11 could be inhibited only by the homologous anti-Id, indicating that the assay is a true measure of binding site-specific interactions. One explanation for the observed differences in the inhibition of antigen binding by anti-7H11 and anti-11D5 Ids is that although they each might contain comparable concentrations of site-specific antiidiotopes, the relative affinities of these antibodies differ significantly. However, the titers of the anti-Ids were identical in a non-site-specific assay, that is, the agglutination of idiotype-coated erythrocytes. Thus, we interpret these results to mean that anti-7H11 Id contains a far greater concentration of antibodies which react with site-related idiotopes.

C. IMPLICATIONS FOR THE INDUCTION OF SPECIFIC IMMUNITY

How might this difference influence the outcome of immunization with these molecules? The idiotopes defined by these anti-Ids should not necessarily be restricted to VATat-1.1-binding antibodies because these are products of certain VDJ and VJ combinations which need not be required for the expression of a particular idiotype (12). Thus, the idiotopes defined by the anti-11D5 Id, which are primarily framework associated, might be found on a large population of clones with different antigen-binding specificities. In contrast, because the idiotopes defined by the anti-7H11 Id appear to be closer to or within the antigen-binding site, a larger proportion of clones which bear these idiotopes might also be expected to be antigen binding. In recent studies by Takemori *et al.* (12), similar results were obtained after immunization with cross-linked monoclonal antiidiotopes. Immunization with a free hapten-inhibitable anti-Id led to the production of idiotope-bearing molecules, essentially all of which were NP binding, and the induction of these molecules was strictly strain specific. In contrast, immunization with a monoclonal antiidiotope defining an idiotope not intimately associated with the NP-binding site resulted in the induction of high levels of idiotope-bearing molecules, only a small fraction of which were NP binding. Clearly, the outcome of idiotypic manipulations in the parasite system described here requires exploration with monoclonal antiidiotopes.

Finally, if site-related anti-7H11 idiotopes are responsible for the induction of Id-bearing, antigen-specific clones, to what extent might some of the antibodies be candidates for internal images of antigen which have been reported in the literature (20,21)? That this is unlikely to be so is indicated by (a) the failure of conventional anti-WRATat-1.1 antisera raised in rabbits to react with anti-7H11 Id, one criterion suggested by Nisonoff (22) as a screen for related epitopes; or, more critically, (b) the fact that anti-7H11 Id-induced immunity and idiotype expression were strictly allotype linked. It is improbable that the response to a related epitope borne by the anti-7H11 Id would be so restricted as to include only 7H11-bearing antibodies; thus, even mouse strains unable to produce 7H11 would be expected to recognize and respond to these epitopes.

VI. Summary

Administration of allogenic antiidiotypic antibodies was found to immunize mice against African trypanosomes independent of antigen. Of three anti-Id antibodies raised against three protective monoclonal antibodies, each with specificity for the VAT of a clone of *T. rhodesiense,* only one (anti-7H11 Id) was effective in immunizing BALB/c mice against homologous challenge. The immunity was associated with the more rapid and enhanced expression of the corresponding Id in serum after infection. The immunity was restricted to mice bearing genes linked to Igh-C^a, which appear to control expression of this Id in response to both infection and anti-Id treatment. Another idiotype, 11D5, appeared to be under similar genetic control. Anti-11D5 Id, however, was ineffective in immunizing mice against infection despite inducing high levels of Id-bearing molecules prior to challenge. The immunizing potential of the respective anti-Ids appeared to be related to their relative concentrations of antibodies reactive with idiotopes near or within the antigen-combining site, which in turn determined the relative proportion of Id-bearing clones activated which had antigen-binding activity.

Acknowledgments

I would like to thank A. Sher, G. Kelsoe, and especially J. Bluestone for helpful discussions and critical review of this chapter, and W. J. Davis for editorial assistance.

References

1. Eichmann, K., and Rajewsky, K. (1975). Induction of T and B cell immunity by anti-idiotypic antibody. *Eur. J. Immunol.* **5**, 661.
2. Julius, M. H., Cosenza, H., and Augustin, A. A. (1978). Evidence for the endogenous production of T cell receptors bearing idiotypic determinants. *Eur. J. Immunol.* **8**, 484.
3. Benca, R. J., Quintas, J., Kearney, J. F., Flood, P. M., and Schreiber, H. (1980). Studies on phosphorylcholine-specific T cell idiotypes and idiotype specific immunity. *Mol. Immunol.* **17**, 823.
4. Miller, G. G., Nadler, P. I., Asano, Y., Hodes, R. J., and Sachs, D. H. (1981). Induction of idiotype-bearing nuclease-specific helper T cells by *in vivo* treatment with anti-idiotype. *J. Exp. Med.* **154**, 24.
5. Cazenave, P.-A. (1977). Idiotypic-anti-idiotypic regulation of antibody synthesis in rabbits. *Proc. Natl. Acad. Sci. U.S.A.* **77**, 5122.
6. Urbain, J., Wikler, M., Franssen, J. D., and Collignon, C. (1977). Idiotypic regulation of the immune system by the induction of antibodies against anti-idiotypic antibodies. *Proc. Natl. Acad. Sci. U.S.A.* **74**, 5126.
7. Trenkner, E., and Riblet, R. (1975). Induction of antiphosphorylcholine antibody formation by anti-idiotypic antibodies. *J. Exp. Med.* **142**, 1121.
8. Sachs, D. H., El-Gamil, M., and Miller, G. (1981). Genetic control of the immune response to staphylococcal nuclease. XI. Effects of *in vivo* administration of anti-idiotypic antibodies. *Eur. J. Immunol.* **11**, 509.
9. Kelsoe, G., Reth, M., and Rajewsky, K. (1980). Control of idiotype expression by monoclonal anti-idiotope antibodies. *Immunol. Rev.* **52**, 75.
10. Bluestone, J. A., Sharrow, S. O., Epstein, S. L., Ozato, K., and Sachs, D. H. (1981). Induction of anti-H-2 antibodies in the absence of alloantigen exposure by *in vivo* administration of anti-idiotype. *Nature (London)* **291**, 233.
11. Epstein, S. L., Masakowski, V. R., Sharrow, S. O., Bluestone, J. A., Ozato, K., and Sachs, D. H. (1982). Idiotypes of anti-IA antibodies. II. Effects of *in vivo* treatment with xenogeneic anti-idiotype. *J. Immunol.* **129**, 1545.
12. Takemori, T., Tesch, H., Kelsoe, G., and Rajewsky, K. (1982). The immune response against anti-idiotypic antibodies. I. Induction of idiotope bearing antibody and analysis of idiotype repertoire. *Eur. J. Immunol.* **12**, 1040.
13. Sacks, D. L., Esser, K. M., and Sher, A. (1982). Immunization of mice against African trypanosomiasis using anti-idiotypic antibodies. *J. Exp. Med.* **155**, 1108.
14. Doyle, J. J. (1977). Antigenic variation in the salivarian trypanosomes. *In* "Immunity to Blood Parasites in Animals and Man" (L. Miller, J. Pine, and J. McKelvey, eds.), p. 27. Plenum, New York.
15. Sher, A., and Cohn, M. (1972). Inheritance of an idiotype associated with the immune response of inbred mice to phosphorylcholine. *Eur. J. Immunol.* **2**, 319.
16. Hiernaux, J., Bona, C., and Baker, P. J. (1981). Neonatal treatment with low doses of anti-idiotypic antibodys leads to the expression of a silent clone. *J. Exp. Med.* **153**, 1004.
17. Bona, C., Heber-Katz, E., and Paul, W. E. (1981). Idiotype-anti-idiotype regulation. I. Immunization with a levan-binding myeloma protein leads to the appearance of auto-anti antibodies and to the activation of silent clones. *J. Exp. Med.* **153**, 951.
18. Primi, D., Juy, D., and Cazenave, P.-A. (1981). Induction and regulation of silent idiotype clones. *Eur. J. Immunol.* **11**, 393.
19. Bluestone, J. A., Epstein, S. L., Ozato, K., Sharrow, S. O., and Sachs, D. H. (1981).

Anti-idiotypes to monoclonal anti-H-2 antibodies. II. Expression of anti-H-2K^k idiotypes on antibodies induced by anti-idiotype or H-2K^k antigen. *J. Exp. Med.* **154**, 1305.

20. Sege, K., and Peterson, P. A. (1978). Use of anti-idiotypic antibodies as cell surface receptor probes. *Proc. Natl. Acad. Sci. U.S.A.* **75**, 2443.

21. Urbain, J., Cazenave, P.-A., Wikler, M., Franssen, J. D., Mariane, B., and Leo, O. (1981). Idiotypic induction and immune networks. *In* "Immunology 80: Progress in Immunology IV" (M. Fougereau and J. Dausset, eds.), Vol. 1. Academic Press, New York.

22. Nisonoff, A., and Lamoyi, E. (1981). Implications of the presence of an internal image of the antigen in anti-idiotypic antibodies; possible application to vaccine production. *Clin. Immunol. Immunopathol.* **21**, 397.

Chapter 22

The Idiotype Network: Theoretical and Practical Implications for Autoimmune Disease

Michael Fischbach and Norman Talal

The University of Texas Health Science Center at San Antonio
Department of Medicine
and
Audie L. Murphy Veterans' Administration Hospital
San Antonio, Texas

I. Introduction

Today there is little doubt that idiotypes exist and can be manipulated *in vivo* to produce sometimes dramatic consequences for immunoregulation. Remarkable progress has been made in recent years toward elucidating how the idiotype network actually works. Other chapters in this volume describe elegant experimental systems documenting the existence of idiotype networks and the role played by various lymphocyte subpopulations in their manipulation.

Autoimmunity, immunodeficiency, and some forms of lymphoproliferation can be viewed as diseases of immunoregulation, and as such might have underlying abnormalities of normal network functions contributing to induce or maintain the disease. These abnormalities could be either positive or negative. For example, B-cell proliferation and/or autoantibody production could arise positively, as a consequence of stimulation or provocation by network derangements, or negatively, as a consequence of immunoregulatory defects or "holes" in the network. By either mechanism, idiotype defects could be pri-

417

mary pathogenetic mechanisms, and therefore of fundamental importance, or secondary manifestations of disease and rather trivial.

Using classic network theory, one idiotype generates a complementary antiidiotypic antibody, which in turn generates an anti-antiidiotypic antibody. Antiidiotypic antibodies share structural similarities with the inducing antigenic epitope (Cazenavé, 1977; Nisonoff *et al.*, 1977; Urbain *et al.*, 1977; Eichmann and Rajewsky, 1975; Cosenza *et al.*, 1977) and thus can trigger B and T cells as if it were antigen. This would be an example of a positive abnormality in which autoantibody-specific B-cell proliferation and autoantibody production result via network derangements without antigen becoming involved.

Idiotypy represents a language by which cells of the immune system communicate. B and T cells interact and influence each other through complementary idiotypic or antiidiotypic membrane receptors (Bona, 1981). A major effect of idiotypic or antiidiotypic antibodies is the generation of suppressor T cells (Sy *et al.*, 1980; Nisonoff *et al.*, 1977; Kohler, 1978). A disease process resulting in the loss of suppressor T cells is an example of a negative defect in the idiotype network. It is easy to image how this could result in lymphoproliferation or production of autoantibodies.

Studies concerned with the role of idiotypy in autoimmunity are still rather primitive and largely descriptive. For the most part, they represent early first attempts at characterization of regulatory pathways. Nonetheless, this approach is important because an idiotype strategy offers therapeutic potential for restoring immunoregulation and controlling disease.

The following are specific examples of clinical situations in which idiotypic strategies are beginning to emerge.

II. Systemic Lupus Erythematosus (SLE)

Antinucleic acid antibodies are important serologic and at times diagnostic markers of SLE. Antibodies to DNA have received the widest study because they are involved in the immune complexes which deposit in the kidney, fix complement, and may lead to severe disease manifestations including death from uremia.

Several approaches have been used to study the heterogeneity of these spontaneously forming antinucleic acid antibodies. These studies are based, in part, on the concept that the degree of restriction reflects the number of clones involved in the response, the marked restriction perhaps reflecting an immunoregulatory abnormality in the idiotype network. Spectrotype analysis by isoelectric focusing shows some antinucleic acid antibodies to be heterogeneous, whereas others are restricted.

Antibodies to DNA are very heterogeneous and similar in human and murine lupus whether they arise spontaneously, following immunization, or after polyclonal stimulation. By contrast, antibodies to polyriboadenylic acid arising under the same circumstances are quite restricted (Fischbach *et al.*, 1981).

Similar conclusions were reached by studying the antigen-binding specificities of monoclonal hybridoma anti-DNA antibodies prepared from spleen cells of lupus mice (Andrezejewski *et al.*, 1981; Marion *et al.*, 1982). The monoclonal antibodies had different isoelectric points and bound different epitopes. Statistical analysis estimated the anti-DNA antibody repertoire to be 80 B-cell clones.

Interestingly, it appears that the pathogenic potential of anti-DNA antibodies may be related to their intrinsic properties. Antibodies eluted from renal glomeruli are quite restricted compared to serum antibodies, and all antibodies have alkaline isoelectric points (Dang and Harbeck, 1982; Ebling and Hahn, 1982).

Although anti-DNA antibodies display large antigenic diversity, antiidiotypic antibodies raised against monoclonal anti-DNA antibodies reveal shared idiotypes (Rauch *et al.*, 1982; Tron *et al.*, 1982). The proportion of spontaneous serum anti-DNA antibodies that express a common idiotype remains to be determined. Likewise, the extent of cross-reactivity between murine and human idiotypes is unknown.

The anti-DNA antibody network appears to be complex. Differences in idiotope recognition were observed by Tron *et al.* (1982). Different murine strains produced different antiidiotypic antibodies to a single monoclonal antibody. One strain, NZB, produced antiidiotypic antibodies that were not ligand modifiable and of "private" idiotypic specificity; however, another strain, A/J, produced antiidiotypic antibodies that were ligand modifiable and recognized "public" idiotypes present in serum from a large number of autoimmune mice. In the studies of Rauch *et al.* (1982), one antiidiotypic serum produced against a monoclonal anti-DNA recognized 40–60% of serum anti-DNA antibodies, but it was even more reactive with non-DNA-binding antibodies, suggesting recognition of a non-ligand-specific conformational determinant.

Very recent work extends the observations in mice to human patients with SLE. Thirty monoclonal anti-DNA antibody hybridomas were produced from peripheral blood mononuclear cells or splenocytes of six SLE patients. These monoclonal antibodies reacted with a wide range of nucleic acids, and some reacted with cardiolipin. The reactivity with the latter was felt to be caused by reactivity with diester phosphate groups present on both DNA and cardiolipin molecules (Shoenfeld *et al.*, 1983).

Solomon *et al.* (1983) obtained serum enriched for anti-DNA antibodies from a patient with SLE. Five mouse monoclonal antiidiotype antibodies were produced, one of which was extensively studied. Although it reacted with the F(ab')$_2$ fragment, the antiidiotype was not antigen binding site specific. Of interest was the fact that the antiidiotypic antibody reacted with sera from 13 unrelated SLE patients. Four of these sera had no DNA-binding activity. This implies that the antiidiotype might react with non-anti-DNA antibodies, or alternatively, that it did bind to anti-DNA antibodies, but antibody activity was not detected because the antibodies were part of DNA–anti-DNA antibody circulating immune complexes.

Additional studies are necessary before we achieve a comprehensive understanding of anti-DNA antibodies. Nonetheless, the existence of a spontaneous DNA-specific idiotype–antiidiotype interaction in human disease has been suggested by the work of Abdou *et al.* (1981). Sera from patients with SLE whose disease was inactive were able to block the binding of DNA to autologous anti-DNA antibodies. The blocking capacity was localized to the F(ab')$_2$ portion of IgG. Sera obtained when the patients' disease was very active were unable to block idiotype-ligand binding. These findings were interpreted as evidence for auto-antiidiotypic antibodies produced by SLE patients at times of remission.

Auto-antiidiotypic antibodies have been shown to play a regulatory role during the immune response of normal mice. They are believed to combine with B-cell surface antigen receptors, which leads to decreased production of idiotypic antibodies. The presence of auto-antiidiotypic antibody can be demonstrated as an increase in the number of plaque-forming cells obtained by displacing the surface-bound antiidiotypic antibody with hapten.

Autoimmune New Zealand mice failed to produce auto-antiidiotypic antibody following immunization with a conventional T cell-dependent antigen, TNP-BGG. Not only was the magnitude of the idiotypic response altered, but the anti-TNP antibodies were of restricted heterogeneity and of higher affinity than those observed in conventional strains. Defective auto-antiidiotypic antibody production in autoimmune mice resulted in both a quantitatively and qualitatively altered immune response (Goidl, 1981).

The spontaneous production of auto-antiidiotypic antibodies has been studied in another autoantibody system associated with SLE. Coombs' antibodies to erythrocytes produces severe hemolytic anemia in New Zealand (NZB) mice and in some patients. The F_1 hybrids of NZB and normal strains develop a milder form of disease with lesser amounts of Coombs' antibodies. This correlates with the presence of auto-antiidiotypic antibodies that specifically recognize the idiotype of the NZB Coombs' antierythrocyte antibody. These auto-antiidiotypic antibodies are not present in NZB mice with severe hemolytic anemia (Cohen and Eisenberg, 1982).

Whether the defective production of auto-antiidiotypic antibodies represents a general immunoregulatory problem in SLE remains to be determined.

III. Cryoglobulins

The isolation of antiidiotypic antibodies in man has proved elusive. One obvious source may be circulating immune complexes or cryoglobulins if they are composed of idiotype–antiidiotype. Most cryoglobulins appear not to be of this variety. For example, mixed cryoglobulins generally contain an IgM (either monoclonal or polyclonal) reactive with polyclonal IgG through the Fc portion. However, in one study of patients with essential mixed cryoglobulinemia, the authors reported that the IgM component was reactive with the $F(ab')_2$ fragment of the IgG. This cryoglobulin contained antibodies to hepatitis B surface antigen. Addition of hepatitis B surface antigen inhibited the binding of the component of the cryoglobulin IgM to the $F(ab')_2$ of IgG. This effect was not observed with cryoglobulins lacking hepatitis antibody (Geltner et al., 1980). This single study implies that a few cryoglobulins may contain circulating idiotype–antiidiotype immune complexes.

IV. Rheumatoid Factor

The most extensively studied human autoantibody is rheumatoid factor (anti-IgG). Monoclonal IgM rheumatoid factors isolated from patients with cryoglobulinemia possess a cross-reactive idiotype which is present on 60% of all monoclonal rheumatoid factors (Kunkel et al., 1973). Cross-reactive idiotypes common to small groups of both monoclonal and polyclonal rheumatoid factors have also been reported (Forre et al., 1979).

Pokeweed-stimulated B cells from the blood or synovial tissue of patients with rheumatoid arthritis produce polyclonal rheumatoid factors. However, among this polyclonal response are numerous B cells (11–18%) expressing the cross-reactive idiotype of the monoclonal cryoglobulin rheumatoid factor (Bonagura *et al.*, 1982). This observation supports the concept of families of idiotypically related rheumatoid factors present within a polyclonal rheumatoid factor response.

A study of rheumatoid factors present in three generations of a single family suggested the inheritance of a common idiotype. There was no apparent relationship between idiotype and histocompatibility antigens.

Rheumatoid factors have an additional order of complexity. Agnello *et al.* (1980) have described a subset of rheumatoid factors that react with antigens present on both IgG and a DNA–histone complex. These rheumatoid factors have distinctive idiotypes that differ from those of other subgroups of rheumatoid factors.

The existence of a rheumatoid factor network is suggested by the studies of Bona *et al.* (1982), in which human monoclonal rheumatoid factor was injected into mice. The mice recognized a series of idiotopes and produced (a) conventional antiidiotypic antibodies directed against idiotopes associated with the antigen-combining site, (b) antiidiotypic antibodies directed against idiotopes associated with the framework of the variable region, and (c) antiidiotypic antibodies that reacted with the Fc region of IgG. Injection of antiidiotypic antibodies into a second set of mice yielded anti-antiidiotypic antibodies that reacted not only with the antiidiotype but also with rheumatoid factors.

These experiments are very similar to those of Sege and Petersen (1978), in which antiinsulin antibodies induce anti-antiinsulin antibodies which mimic the action of insulin. Studies should now be directed at determining if similar antibody cascades exist in man.

V. Antitetanus Toxoid Antibodies

Attempts to regulate a human immune response through idiotype–antiidiotype manipulations have yielded interesting results. Normal human subjects immunized with tetanus toxoid have been extensively studied. Antibodies to tetanus toxoid do not contain a cross-reactive idiotype, but shared idiotypes are present on antibody molecules of the IgG, IgM, and IgE classes. Rabbit antiidiotypic antibody recognizes non-antigen-binding idiotypic determinants (Geha and Weinberg, 1978). Antiidiotypic antisera added to *in vitro* cultures of peripheral blood mononuclear cells specifically suppress the production of antitetanus toxoid antibody of the IgG and IgE classes. Other antibodies are not affected. This inhibition occurs via direct suppression of B cells, as well as by induction of idiotypic-specific suppressor T cells. Both B and T cells have surface receptors of similar idiotype (Geha and Comunale, 1983).

Regulation of serum IgE antibodies has potential importance for the control of allergic reactions. The fact that IgG antiidiotypic antibodies control both IgG and IgE antitetanus toxoid antibodies suggests that IgE B cells share immunoglobulin variable-region genes with IgG B cells. Similar interactions have been observed *in vivo* as well. Rabbit antiidiotypic antibodies directed against antitetanus toxoid antibodies can elicit a Prausnitz–Kustner reaction in normal human skin that was sensitized 48 h earlier with IgE antitetanus toxoid antibodies (Geha, 1982a).

Auto-antiidiotypic antibodies occur following booster immunization with tetanus toxoid. Auto-antiidiotypic antibodies, like xenogeneic antiidiotypic antibodies, are specific, reacting only with idiotypes of the same individual. There is no reactivity with antitetanus toxoid antibodies from other individuals.

As with SLE, auto-antiidiotypic antibodies appear to evert a regulatory influence. The predominant antitetanus toxoid idiotype observed shortly after primary immunization decreases concomitantly with the appearance of auto-antiidiotypic antibodies and remains reduced throughout the time that auto-antiidiotypic antibodies are present (Geha, 1982b). Long-term observations were not made.

A physiologic role for auto-antiidiotypic antibodies may explain certain observations in a patient with hypogammaglobulinemia. This patient developed an IgG kappa paraprotein without evidence of multiple myeloma. A rabbit antiidiotypic antibody raised against the patient's paraprotein inhibited the *de novo* synthesis of the paraprotein by the patient's peripheral blood lymphocytes *in vitro*. One examination for the appearance of this paraprotein in the setting of hypogammaglobulinemia would be the inability to produce auto-antiidiotypic antibody, allowing a particular protein to express itself (Mudawwar *et al.*, 1980). This could be an example of the immunoregulatory defect or hole in the network discussed in Section I.

VI. Leukemia and Lymphoma

Certain neoplastic lymphoproliferative disorders may also lend themselves to idiotypic regulatory maneuvers. Chronic lymphocytic leukemia cells of B-cell origin have IgM and IgD on the cell surface. These immunoglobulins can be eluted by papain treatment. Antiidiotypic sera demonstrate a similar idiotype on both IgM and IgD (Hough *et al.*, 1976; Stevenson *et al.*, 1980).

Antiidiotypic antibodies can regulate leukemic cell activity. Bona and Fauci (1980) studied a patient with chronic lymphocytic leukemia whose B cells had surface IgM with antisheep erythrocyte specificity and whose serum had a monoclonal IgM with the same reactivity. An antiidiotype prepared against the serum monoclonal IgM demonstrated common idiotypes on both the serum and cell surface IgM. The antiidiotypic antibody suppressed *in vitro* both spontaneous and mitogen-induced antisheep erythrocyte antibodies produced by peripheral blood cells. The mechanism of suppression appeared to be by direct action on the leukemic cells.

Other investigators used xenogeneic antiidiotypic antibody *in vivo* to treat a patient with chronic lymphocytic leukemia. There was a transient fall in circulating leukemic cells, but this was associated with considerable toxicity (Hamblin *et al.*, 1980).

Using a different methodology, monoclonal antibody was obtained by fusing non-immunoglobulin-secreting nodular lymphoma cells with mouse myeloma cells NS-1 by standard hybridoma technology. An antiidiotype was prepared. The enumeration of idiotype-positive cells in circulation correlated with the patient's clinical status. Idiotype-positive cells fell during disease remissions and rose during exacerbations. No spontaneous antiidiotypic antibody was found in the serum, nor did the patient's T cells express or bind idiotype (Hatzubai *et al.*, 1981). One must consider the possibility that the lymphoma developed as a consequence of absent auto-antiidiotypic regulation.

In addition to studying the biology of B-cell malignancies, the high degree of specificity of antiidiotypic antibodies makes them therapeutically attractive reagents. Monoclonal idiotypic antibody from a patient with poorly differentiated lymphocytic lymphoma was prepared following fusion with mouse myeloma cells. Monoclonal antiidiotypic antibodies were prepared by injection of the monoclonal idiotype into mice, followed by fusion of reactive spleen cells with NS-1 myeloma cells. The monoclonal antiidiotypic antibody reacted with the surface immunoglobulin of the lymphoma cells and was used to treat the patient. Remarkable regression in tumor mass and normalization of hematologic values occurred. The patient remained in clinical remission for 6 months without any further treatment at the time the study was reported (Miller *et al.*, 1982). There was no treatment-associated toxicity, although the antiidiotypic antibody was of murine origin. The lack of toxicity was attributed to the monoclonal nature of the antiidiotype. Because the tumor continued to regress after treatment was stopped, a search for antiidiotype production by the patient was undertaken. Unfortunately, none was found. The mechanism of tumor control was not studied. Extrapolation from work with mice suggests that probable control is via the development of idiotype-specific suppressor T cells (Abbas *et al.*, 1980). This experience in humans supports the finding from the work in mice: Malignant lymphocytes may be subject to the same immunological controls as normal lymphocytes (Abbas *et al.*, 1982; Lynch *et al.*, 1979).

VII. Conclusions

Work directed at the theoretical and practical implications of the idiotype network for autoimmune disease is still in its infancy. It is clear, however, that an idiotype network can be studied in disease states. Furthermore, autoimmune and abnormally proliferating lymphocytes can be regulated by antiidiotypic antibody in a manner similar to that of normal cells. No clear understanding of regulation has emerged from the well-conceived and relatively simple experimental systems of mice. Antigenic systems vary from one another in important regulatory details (Paul, 1981). Lymphocyte populations are in constant flux, with some populations arising and others declining (Bona, 1981). Precise study of network immunoregulation in diseases will be difficult because autoimmune reactions occur spontaneously and for unknown reasons. Furthermore, cellular relationships observed at one point in a dynamic disease process may be different from those occurring at later times. Finally, immunological dysregulation may arise from different pathological mechanisms all producing an array of network abnormalities.

It is becoming clear that auto-antiidiotypic antibodies are important regulatory molecules. Suggestive evidence for defective production of auto-antiidiotypic antibody is found in several diseases. Decreased auto-antiidiotypes are associated with the presence of abnormal autoantibodies. The cellular mechanisms responsible for decreased auto-antiidiotypic production are not known, any more than the mechanisms underlying autoantibody formation are known. Is there a causal relationship between the two, and if so, precisely how does it happen?

The elegant studies of Greene and colleagues in mice predict that an auto-antiidiotypic antibody can suppress idiotype by stimulating the generation of suppressor T cells. These suppressor T cells and their secreted suppressor factors would be both idiotype and MHC restricted (Greene and Benacerraf, 1980).

The exact mode of interaction of idiotype and MHC determinants to mediate immunoregulation is a key issue in contemporary immunology. The important suppressor cell interactions in mice that lead to idiotype suppression of delayed hypersensitivity require both idiotype and MHC elements (Germain *et al.*, 1981).

Study of this association has clinical relevance. Solinger and Stobo (1982) studied the reactivity of T cells to denatured collagen. They found that T-cell reactivity was associated with the presence of an *HLA-DR4* gene. Individuals who possessed the *DR4* gene had T cells that could respond to collagen, whereas those individuals who were $DR4^-$ were incapable of responding to collagen. Unresponsiveness was caused by the presence of collagen-specific suppressor T cells. Whether these suppressor cells correspond to idiotype-induced suppressors in mice is unknown at present.

Clearly, more descriptive and quantitative work remains to be done. Careful cellular and molecular analyses to determine the extent of network and nonnetwork lymphocyte interactions must be completed before immunoregulatory defects can be understood.

Nevertheless, therapeutic modifications using idiotype strategies may be successful without a complete biological understanding. The encouraging work with lymphomas suggests that this might be the case. However, optimism must be tempered by the realization that control of spontaneous autoantibodies may be difficult. Restoration of immunological control by administration of antiidiotypic antibody may not mirror the control achieved by spontaneous auto-antiidiotypic antibody production. In normal mice, the addition of antiidiotypic antibodies to an ongoing immune response produces little idiotype suppression compared to the excellent suppression noted when antiidiotype is administered prior to immunization.

The ability to clone large numbers of specific T cells provides another potential avenue for treatment based on idiotype network considerations. Antiidiotype-induced T-cell clones or regulatory molecules from T-cell hybridomas could be administered to patients. This approach eliminates the need to induce such cells in patients whose immunological defect may preclude the ability to produce such regulatory T cells. A highly perturbed network may require the outside addition of functional cells or their specific products to restore physiological immunoregulation.

In conclusion, the implications and benefits of the idiotype network for autoimmune disease have been more theoretical than practical before now. More work in this promising area needs to be done before one can decide its relevance for understanding human disease mechanisms and its potential for a more rational approach to these disorders of immunoregulation.

References

Abbas, A. K., Perry, L. L., Bach, B. A., and Greene, M. I. (1980). *J. Exp. Med.* **152**, 968–973.

Abbas, A. K., Takaoki, M., and Greene, M. I. (1982). *J. Exp. Med.* **155**, 1216–1221.

Abdou, N. I., Wall, H., Lindsley, H. B., Halsey, J. F., and Suzuki, T. (1981). *J. Clin. Invest.* **67**, 1297–1304.

Agnello, V., Arbetter, A., DeKasep, G. I., Powell, R., Tan, E. M., and Joslin, F. (1980). *J. Exp. Med.* **151**, 1514–1527.

Andrzejewski, C., Rauch, J., Lafer, T., Stollar, B. D., and Schwartz, R. S. (1981). *J. Immunol.* **126**, 226–231.

Bona, C. A. (1981). "Idiotypes and Lymphocytes," pp. 76–156. Academic Press, New York.

Bona, C. A., and Fauci, A. S. (1980). *J. Clin. Invest.* **65**, 761–767.

Bona, C. A., Finley, S., Waters, S., and Kunkel, H. G. (1982). *J. Exp. Med.* **156**, 986–999.

Bonagura, U. R., Kunkel, H. G., and Pernis, B. (1982). *J. Clin. Invest.* **69**, 1356–1365.

Cazenave, P.-A. (1977). *Proc. Natl. Acad. Sci. U.S.A.* **74**, 5122–5125.

Cohen, P. L., and Eisenberg, R. A. (1982). *J. Exp. Med.* **156**, 173–180.

Cosenza, H., Julius, M. H., and Augstin, A. (1977). *Immunol. Rev.* **34**, 3–97.

Dang, H., and Harbeck, R. J. (1982). *J. Clin. Lab. Immunol.* **9**, 139–145.

Ebling, F., and Hahn, B. H. (1980). *Arthritis Rheum.* **23**, 392–403.

Eichmann, K., and Rajewsky, K. (1975). *Eur. J. Immunol.* **5**, 661–665.

Fischbach, M., Rabbie, J., and Talal, N. (1981). *J. Clin. Invest.* **68**, 1036–1043.

Forre, O., Dublong, J. H., Michaelsen, T. E., and Natvig, J. B. (1979). *Scand. J. Immunol.* **9**, 281–289.

Geha, R. S. (1982a). *J. Clin. Invest.* **69**, 735–741.

Geha, R. S. (1982b). *J. Immunol.* **129**, 139–144.

Geha, R. S., and Comunale, M. (1983). *J. Clin. Invest.* **71**, 46–54.

Geha, R. S., and Weinberg, R. P. (1978). *J. Immunol.* **121**, 1518–1523.

Geltner, D., Franklin, E. C., and Frangisne, B. (1980). *J. Immunol.* **125**, 1530–1535.

Germain, R. N., Sy, M. S., Rock, K., Dietz, M. H., Greene, M. I., Nisonoff, A., Weinberger, J. Z., Ju, S. T., Dorf, M. C., and Benacerraf, B. (1981). *In* "Immunoglobulin Idiotypes" (C. Janeway, E. E. Sercarz, and H. Wigzell, eds.), pp. 709–723. Academic Press, New York.

Goidl, E. A. (1981). *In* "Immunoglobulin Idiotypes" (C. Janeway, E. E. Sercarz, and H. Wigzell, eds.), pp. 779–784. Academic Press, New York.

Greene, M. I., and Benacerraf, B. (1980). *Immunol. Rev.* **50**, 163–180.

Hamblin, T. J., Abdul-Ahad, A. K., Gordon, J., Stevenson, F. K., and Stevenson, G. I. (1980). *Br. J. Cancer* **42**, 495–502.

Hatzubai, A., Maloney, D. G., and Levy, R. (1981). *J. Immunol.* **126**, 2397–2402.

Hough, D. W., Eady, R. P., Hamblin, T. J., Stevenson, F. K., and Stevenson, G. T. (1976). *J. Exp. Med.* **144**, 960–969.

Kohler, H. (1978). *Immunol. Rev.* **27**, 24–56.

Kunkel, H. G., Agnello, V., Joslin, F. G., Winchester, R. J., and Capra, J. D. (1973). *J. Exp. Med.* **137**, 331–342.

Lynch, R. G., Rohrer, J. W., Odermatt, B., Gebel, H. M., Autry, J. R., and Hoover, R. G. (1979). *Immunol. Rev.* **48**, 45–80.

Marion, T. N., Lawton, A. R., Kearney, J. F., and Briles, D. E. (1982). *J. Immunol.* **128**, 668–674.

Miller, R. A., Malone, D. G., Warnke, R., and Levy, R. (1982). *N. Engl. J. Med.* **306**, 517–522.

Mudawwar, F., Awdeh, Z., Ault, K., and Geha, R. S. (1980). *J. Immunol.* **65**, 1202–1209.

Nisonoff, A., Ju, S.-T., and Owen, F. L. (1977). *Immunol. Rev.* **34**, 89–118.

Pasquali, J. L., Fong, S., Tsoukas, C., Vaughan, J. H., and Carson, D. A. (1980). *J. Clin. Invest.* **66**, 863–866.

Paul, W. E. (1981). *In* "Immunoglobulin Idiotypes" (C. Janeway, E. E. Sercarz, and H. Wigzell, eds.), pp. 851–860. Academic Press, New York.

Rauch, J., Murphy, E., Roths, J. B., Stollar, D., and Schwartz, R. S. (1982). *J. Immunol.* **129**, 236–241.

Sege, K., and Petersen, P. A. (1978). *Proc. Natl. Acad. Sci. U.S.A.* **75**, 2443–2446.

Shoenfeld, Y., Rausch, J., Massicotte, N., Dotta, S., Schwartz, J. A., Solinger, A. M., and Stobo, J. D. (1982). *J. Immunol.* **129**, 1916–1920.

Solomon, G., Schiffenbauer, J., Keiser, H. D., and Diamond, B. (1983). *Proc. Natl. Acad. Sci. U.S.A.* **80**, 850–854.

Stevenson, F. K., Hamblin, T. J., Stevenson, G. T., and Tuh, A. L. (1980). *J. Exp. Med.* **152**, 1484–1496.

Stollen, B. D., and Schwartz, R. S. (1983). *N. Engl. J. Med.* **386**, 414–420.

Sy, M. S., Brown, A. R., Benacerraf, B., and Greene, M. I. (1980). *J. Exp. Med.* **151**, 896–909.

Tron, F., LeGuern, C., Cazenave, P.-A., and Bach, J. F. (1982). *Eur. J. Immunol.* **12**, 761–766.

Urbain, J., Wikler, M., Fraussen, J. D., and Collignon, C. (1977). *Proc. Natl. Acad. Sci. U.S.A.* **74**, 5126–5130.

Chapter 23

Human Antiidiotypic Antibodies

H. G. Kunkel

The Rockefeller University
New York, New York

I. Introduction

A number of investigators have been intrigued by the possibility that naturally developing antiidiotypic antibodies might be involved in disease. Such a possibility should be particularly relevant to immune complex disease, which increasingly is being recognized as a dominant aspect of immune injury. Antiidiotypic antibodies and various parts of the immune network have to be considered as part of this problem because the formation of complexes is an integral part of the network hypothesis. Possible evidence on this point comes from work on certain of the immune complexes found in the sera of patients with systemic lupus erythematosus (SLE). Isolation of these complexes has frequently failed to reveal any distinct antigens, and only Igs that appear to associate among themselves have been found. Direct analyses of such complexes have thus far revealed only suggestive evidence for antiidiotypic antibodies, but technical problems have hampered a resolution. Anti-γ globulins of other types, such as rheumatoid factors, are clearly involved in many of these complexes, and those against the F(ab) portion of IgG are especially difficult to separate from antiidiotypic antibodies. Perhaps these too should be considered part of the network.

Antiidiotypic antibodies may also play an important role in disease when antireceptor antibodies have been implicated in causation, as in

Graves' disease and myasthenia gravis. These antibodies may have arisen as antiidiotypic antibodies and reacted secondarily with receptors for the primary antigen. This field of investigation has become very active, although it is usually unclear just how the antireceptor antibodies arise.

In this chapter, an attempt will be made to summarize the work on these disease relationships and describe various other auto-antiidiotypic systems unrelated to disease, especially those that appear in the maternal–fetal situation.

II. Auto-Antiidiotypic Antibodies

In the human system, only a few well-documented examples have been described demonstrating auto-antiidiotypic antibodies. One of the best examples is in the casein system of Cunningham–Rundles (1982), where individuals with IgA deficiency and antibodies to BSA derived from food also develop secondary antiidiotypic antibodies. In these studies, antibodies to casein were isolated from two individuals, and anti-anticasein antibodies were isolated on affinity columns of the anticasein antibodies. Inhibition studies of these isolates showed specificity that was strongly inhibited by casein. Some cross-specificity was observed between the systems of the two patients, so the exact idiotypy in this system was not totally defined. Geha (1982) described auto-antiidiotypic antibodies found after tetanus toxoid immunizations. Clear evidence for such antibodies was obtained, beginning 10 days after booster immunization. This system proved to be highly specific, and no cross-reactions between different individuals were observed. Some evidence of modulation of idiotypes was observed after the development of antiidiotypes. G. W. Siskind and associates (personal communication, 1983) recently described antiidiotypic antibodies against allergen antibodies. Isolated ragweed antibodies were shown to absorb antibodies from autologous sera that showed idiotypic specificity. These may play an important role in regulating the allergic antibodies as well as the blocking antibodies.

The possibility of developing antiidiotypic antibodies that may play a significant role in disease has been raised by a number of investigators. This is especially true of immune complex disease, and extensive studies were carried out in the author's laboratory seeking antiidiotypic antibodies in complexes that fail to show evidence of specific antigens; IgG and IgM totally dominate the components of such isolated complexes. Antibodies to the $F(ab')_2$ fragment of IgG are demonstrable in such complexes, but these antibodies do not show clear specificity and can be absorbed on F(ab')$_2$ fragments of any IgG myeloma protein (H. G. Kunkel *et al.*, unpublished observations, 1982). They thus resemble the antibodies described many years ago and termed "pepsin IgG agglutinators" (Osterland *et al.*, 1963) and not "antiidiotypic antibodies." Other anti-γ globulins of the rheumatoid factor type are also found in these complexes and appear to be significant constituents (Agnello *et al.*, 1971). Furthermore, we recently delineated a new category of antiidiotypic antibodies designated "epibodies" (Bona *et al.*, 1982) which bind to human Fcg fragment and which can play an important role in activation of clones producing rheumatoid factors.

Several studies have concluded that anti-anti-DNA idiotypic antibodies appear in SLE. The evidence for this is not completely conclusive, again primarily because of the presence of anti-Fab antibodies of the nonspecific type revealed by enzymatic digestion of IgG. Abdou and associates (1981) showed that certain SLE sera contained Igs that blocked the DNA–anti–DNA reaction. These were thought to be antiidiotypic antibodies, but specific adsorption on isolated DNA antibodies was not demonstrated. In addition, some normal sera inhibited the DNA system. Inactive SLE sera were most active, especially in an autologous system. The latter specificity, if confirmed in further experiments, is certainly suggestive of antiidiotypic antibodies. Nasu *et al.* (1982) purified antibodies from SLE sera on columns coated with FrII F(ab')$_2$ fragments. These antibodies were thus purified from normal IgG columns. They showed inhibition of the reaction of DNA antibodies with DNA in a radioimmunoassay, which was not seen with similarly purified antibodies from rheumatoid arthritis sera. These were called antiidiotypic antibodies, but their character remains to be elucidated. Immune complexes containing DNA were not ruled out, and this and other explanations might be involved. The antibodies were also shown to inhibit the mouse DNA–anti-DNA system. Further studies regarding specificity are required in this system, which still may be of considerable interest.

Perhaps the best evidence for antiidiotypic antibodies to autoantibodies comes from the work with myasthenia gravis sera by Dwyer and associates (1983). Such antibodies were detected through the use of mouse monoclonal antibodies to the acetylcholine receptor and were isolated on affinity columns of the monoclonal antibody. These antiidiotypic antibodies were inhibited by receptor and were shown to react with antireceptor antibodies of different patients but not with other human or mouse Igs. The exact role of these antibodies in the disease remains unclear; they may play a beneficial role in suppressing the harmful antibody or T-cell mediated responses.

A number of additional autoantibody systems (Birdsall and Rosen, 1982; Lewis *et al.*, 1976) were described in which anti-IgG antibodies appear to be involved, but the question of whether these antibodies are antiidiotypic was not definitively answered. The ubiquitous anti-Fc anti-γ globulins and the anti-F(ab) types without specificity were not ruled out.

III. Antiidiotypic Antibodies against Stimulated T Cells

A number of investigators have obtained evidence of antiidiotypic antibodies against maternal T cells stimulated against paternal MHC antigens from the fetus. These may be of considerable importance in the protection of the fetus against immune rejection. Miyagawa and associates (1981, 1982, 1983) carried out a series of studies on such antibodies synthesized by the fetus that are found in the IgM fraction of the cord blood. The latter is known to be synthesized by the fetus and not transferred from the mother. The most striking finding in their later publications is that at least certain of these antibodies are specific for maternal T-cell blasts stimulated in MLC reactions with paternal cells. Specific inhibition of these MLC reactions is obtained, but not inhibition of MLC reactions stimulated by other stimulators of the maternal cells. Fluorescence studies also demonstrated specific staining of the appropriate MLC blasts. Cytotoxic T cells formed in these MLC reactions are inhibited by the homologous fetal IgM. These studies all emphasized the fetal IgM as the source of these anti-idiotypic antibodies.

Suciu-Foca and associates (1982) found similar antibodies in maternal sera. These are specific for MLC blasts of the mother which are stimulated *in vitro* by paternal lymphocytes. Fluorescent antibody analyses showed this specificity, as did the inhibition of the MLC. Maternal blasts stimulated by lymphocytes of other individuals were negative. Some cross-specificity was observed where similar DR types were involved. In addition, evidence was obtained indicating that these antibodies reacted both with the T-cell blasts and with anti-DR antibodies. In a separate study, these workers (Suciu-Foca *et al.*, 1983) showed that antiidiotypic T cells can be generated *in vitro* and directed against idiotypes of the DR-receptor sites on T-cell blasts. It is unclear whether these cells also recognize anti-DR antibodies.

Studies of our own group (Patarroyo and Kunkel, 1983) also demonstrated antibodies in maternal sera that react with T-cell blasts generated *in vitro* against paternal lymphocytes. Bright staining of 10–30%

of the MLC blasts was observed with the sera of all of a group of sera from multipara. Each of the sera reacted with the autologous blasts but not with others, clearly showing specificity. However, all reactivity disappeared after absorption of the sera with paternal cells. These results suggest that the maternal T-cell blasts had acquired MHC determinants from the stimulating paternal cells and the reaction was caused not by antiidiotypic antibodies in the maternal sera but by alloantibodies. We had shown previously that this occurs for DR antigens in MLC reactions (Yu *et al.*, 1980). Thus, the question of antiidiotypic antibodies in this situation remains unsettled.

IV. Antiidiotypic Antibodies against Maternal Antibodies

It is well known that human antiallotype antibodies develop in the newborn stimulated by maternal Igs that cross the placenta (Speiser, 1966). These usually appear later than 6 months after birth, at the time when maternal Ig has disappeared from the blood of the offspring. This was a surprising finding because tolerance to the maternal allotype would have been expected. It therefore appeared quite conceivable that the child might also develop antiidiotypic antibodies in a similar fashion. Some evidence for this possibility was obtained in our laboratory a number of years ago, when large-scale screening of normal sera was carried out in adults in the search for good antiallotype reagents. A few sera were found which showed an agglutination pattern that was idiotypic rather than allotypic. These sera were specific for anti-Rh antibodies, reacting with some anti-Rh coats and not others. They failed to agglutinate red cells coated with FrII γ globulin. It appeared that these sera contained antibodies originally produced against maternal anti-Rh antibodies and showed cross-idiotypic specificity to certain other anti-Rh antibodies used in our screening. We know that the anti-Rh coat on red cells is a very good system for the detection of antiidiotypic antibodies because only one of the two combining sites of the anti-Rh antibodies is adherent to the red cell and the other is available for reaction with combining-site antibodies (Kunkel *et al.*, 1976). In addition, the anti-Rh coat on the red cell represents an isolated antibody. Table I shows the agglutination pattern of one such serum, E.S. Inhibition assays were also carried out, and FrII failed to inhibit the agglutination of anti-Rh 66-coated red cells. The Ri coat, which is known to be extremely heterogeneous, showed some agglutination and thus appeared to have a minor population of antibodies that cross-reacted.

TABLE I

Agglutination Pattern of Dilutions of Normal E.S.
Serum against Red Cells Coated with Various
Anti-Rh Antibodies and FrII

	1/2	1/4	1/8	1/32	1/64	1/128
Anti-Rh 66	3	3	3	3	1	0
Anti-Rh Ri	2	2	1	0	0	0
Anti-Rh 17	0	0	0	0	0	0
Anti-Rh 22	0	0	0	0	0	0
FrII	0	0	0	0	0	0

These results were not published previously because the presumed immunizing anti-Rh antibody was not available for testing. More recently, however, we found an instance of similar antibodies developing in a child who shows specificity for the maternal anti-Rh antibody. This child had hemolytic disease of the newborn caused by anti-Rh incompatibility, and the mother had a high titer of anti-Rh antibody. Serum specimens were obtained from the child at 6 and 9 months after birth. Both specimens agglutinated red cells coated with the maternal antibody in a highly specific fashion. Table II shows these agglutination patterns for this S.B. family. Some cross-idiotypic specificity appeared to be present, and slight agglutination of the Hey and the 17 coat was observed. The IgG fraction of S.B. maternal serum was subjected to pepsin digestion. This F(ab')$_2$ fragment, containing anti-Rh antibodies, coated cells that were agglutinated by anti-light chain antibodies but not by anti-IgG Fc antibodies. This coat was strongly agglutinated by S.B. child serum. Inhibition studies also confirmed the idiotypic specificity. The agglutination by S.B. child serum was inhibited only by S.B. maternal serum and no other, including the Ri serum, which showed some agglutination. Antiallotype antibodies were ruled out as being responsible for the agglutination because removal of anti-Rh antibodies from the maternal serum eliminated the inhibition. Another S.B. child serum was obtained 3 months later, and the same agglutination pattern was observed, although the agglutination was weaker.

Two other families were studied in which the mother had significant anti-Rh antibodies, but no agglutination was observed with single specimens of offspring sera obtained at 6 months of age. Further studies have been hampered by the current therapy using pooled anti-Rh antibody injection. Studies with other maternal antibody systems

TABLE II

Agglutination Pattern of the Serum from an S.B. Child against Red Cells
Coated with Various Anti-Rh Antibodies[a]

	S.B. child serum							
	1/2	1/4	1/8	1/16	1/32	1/64	1/128	1/256
Anti-Rh SBm	4	4	4	4	4	4	2	0
Anti-Rh Ri	0	0	0	0	0	0	0	0
Anti-Rh Hey	3	2	2	1	0	0	0	0
Anti-Rh 5214	0	0	0	0	0	0	0	0
Anti-Rh 66	0	0	0	0	0	0	0	0
Anti-Rh 09	0	0	0	0	0	0	0	0
Anti-Rh 17	2	1	0	0	0	0	0	0
Anti-Rh 07	0	0	0	0	0	0	0	0
Anti-Rh 50	0	0	0	0	0	0	0	0
Anti-Rh 73	0	0	0	0	0	0	0	0

[a] S.B. child serum specifically agglutinated cells coated with S.B. maternal anti-Rh antibodies.

are currently in progress, looking for further examples of offspring antiidiotypic antibodies to maternal antibodies. The need for isolation of the maternal antibody, as well as antibody from controls, has slowed this work, and few other systems are as definitive as the anti-Rh system.

V. Summary

Various antiidiotypic antibody systems that have been described in the human have been reviewed. It is evident that auto-antiidiotypic antibodies are widely produced following the antibody response to external antigens. Also, some evidence for such antibodies against several autoantibodies has been obtained; this is most clearly demonstrated in the myasthenia gravis system. Direct involvement of such antiidiotypic antibodies in disease processes has not been proven. This has been looked for particularly with respect to immune complexes in which no antigen is detectable, and some positive results obtained; however, nonspecific antibodies to the Fab portion of IgG have hampered these studies.

Results of special interest have been obtained in various maternal–fetal situations. Antiidiotypic antibodies against T-cell blasts have been demonstrated in both maternal and cord blood sera. These show specificity for blasts formed against fetal MHC determinants and may play a role in the protection of the fetus from immune rejection. Data are presented showing that the child can also form antiidiotypic antibodies against maternal antibodies.

References

Abdou, N. I., Wall, H., Lindsley, H. B., Halsey, J. F., and Suzuki, T. (1981). *J. Clin. Invest.* **67**, 1297.

Agnello, V., Koffler, D., Eisenberg, J. W., Winchester, R. J., and Kunkel, H. G. (1971). *J. Exp. Med.* **134**, 228s.

Birdsall, H. H., and Rosen, R. D. (1982). *J. Clin. Invest.* **69**, 75–84.

Bona, C., Finley, S., Waters, S., and Kunkel, H. G. (1982). *J. Exp. Med.* **156**, 986–999.

Cunningham-Rundles, C. (1982). *J. Exp. Med.* **155**, 711–719.

Dwyer, D. S., Bradley, R. J., Urquhart, C. K., and Kearney, J. F. (1983). *Nature (London)* **301**, 611–614.

Geha, R. S. (1982). *J. Immunol.* **129**, 139–144.

Kunkel, H. G., Joslin, F., and Hurley, J. (1976). *J. Immunol.* **116**, 1532–1535.

Lewis, M. G., Hartman, D., and Jerry, L. M. (1976). *Ann. N.Y. Acad. Sci.* **276**, 316.

Miyagawa, Y., Komiyama, A., and Akabane, T. (1981). *Eur. J. Immunol.* **11**, 106–109.

Miyagawa, Y., Komiyama, A., Akabane, T., Uehara, Y., and Yano, A. (1982). *J. Immunol.* **129**, 1983.

Miyagawa, Y., Komiyama, A., Akabane, T., Uehara, Y., and Yano, A. (1983). Submitted for publication.

Nasu, H., Chia, D. S., Taniguchi, O., and Barnett, E. V. (1982). *Clin. Immunol. Immunopathol.* **25**, 80–90.

Osterland, C. K., Harboe, M., and Kunkel, H. G. (1963). *Vox Sang.* **8**, 135–152.

Patarroyo, M., and Kunkel, H. G. (1983). In preparation.

Speiser, P., Pausch, V., and Mayr, W. R. (1970). *Wenner-Gren Cent. Int. Symp. Ser.* **17**, 151–160.

Suciu-Foca, N., Rohowsky, C., Kung, P., and King, D. W. (1982). *J. Exp. Med.* **156**, 283–288.

Suciu-Foca, N., Reed, E., Rohowsky, C., Kung, P., and King, D. W. (1983). *Proc. Natl. Acad. Sci. U.S.A.* **80**, 830–834.

Yu, D. T. Y., McCune, J. M., Fu, S. M., Winchester, R. J., and Kunkel H. G. (1980). *J. Exp. Med.* **152**, 89s–92s.

Index

A

T

V

X